THALLIUM-201 AND
TECHNETIUM-99m-PYROPHOSPHATE
MYOCARDIAL IMAGING
IN THE
CORONARY CARE UNIT

DEVELOPMENTS IN CARDIOVASCULAR MEDICINE

VOLUME 9

1. C.T. Lancée, *Echocardiology*, 1979. ISBN 90-247-2209-8.
2. J. Baan, A.C. Arntzenius, E.L. Yellin, *Cardiac Dynamics*. 1980. ISBN 90-247-2212-8.
3. H.J.Th. Thalen, C.C. Meere, *Fundamentals of Cardiac Pacing*. 1979. ISBN 90-247-2245-4.
4. H.E. Kulbertus, H.J.J. Wellens, *Sudden Death*. 1980. ISBN 90-247-2290-X.
5. L.S. Dreifus, A.N. Brest, *Clinical Applications of Cardiovascular Drugs*. 1980. ISBN 90-247-2295-0.
6. M.P. Spencer, J.M. Reid. *Cerebrovascular Evaluation with Doppler Ultrasound*. 1980. ISBN 90-247-2384-1.
7. D.P. Zipes, J.C. Bailey, V. Elharrar. *The Slow Inward Current and Cardiac Arrhythmias*. 1980. ISBN 90-247-2380-9.
8. H. Kesteloot, J.V. Joossens. *Epidemiology of Arterial Blood Pressure*. 1980 ISBN 90-247-2386-8.

series ISBN 90-247-2336-1

THALLIUM-201 AND TECHNETIUM-99m-PYROPHOSPHATE MYOCARDIAL IMAGING IN THE CORONARY CARE UNIT

edited by

FRANS J.TH. WACKERS

Yale University School of Medicine
Department of Medicine
Cardiology Section
New Haven, Connecticut

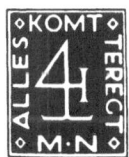

1980

MARTINUS NIJHOFF PUBLISHERS
THE HAGUE / BOSTON / LONDON

Distributors:

for the United States and Canada

Kluwer Boston, Inc.
190 Old Derby Street
Hingham, MA 02043
USA

for all other countries

Kluwer Academic Publishers Group
Distribution Center
P.O. Box 322
3300 AH Dordrecht
The Netherlands

ISBN-13:978-94-009-8906-1   e-ISBN-13:978-94-009-8904-7
DOI: 10.1007/978-94-009-8904-7

To my wife Marjan
   and my sons, Michiel and Paul
   who had to tolerate and cope with my schedule

CONTENTS

CONTRIBUTORS

FREDERICK J. BONTE, M.D., Professor of Radiology. Dean, Southwestern Medical School. The University of Texas Health Science Center, Dallas, Texas.

ELLINOR BUSEMANN SOKOLE, M.S., Department of Nuclear Medicine, Wilhelmina Gasthuis, The University of Amsterdam, Amsterdam, The Netherlands.

L. MAXIMILIAN BUJA, M.D., Associate Professor of Pathology, The University of Texas Health Science Center, Dallas, Texas.

SAMUEL E. LEWIS, M.D., Assistant Professor of Radiology, Director of Nuclear Medicine, The University of Texas Health Science Center, Dallas, Texas.

K.I. LIE, M.D., Director, Coronary Care Unit, Department of Cardiology, Wilhelmina Gasthuis, The University of Amsterdam, Amsterdam, The Netherlands.

ROBERT W. PARKEY, M.D., Professor and Chairman, Department of Radiology, The University of Texas Health Science Center, Dallas, Texas.

GERARD SAMSON, Ph.D., Department of Nuclear Medicine, Wilhelmina Gasthuis, The University of Amsterdam, Amsterdam, The Netherlands.

JAN B. VAN DER SCHOOT, M.D., Professor of Nuclear Medicine, Chief, Department of Nuclear Medicine, Wilhelmina Gasthuis, The University of Amsterdam, Amsterdam, The Netherlands.

ERNEST M. STOKELY, Ph.D., Assistant Professor of Radiology, The University of Texas Health Science Center, Dallas, Texas.

FRANS J. TH. WACKERS, M.D., Assistant Professor of Medicine and Diagnostic Radiology, Department of Medicine, Cardiology Section, Yale University School of Medicine, New Haven, Connecticut.

HEIN J.J. WELLENS, M.D., Professor of Cardiology, Department of Cardiology, Annadal Hospital. The University of Limburg, Maastricht, The Netherlands.

JAMES T. WILLERSON, M.D., Professor of Medicine, Chief, Cardiology Service, Director of Ischemic Heart Center, The University of Texas Health Science Center, Dallas, Texas.

PREFACE

Noninvasive visualization of myocardial infarction using radionuclides dates back over eighteen years. Edward A. Carr and William H. Beierwaltes were first to report (1962) successful external imaging of myocardial infarcts in dogs and in man using an Anger scintillation camera. They demonstrated that after intravenous administration of ^{86}Rb or ^{131}CS an infarct was visualized as a "cold spot", while ^{203}Hg-labeled-chlormeridin resulted in a "hot-spot" image of the infarct.

Since then, there have been major developmental improvements in available radionuclides, scintillation cameras and computer processing capabilities. In particular, the development of mobile gamma cameras opened the possibility to obtain high quality images even at the bedside of critically ill patients.

Since the development in 1974 of a new radiopharmaceutical, ^{201}Tl and the application of ^{99m}Tc-pyrophosphate for myocardial imaging, these imaging agents are widely used for the detection of acute myocardial infarction. However, for practical application, frequently there appears to be uncertainty or even confusion concerning the relative merits of each method.

In this volume an up-to-date review of the clinical value and limitations of both imaging techniques is presented. After an introduction on technical aspects and instrumentation, successively in a back-to-back fashion the mechanisms of myocardial accumulation, the results in acute myocardial infarction, unstable angina and in patients with atypical chest pain of ^{201}Tl and ^{99m}Tc-pyrophosphate scintigraphy are discussed. It is emphasized that rather than being competitive both techniques provide different and unique information, which is not readily obtainable by more conventional approaches, either invasive or noninvasive.

The purpose of this book is to place in proper perspective the practical characteristics of the two myocardial imaging methods. Provided that the choice of imaging agent, timing and technique of scintigraphy are correct, important clinical information can be derived from the images.

This book is not meant to be a textbook on nuclear cardiology. Other techniques, such as myocardial perfusion imaging following exercise, assessment of cardiac performance at rest and exercise or single photon and positron tomography, are important additional modes to evaluate patients with heart disease, but are beyond the scope of this book.

It is our hope that this volume will be a useful and practical guide for students, house officers and practicing physicians to use both imaging techniques in the most efficient and most effective way in the coronary care unit or emergency room.

We would like to express our gratitude to Ruth Rosen, Laurie Grey and Belinda Lambert for their invaluable secretarial assistance.

FRANS J. TH. WACKERS, M.D.

1. INSTRUMENTATION FOR RADIONUCLIDE CARDIOLOGY

SAMUEL LEWIS, ERNEST STOKELY and ROBERT PARKEY

INTRODUCTION

Radioactive tracers have been employed for the evaluation of cardiac structure and function for over 50 years. The discipline had its genesis in 1927 with the innovative experiments of Blumgart and Weiss[1]. These investigators, utilizing the principles of the radioactive tracer method devised by Hevesy[2], measured circulation in man by injecting a dose of radium C-salt (radon) into an antecubital vein detecting its arrival in the contralateral brachial artery with a Wilson cloud chamber. This technique was revived by Prinzmetal and associates[3] in 1948 with the advent of atomic age technology. Using a Geiger-Muller counter and the artifical radionuclide ^{24}Na, these investigators repeated the Blumgart and Weiss determination of circulation time also recording temporal changes in the radioactivity over the heart and lungs. The radionuclide angiocardiogram was thus discovered. Many improvements in instrumentation and radiopharmaceuticals have since been introduced to facilitate evaluation of the central circulation. Cardiovascular nuclear medicine procedures today encompass a myriad of qualitative and quantitative techniques including: (1) detection and quantitation of intracardiac shunts, (2) measurements of regional myocardial blood flow, (3) visualization of anatomic relationships of major cardiovascular structures – such as chamber dilatation, ventricular or septal hypertrophy, pericardial effusion, or ventricular aneurysm, (4) identification of intracardiac clot or mass, (5) evaluation of heart mechanical function, (6) identification, anatomic localization, and sizing of acute myocardial infarcts, (7) noninvasive assessment of myocardial perfusion at rest and during exercise or pharmacologic stress, (8) assessment of severity of valvular regurgitation, and (9) evaluation of regional myocardial metabolism.

The progress of nuclear cardiology over the last 50 years is due to complimentary evolutions in radiopharmaceuticals and instrumentation. The purpose of this chapter is to present the fundamental concepts and instrumentation useful for cardiovascular studies.

BASIC ATOMIC STRUCTURE

Recall that all matter is composed of atoms and that an atom can be considered to be composed to a cloud of electrons surrounding a central nucleus. The nucleus contains many types of particles but protons and neutrons are most important. The mass of the proton is arbitrarily defined as one atomic mass unit. The proton possesses an electrical charge of 1.6×10^{-19} coulomb, which is defined as one unit of positive charge. The mass of the neutron is slightly greater than that of the proton and the neutron possesses zero electrical charge. The nucleus will always contain one or more protons. The number of protons in the nucleus is termed the atomic number of the atom and specifies its chemical identity and relative position in the periodic table. Atoms of different atomic number and therefore different chemical identities are called elements. Each element has a unique atomic number. Different types of nuclei are termed nuclides. A nuclide is characterized both by its number of protons (atomic number) and by its total number of nuclear particles (mass number = number of protons + number of neutrons). Some categories of nuclides have been given special terminologies. For instance, nuclides which have the same number of protons are termed isotopes.

The electrons revolve about the nucleus in fairly well defined orbits of different radii. The mass of the electron is approximately 1/1800th the mass of the proton and the electron possesses an electrical charge equal to but opposite to that of the proton. Electron orbits of similar radii form a band which is termed an orbital shell. The shell that is located closest to the nucleus is termed the " K " shell. The second shell distant from the nucleus is the " L " shell. The third shell is the " M " shell, and so forth. Each electron is bound to the nucleus by a relatively fixed amount of energy. This energy is called the binding energy of the electron and is virtually identical for electrons in the same orbital shell. Under normal conditions, electrons occupy only those sites which are located in the lowest possible orbital shells. In this condition, termed the ground state of the atom, the minimum possible energy is required to bind the electrons to the nucleus.

THE RADIONUCLIDE

Cardiovascular nuclear medicine procedures employ the radioactive tracer method. By measuring the distribution of body radioactivity following the injection of selected radioactive tracers, these procedures can provide considerable data regarding cardiac mechanical function, myocardial blood flow, and myocardial metabolism. The radioactive tracers are injected into patients as ions or as atoms incorporated into naturally occurring compounds or pharmaceutical molecules, thus the term radiopharmaceuticals. Usually the injected elements or compounds are of specific biological importance; however, some radionuclides have no important biological function but are used because the half-life and energy of the photons released during radioactive decay are appropriate for the available detection instruments.

The measurement of the distribution of body radioactivity requires the detection of high energy gamma rays emitted during the process of radioactive decay when the nucleus of an isotope undergoes a transformation from one energy level to a lower one. Radioactivity is a phenomenon of unstable nuclei. Most naturally occurring substances are composed of atoms with stable nuclei. Such nuclei are nonradioactive. Other nuclei possess an inherent physical instability due to the geometry or relative numbers of nuclear particles. These unstable nuclides are termed radionuclides. Radionuclides may attain more stable configurations via the emission of electromagnetic radiation or charged particles, a process known as radioactive decay.

Gamma rays are a form of electromagnetic radiation and are best characterized as discrete bundles of energy traveling at the speed of light. Each of these bundles of energy is called a photon. Radiowaves and visual light are also photons, distinguishable from X-ray and gamma radiations by their energy. Since all photons travel at the same velocity, they are distinguished by their energy. The unit used to measure the energy of photons is the electron volt (eV). The eV is the amount of energy gained by an electron when it is accelerated through an electric field with a potential difference of 1 V. Since the eV is a very small unit of energy, gamma ray energies are usually measured in terms of the kilo-electron volt (keV), which is equal to 1000 eV. Gamma photons emitted from radionuclides can thus be visualized as tiny bullets traveling at the velocity of light with an energy measured in terms of kilo-electron volts.

Radionuclides useful for cardiovascular studies decay by either single photon or positron emission.

SINGLE PHOTON EMISSION

Radionuclides whose photons arise from electron capture (EC), electron emission (β^-) or isomeric transition (IT) are said to decay by single photon emission. The single photon radionuclides often emit several photons at different energies, but only one photon is normally used for detection and hence the name single photon emitter.

Electron capture

Electron capture is a phenomenon of large nuclei which possess a relative excess of positive charge. An illustrative example of electron capture is the decay of ^{201}Tl. Stable, that is nonradioactive, thallium has a nuclear component of 81 protons and 123 neutrons. The positive charge of 81 protons balances the negative charge of 81 orbital electrons. The radionuclide ^{201}Tl has only 120 neutrons and thus has a relative excess of positive nuclear charge. Sometime during the life of one atom of ^{201}Tl a "K" orbit electron will fly close enough to the nucleus to be captured. The resultant electron-proton interaction creates a neutron and cancels the excess positive nuclear charge. With the loss of a proton, the atom becomes mercury (80 protons, 121 neutrons). The "K" shell vacancy is subsequently filled by a free electron and energy is released as a characteristic X-ray. This 80 keV photon is known as a mercury X-ray. In addition, about 8% of the time, a mercury atom will be left in an excited state, a state wherein the nuclear energy is greater than that of a stable nucleus having the same atomic electron configuration. This excess nuclear energy places the atom 135 or 167 keV above its ground stage. Stability is achieved by emission of a gamma ray bearing off the excess nuclear energy. Thus, 8% of all ^{201}Tl decays result in a 135 or 167 keV photon in addition to the 80 keV photon of the mercury X-ray. Since far more 80 keV photons are available than are 135 or 167 keV photons, one usually confines the detection devices to accept only the "single" 80 keV photon.

Electron emission(β^-)

Some nuclides are unstable because they contain an excess number of neutrons. Radionuclides such as ^{86}Rb and ^{133}Xe decay by the emission of a negatively charged electron thereby converting a neutron to a proton. The resultant atom has an increase in atomic number by one and is usually left in an excited state. This excess nuclear energy is released via the emission of one or more gamma photons, some of which may be detectable. It is these photons that are important for cardiovascular studies.

The emitted electron is not detected since its range in tissue is less than 1 cm. However, the interaction of this particulate radiation with tissue contributes heavily to the total radiation dose delivered to the patient. In order to keep the patient radiation dose within acceptable limits, the amount of radioactivity injected must be kept small. This means that fewer photons will be available for detection and thus limits the utility of such radionuclides for many cardiovascular procedures.

Isomeric transition

A nucleus can be excited to a higher energy level by the absorption of energy. The decay of an excited nucleus to a lower energy level by the emission of high energy gamma radiation is known as isomeric transition. Nuclear components are unaltered by this transformation. The higher energy states of nuclides are called excited states and are generally quite unstable. Most excited states are of very brief duration with stability being achieved by decay to the ground state or states of even lower energy via the emission of high energy radiation. Excited states of nuclides have the same mass number, same atomic number and same number of neutrons as the ground state and are called isomers. If the excited state of a nuclide has a measurable lifetime of minutes or hours, they are designated metastable states. An important isotope in radionuclide cardiology that decays via isomeric transition is a form of technetium, ^{99m}Tc. The "m" designates a metastable state. Technetium-99m is produced by the decay of ^{99}Mo. The daughter nucleus, ^{99m}Tc, has uniquely desirable characteristics for use in clinical studies. This isotope decays via the emission of a 140 keV gamma photon. This photon is easily detected by most commercially available instruments. This transformation is also important since it releases no particulate radiation and has a half-life of 6 hr.

Positron emission (β^+)

Positron emission occurs when a nucleus has relative excess of protons. Radionuclides such as ^{11}C, ^{15}O, ^{13}N, ^{38}K, ^{82}Rb, and ^{68}Ga decay by the emission of a positively charged electron (positron), thereby converting a proton to a neutron. The positron travels a short distance after its ejection

Table 1-1. Decay characteristics of radionuclides useful for cardiovascular studies

Tracer	Half-life	Decay mode	Principal photons (keV) with intensity (%)
^{99m}Tc	6.0 hr	IT	140 (90%)
^{201}Tl	73.0 hr	EC	73-80 (93%), 135 (2%), 167 (8%)
^{133}Xe	5.3 days	β^-	81 (35%)
^{127}Xe	36.0 days	EC	172 (21%), 203 (61%), 375 (18%)
^{11}C	20.5 min	β^+	511 (200%)
^{15}O	2.0 min	β^+	511 (200%)
^{13}NH$_3$	9.96 min	β^-	511 (200%)
^{113m}In	100.0 min	IT	393 (64%)
^{38}K	7.7 min	β^+	511 (200%), 2170 (100%)
^{42}K	12.4 hr	β^-	1525 (18%)
^{43}K	22.2 hr	β^-	373 (85%), 618 (81%)

from the nucleus and then combines with any nearby electron. This "annihilation" reaction releases 1.022 MeV of "pure" energy (in accordance with $E = mc^2$) which is equally divided between two photons emitted in opposite directions at a 180° angle. Each photon thus has an energy of 511 keV. The production of these photon pairs makes positron emitting radionuclides especially useful for cardiovascular imaging, particularly computed tomography.

The decay characteristics of radionuclides most useful for cardiovascular studies are given in Table 1-1.

RADIOACTIVITY

The number of disintegrations per unit time is called the "radioactivity" or simply the activity of a given sample of radionuclide. The unit of radioactivity is the curie (Ci) defined as radioactivity of a sample decaying at a rate of $3.7 \cdot 10^{10}$ disintegrations per second. Smaller units of radioactivity are derived from the curie via common metric methodology. The millicurie (mCi) is a particularly useful measure for radionuclide cardiology studies and is equal to $3.7 \cdot 10^7$ disintegrations per second.

For every radionuclide there exists a probability of decay. The parameter which is most useful for characterizing the decay of a given radionuclide is the half-life ($T^{1/2}$). The half-life is defined as the time required for one-half of a given number of nuclei to decay. The activity of the radionuclide at any time "T" is related to the initial radioactivity by:

$$R_t = R_0 \cdot E^{0.693} \cdot t \div T^{1/2},$$

where R_t is the radioactivity at anytime t, R_0 is the sample activity at time 0, and $T^{1/2}$ the half-life.

SCATTERING AND ABSORPTION

The basic technique in nuclear cardiology is the measurement of the distribution of body radioactivity following the injection of various radiopharmaceuticals. The determination of how much radionuclide resides in some part of the body is made by detecting the number of photons emitted from that region. Problems arise because only a very few emitted photons ever reach an external detector as there are two alternative possible fates: (1) photons may be emitted in directions other than that in which the detector is aimed, or (2) photons may interact with tissue atoms between the radionuclide and the detector and be scattered.

The first problem is primarily one of detector geometry and the necessity to focus most detectors with lead collimation. The combined effects leads to a transmission of about 1 in 10,000 emitted photons from radionuclides such as ^{201}Tl and ^{99m}Tc.

The second problem, scatter and attenuation, results in a loss of 50-80% of emitted photons depending upon source of depth within the body and photon energy. Scatter or deflection of emitted photons in tissue, a process known as Compton scattering, is very important in cardiovascular procedures. Compton scattering occurs most often with photons of intermediate energy and thus accounts for practically all tissue attenuation for photons emitted by radionuclides useful for cardiovascular studies. In a Compton interaction a photon collides with a tissue electron striking it with a glancing blow. This results in the ejection of the electron from the atom. A portion of the photon's energy is imparted to the electron. The remaining energy is given to a new photon of lower energy in different direction from the original photon. The energy of the " scattered" photon and the magnitude of the secattering angle are related to the energy of the incident photon and to the energy "lost" to the electron. This is shown in Figure 1-1. The scattering angle can be calculated by converting the energies of the incident photon and the scattered outgoing photon to their Compton wave lengths by dividing these energies in keV into 511. Then angular deflection is given by $\theta = \cos^{-1}(1 - \lambda^1 + \lambda)$, where λ^1 is the Compton wavelength of the scattered photon, λ is the Compton wavelength of the incident photon, and θ is the scattering angle. This dependence of scattering angle on incident photon energy is extremely important in the clinical setting. For example, a 1% energy loss in a Compton interaction would be associated with a 20° deflection for an 80 keV photon from ^{201}Tl but only with an 8° deflection for the 373 keV photon of ^{43}K. Low energy photons that lose only small amounts of energy in a Compton event are thus

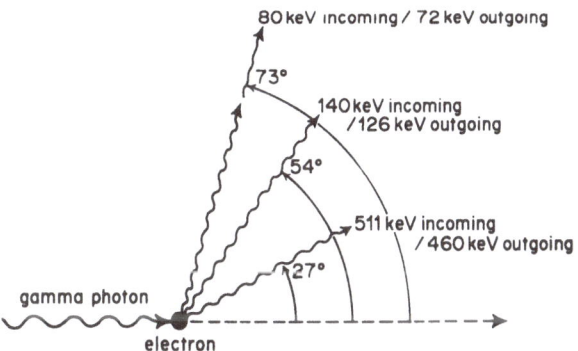

Figure 1-1. The angular distribution of Compton scattered photons is dependent on the energy of the incoming photon before scattering. Illustrated are the angular deflections for incoming photons of 80, 140, and 511 keV which lose 10% of their kinetic energy in a compton interaction. Note that lower energy photons that lose only small amounts of energy in a Compton event are deflected by greater angles than high energy photons that have experienced a larger absolute energy loss.

deflected by greater angles than high energy photons that have experienced a larger absolute energy loss. This is important because the elimination of unwanted scattered photons from scintigraphic images is primarily a process of energy discrimination. If this « energy selection " is to be useful for low energy photons, it must be relatively more precise than is necessary for high energy photons.

The loss of photons between source and detector can be considered a partial absorption phenomenon, with the amount of absorption dependent upon photon energy. As illustrated in Figure 1-2, the transmission of 80 keV photons from ^{201}Tl through 10 cm of water is less than one-half that of 511 keV photons from ^{11}C or other positron emitters. Attenuation is a serious problem in quantitative nuclear cardiology. As shown in Figure 1-3, only about 25% of 80 keV ^{201}Tl protons emitted from the posterior myocardium will reach the chest wall. The effects of attenuation on photons in different tissues is even more dramatically illustrated in Figure 1-4. If a radionuclide is distributed in the myocardium with a tissue concentration of 4:1 relative to

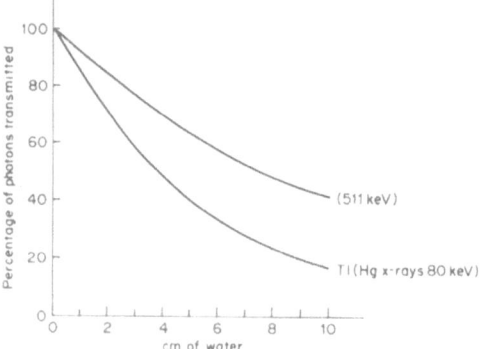

Figure 1-2. Effect of the attenuation of photons emitted from different depths in tissue (water). Note that only half as many 80 keV photons as compared to 511 keV photons will penetrate 10 cm of water.

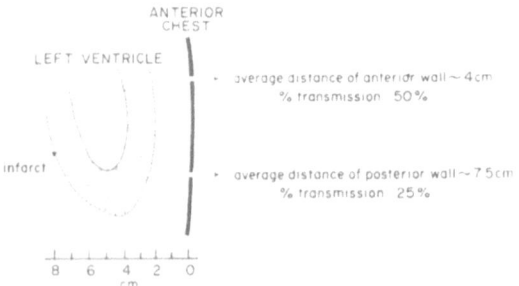

Figure 1-3. Effect of distance on the attenuation of photons emanated by anterior and posterior wall of the left ventricle.

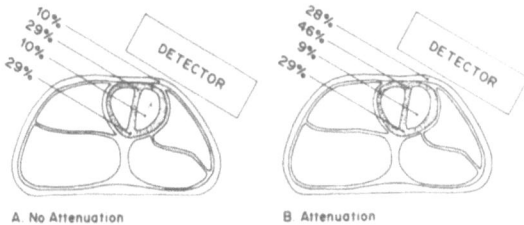

Figure 1-4. Effect of attenuation of ²⁰¹Tl photons in different tissues and relative contribution to an image from different portions of the heart.

blood in lung and there is no attenuation, various regions of the thorax contribute to the two-dimensional projection image as shown in Figure 1-4. Note that in this case, photons from posterior and anterior myocardium would contribute equally to both total and myocardial activity in the projected image. However, when realistic attenuation coefficients and values are considered, the fractional contribution of the posterior myocardium to the projected images decreased significantly, while the fractional contribution from the anterior myocardium increases (Figure 1-4B). It can be appreciated from these examples that the existence of attenuation and the effect of attenuation on photons of various energies is extremely important for imaging procedures and attempts at quantitation.

PHOTON DETECTION

Following the injection of a radiopharmaceutical, photons are emitted from a large number of source nuclei in the body. These photons are emitted randomly in all directions. Some photons are absorbed by tissue. Others are deflected from their course and degrade in energy. Only a small percentage of all emitted photons actually pass through the body unscathed. A very few of these "primary" photons will actually reach the detector along with some scattered photons and some background photons not related to the radiopharmaceutical injected. The detector should: (1) detect only primary photons and reject all others, and if images are to be obtained (2) localize the site of photon interaction with the detector.

Most photon detection instruments employ a sodium iodide crystal doped with a small amount of thallium impurity as a detector. The collision of a photon produces blue light, a process known as scintillation. Intensity of the light produced in the crystal is proportional to the energy lost in the crystal by the incident photon. Visual photons emitted by the scintillation crystal are converted to a usable electronic signal by a photo-electron multiplier tube (PMT). This photomultiplier tube is optically coupled to the crystal and performs as an energy transformation amplifier. The operation of this device is shown in Figure 1-5. Light photons emitted from the crystal strike a glass plate (photocathode) which is coated with a rare earth material. Each collision of a visual light photon with a photocathode releases an electron. Inside the photomultiplier tube, the released electron is accelerated through an electric field toward a metal plate (dynode). Upon striking the dynode, more electrons are released which are in turn accelerated to another dynode where even more electrons are released; thus the name photomultiplier tube. The end result is that for each light photon which strikes the photocathode, a million or more electrons are sent out from the photomultiplier tube. The current generated by the photomultiplier tube is then obviously proportional to the number of light photons which strike the photocathode. Since the number of light photons released by the scintillation process is proportional to the energy of the incoming photon, the instantaneous signal arising from the photomultiplier tube is also proportional to the energy of the incident photon.

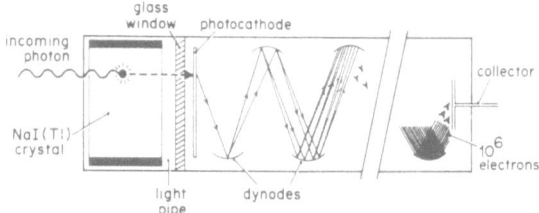

Figure 1-5. The basic photon detector consists of a sodium iodide crystal optically coupled to a photomultiplier tube. The collision of an incoming gamma photon with the crystal produces blue light with intensity proportional to the energy lost by the incident photon. Light photons from the crystal strike the photocathode releasing photoelectrons. These electrons are multiplied while cascading through a series of metal grids (dynodes). For each light photon which strikes the photocathode, a million or more electrons is sent out from the photomultiplier tube.

An important function of the detector electronics involves selecting only those signals corresponding to unscattered photons from the injected radionuclide. Other signals arise from photons scattered in the patient or from failure of some photons to transfer all of their energy to the crystal. For high resolution imaging of the myocardium this energy selection is essential since the detection of scattered photons would result in blurring of the final image.

The electron current generated by the photomultiplier tube is converted to a usable signal by special electronic circuitry. Those signals arising from unscattered photons that transfer all of their energy to the crystal create a sharply defined peak in the output spectrum. This is illustrated in Figure 1-6. The pulse height analyzer is the electronic device that differentiates these photopeak events from pulses corresponding to Compton scattered radiation in the patient and radiation from isotopes other than the one being measured.

PULSE HEIGHT SPECTRUM

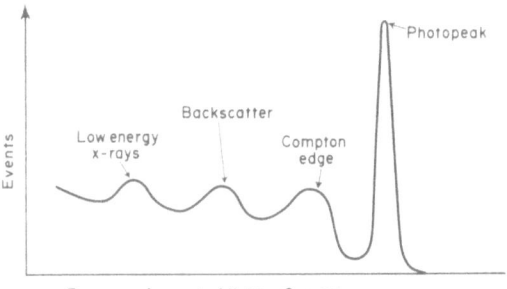

Figure 1-6. Signals arising from unscattered photons that transfer their energy to a crystal create a sharply defined peak in the output spectrum.

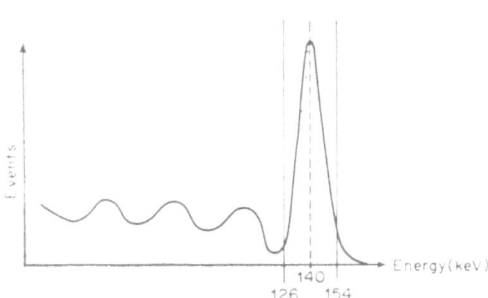

A. Setting a "window" about the photopeak

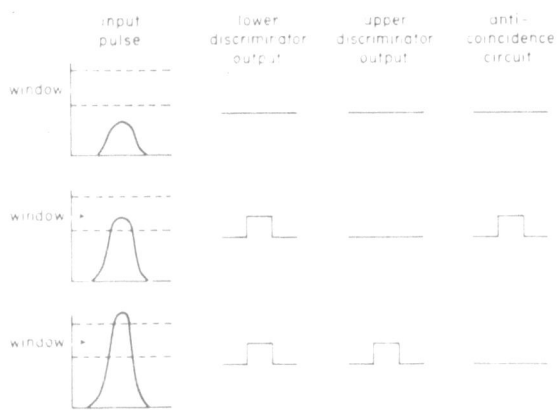

B. Operation of the anticoincidence circuit

Figure 1-7. Energy discrimination is accomplished by using two discriminators coupled via an anticoincidence circuit.

Energy discrimination is accomplished by the use of two discriminators coupled via an anticoincident circuit. This is shown in Figure 1-7. The barrier height of each discriminator is set by selecting an energy window which is some percentage of the photopeak energy. For example, a 20% acceptance window for the 80 keV photon of ^{201}Tl would be 16 keV wide and centered about the photopeak. This setting would thus accept photons ranging in energy from 72 to 88 keV. Only pulses of greater magnitude than the first barrier and lesser magnitude than the second barrier will be accepted by this discriminator circuit. Pulses of lesser height than the initial barrier or greater height than the second barrier will be discarded. Pulse height discrimination allows the use of different radioisitopes for various studies to be performed during a single examination. For instance, the ^{99m}Tc first transit angiocardiogram can be performed following a ^{201}Tl myocardial perfusion study by simply changing the window setting of the detector from a 20% window about an 80 keV photopeak to a 20% window about the 140 keV photopeak of ^{99m}Tc.

Solid state (semi-conductor) detectors convert incoming photons directly to an electronic signal instead of to visual photons (scintillation). High purity germanium, cadmium telluride, and mercuric iodide are candidates for this application. The major advantage of these devices is that they have extremely good energy resolution and can thus exclude much scattered radiation by electronic energy discrimination. Cadmium telluride detectors have recently become commercially available. Solid state detector schemes are potentially extremely valuable in cardiovascular research. The small physical dimensions of these detectors and the ability to interface these devices to small microcomputers may prove to be extremely valuable in the future. For instance, such devices might be used for continuous evaluation of ventricular ejection performance in ambulatory patients or in providing valuable information concerning the beat-to-beat variation in ventricular performance.

THE ANGER CAMERA

The Anger (scintillation) camera consists of a large flat sodium iodide crystal with between 9 and 91 photomultiplier tubes optically coupled and packed over the crystal. In most commercially available versions, crystal thickness varies from 0.64 to 1.27 cm and crystal diameter ranges from 27.9 to 53.5 cm. As with the simple crystal – single photomultiplier tube detection system, incoming photons lose their energy in the crystal producing light photons whose numbers are directly proportional to the total photon energy absorbed. The crystal is optically coupled to a series of photomultiplier tubes which are arranged in an hexagonal array. This is shown in Figure 1-8. Each photomul-

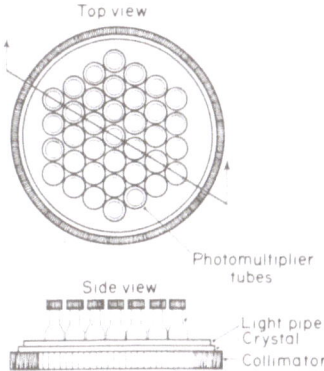

Top view

Photomultiplier
tubes

Side view

Light pipe
Crystal
Collimator

Figure 1-8. Basic concept behind the Anger camera. Photomultiplier tubes, arranged in hexagonal array, are closely packed over a large flat NaI (Tl) crystal.

tiplier tube absorbs the light photons produced within its field of view releasing electrons from its photocathode. Each electron released from the photocathode is then multiplied to 10^6 or 10^7 electrons to produce an output signal which is directly proportional to the total photon energy absorbed within the field of view of the photomultiplier tube. The output of all photomultiplier tubes is summed to produce a " Z " signal which is proportional to the energy lost by the incoming photon. This signal is fed to the pulse height analyzer which allows only those photons producing " Z " pulses with amplitudes within the previously selected range to pass through to the data recording portions of the system. If the " Z " pulse is rejected, that photon is discarded. The X-Y location of each photon-crystal interaction is determined from relative light intensity seen by each of the photomultiplier tubes. For those photons with acceptable " Z " pulses a special computing circuit determines X and Y deflection signals which are fed to an oscilloscope to reproduce the scintillations as point flashes of light at the corresponding X-Y location on an oscilloscope screen. These operations are illustrated in Figure 1-9.

For practical imaging the gamma camera is equipped with a collimator. The basic purpose of a collimator is to exclude from the detector those photons

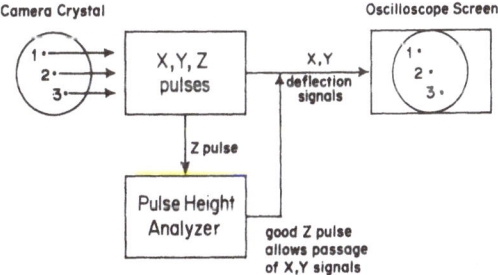

Camera Crystal

Oscilloscope Screen

X,Y,Z
pulses

X,Y
deflection
signals

Z pulse

Pulse Height
Analyzer

good Z pulse
allows passage
of X,Y signals

Figure 1-9. Schematic representation of the operation of a gamma scintillation camera.

which are traveling in some direction other than a straight line from the organ or region of interest. Thus, a collimator is a type of lens to focus on the organ or region of interest. Usually lead is used for collimation to stop unwanted photons. The simplest collimator is a block of lead with a single hole. For myocardial imaging with ^{201}Tl or ^{99m}Tc-pyrophosphate a 16000-parallel-hole, high-resolution or all purpose collimator is used. Other types of collimators include diverging, converging and (multi) pinhole collimators.

Anger camera data are often recorded photographically. The phosphor of the oscilloscope screen is designed to have low persistence, meaning that the point flashes of light produced on the screen disappear almost instantaneously. Permanent images can be recorded by exposing film to the screen scintillation for some period of time, thereby creating a composite photographic image corresponding to the body distribution of radioactivity during that time period. Various recording systems are currently available for photographic recording including polaroid cameras, 35 or 70 mm transparencies, and multiformat imagers which allow recording of a number of different images on special X-ray type film.

Anger cameras are characterized by their spatial resolution, speed or count rate capability, field uniformity, and image quality. Spatial resolution is limited mainly by collimator characteristics, scatter, and the accuracy of the computing circuitry in determining the point in the crystal where each scintillation occurs. In general photons with energies below about 70 keV do not produce sufficient light when they strike the crystal to be accurately recorded and therefore resolution is degraded. Above 70 keV, resolution improves steadily to approximately 250 keV where it again deteriorates. The crystal thickness has a considerable bearing on the useful energy range and overall camera performance as specific energies. Anger camera resolution characteristics can be measured in a number of ways. Manufacturers generally measure resolution by imaging a line source, either with or without a collimator attached to the detector. If a collimator is not used, the measurement is said to indicate the intrinsic characteristics of the system, while the use of a collimator provides data on extrinsic resolution. A diagramatic representation of how to measure the spatial resolution of a gamma camera with a line source is shown in Figure 1-10. The recorded activity across the line source image is plotted as a function of distance. The resulting curve has the typical bell shape. The maximum amplitude of the curve (corresponding to the center of the line source) is determined. Resolution is then measured in terms of the width (in millimeters) of the curve at a point which is one-half the maximum amplitude. Resolution is thus specified as the full width at half maximum (FWHM) of the line spread function.

A more practical method of measuring resolution in the clinical laboratory involves imaging a bar phantom. The bar phantom is normally of the form

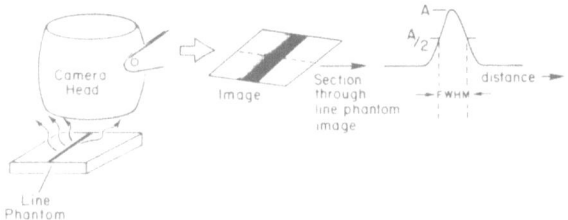

Figure 1-10. Measurement of spatial resolution of a gamma camera using a line phantom. Resolution is measured in terms of the width (in cm) of the curve at a point which is one-half of the maximum amplitude (FWHM).

shown in Figure 1-11 and consists of a square sheet of plastic with four sets of lead bars spaced equal distance to their width embedded in the plastic. Intrinsic resolution is typically obtained by placing the bar phantom in contact with the crystal cover and radiating it either with a uniform flood source or with a point source located along the crystal axis at least 4.5 crystal diameters distance. There is approximately a factor of 2 between the full width half maximum of the line spread function and a systems ability to resolve lead bars. The full width half maximum is approximately twice the width of the smallest lead bars that may be resolved.

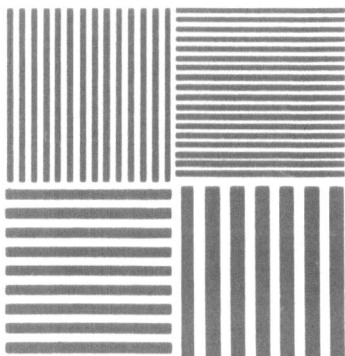

Figure 1-11. Typical bar phantom used for assessment of spatial resolution.

Field uniformity is a problem inherent in the design of single crystal cameras. Figure 1-12 shows images of a uniform flood source from a well tuned camera and one with obvious uniformity problems. Field uniformity is most often specified as the maximum percentage variation across the image of a uniform flood source. Field uniformity may be difficult to achieve. A camera that is tuned to produce a uniform flood image will often have significant spatial nonlinearity. Adjustments to decrease the spatial distortion will, unfortunately, often result in a non-uniform flood field. Because of these difficulties, many manufacturers have elected to offer special micro-computer

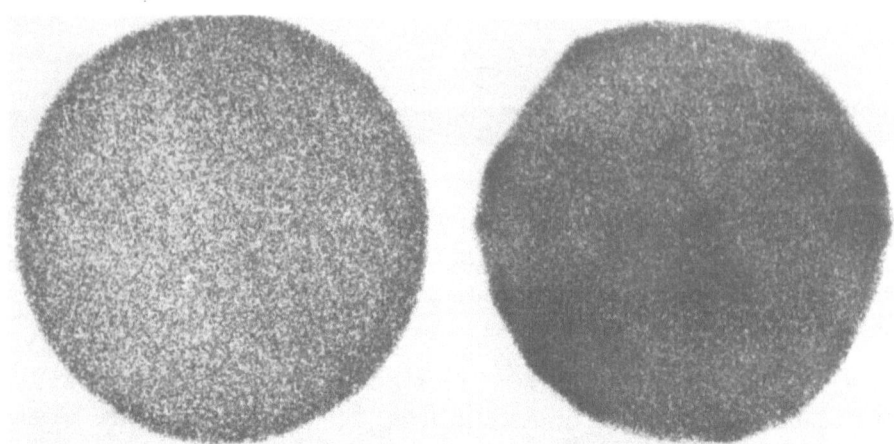

Figure 1-12. Image of a uniform flood source obtained with a well tuned camera (left) and the image obtained with a gamma camera with obvious uniformity problems (right).

controlled uniformity correction circuits. The operation of a typical correction circuit is illustrated in Figure 1-13. In this particular device, uniformity correction is performed by randomy deleting incoming gamma events in regions of increased count rates. Events in other regions are not affected. It is important to note while the appearance of static images may be improved by such uniformity correction techniques, the use of flood correction for quantitative analysis in dynamic studies may adversely effect the results. The best procedure in the clinical laboratory is to use uniformity correction for minor variations in the field uniformity. When significant aberrations appear in the flood image, the camera should be retuned.

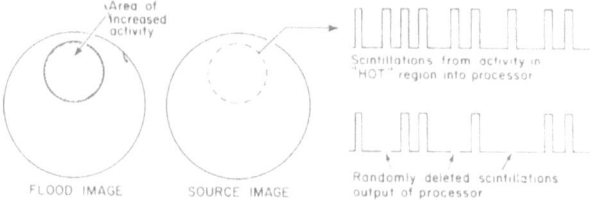

Figure 1-13. The operation of a typical correction circuit for flood field correction. Correction is done by random deletion of incoming gamma events in regions of increased count rate (shaded area). Other regions are not affected.

The count rate capability of an imaging system is especially important for dynamic cardiac studies. All currently available imaging systems will saturate if enough activity is placed within the field of view. This simply means that some primary photons which strike the crystal will not be counted by the imaging system. Dead time is the parameter usually given for characterizing the speed of an imaging system and represents that time interval during

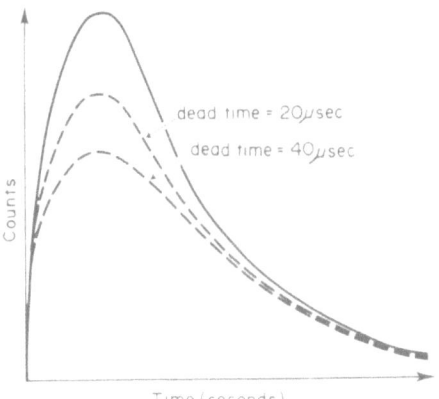

Figure 1-14. Changes in uptake-washout curves due to camera deadtime.

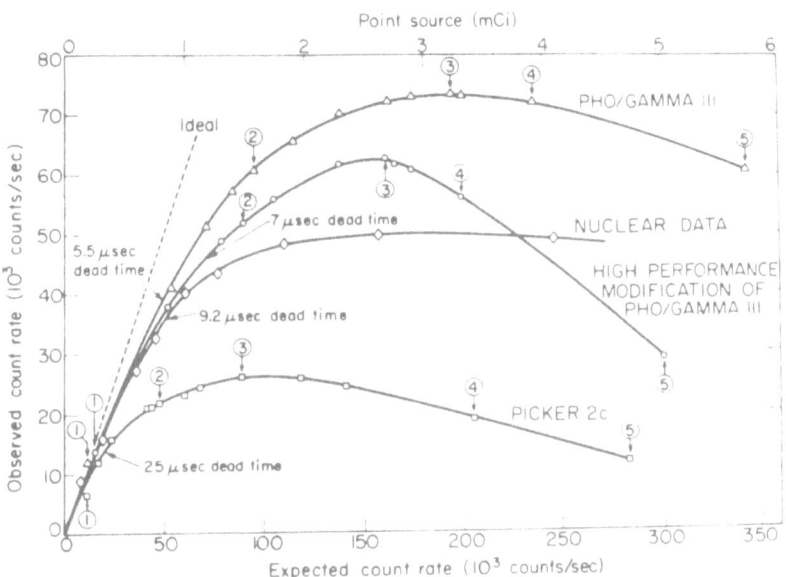

Figure 1-15. Count rates observed with different instruments with increasing radioactivity. Dead time effects obtained by recording a curve of recorded count-rate as opposed to actual count-rate data are shown.

which some primary photons which strike the crystal would be lost. Usually the smaller the dead time, the better the system. A long dead time will cause the data from a dynamic flow study to be seriously distorted. This is illustrated in Figure 1-14. Note that the distortion of the washout phase of the curve results in an inaccurate calculation of myocardial blood flow. A more pratical measure of dead time effects is obtained by recording a curve of recorded count-rate versus actual count-rate. This is illustrated in Figure 1-15. Since most cameras have paralyzable circuits, the recorded count-rate can actually decrease as the activity within the field of view is increased past a given count. The count-rate capability of the system can be characterized as the maximum number of detectable events per second without significant data loss. The camera setting during measurement of count-rate capability must be carefully scrutinized. Count-rate capability is very dependent on window settings. Manufacturers often state maximum count-rate capability at energy windows of 100%, a situation obviously not present in most clinical procedures.

SELECTING AN ANGER CAMERA FOR NUCLEAR CARDIOLOGY

The selection of an Anger camera for cardiovascular procedure is of some importance. Decisions regarding the appropriateness of large field of view cameras versus small field of view cameras and requirements for camera portability must be evaluated for individual situations. Some considerations, however, are of primary importance: (1) what is the record of both manufacturer and the specific instrument in the clinical setting? and (2) can service be easily and reliably obtained when required? The finest instrument is of no use when it is not working properly. Company reputation should be considered, but more important are questions regarding quality of a particular line and responsiveness of local company representatives. This can be evaluated by the experience of local colleagues or other references. The inclusion of a service agreement in the final purchase order is often a good decision.

Technical specifications should not be ignored when evaluating a camera for cardiac applications. As we have noted earlier, important considerations are spatial resolution, speed or count-rate capability, field uniformity, and subjective image quality. The spatial resolution of currently available Anger cameras is limited to a large degree by collimator characteristics. Resolution should therefore be measured with those collimators which will be most often used in the clinical setting. Field uniformity may be evaluated subjectively by viewing an image of the uniform flood source. Alternatively, profiles of detected activity versus distance across the diameter of the crystal can provide a more quantitative display of the same information. Data should be scrutinized under conditions of uniformity correction and without such correction. Count-rate losses are important for many cardiovascular studies such as the high temporal resolution first-transit studies where time activity curves must be corrected for dead time losses and high count-rate. Once again, count-rate capability should be measured with window settings appropriate for clinical procedures. It is helpful to obtain an impression of the clinical performance of the camera system by examining clinical images or images from phantom studies. Nothing can replace the impression gained by looking at the end product. However, one should take special care to note the conditions under which the image was generated – isotope employed, window settings, amount of activity imaged, acquisition time, number of image events, collimation, presence or absence of scatter, and whether the image was enhanced optically, photographically or with computer processing.

MULTI-CRYSTAL CAMERA

Multi-detector cameras are attractive for high count-rate dynamic studies because of their speed and uniformity. The concept of a multi-crystal camera was described by Bender and Blau in 1963 [4]. A modified version of their "autofluoroscope" is currently commercially available as the Baird Atomic System-77. This device consists of 294 individual sodium iodide crystals, each measuring 8 mm-square and 3.8 cm thick, arranged in a rectangular array of 14 columns in 21 rows. The crystals are optically coupled to 35 photomultiplier tubes by a light piping scheme that splits the light from each crystal into two equal parts. Each crystal is thus coupled to two photomultiplier tubes, one shared by all crystals in the same row and another shared by all crystals in the same column. Events occurring in a given crystal produce an output pulse in each of the two photomultiplier tubes coupled to that crystal. One pulse localizes the X coordinate of the crystal and the other pulse localizes the Y coordinate. The output from all photomultiplier tubes is summed to produce the Z signal sent to the single channel analyzer for pulse height analysis.

Multiple detectors permit the completely independent operation of event detection and event localization circuit. This is because each crystal can detect only those photons that pass through the appropriate collimator hole. The collimator then defines the spatial resolution of the system. This design allows the system to operate at up to 400,000 counts per second without significant data loss. The trade off is loss of spatial resolution with only 294 resolution cell per scene.

Multi-detector cameras are characterized by high input count-rate capability, higher sensitivity when compared to Anger cameras, poor energy discrimination caused by pulse stretching in the light-piping scheme, and poor intrinsic spatial resolution. In addition, all multi-detector systems are dependent upon a computer to gather data, and the computer system is an integral part of the imaging system. This necessary expense makes multi-crystal cameras more expensive than an Anger camera of comparable size.

The multi-crystal camera has high temporal resolution for cardiac flow studies and is ideally suited for myocardial blood flow determinations by the radioactive xenon washout technique and for many first-transit applications.

Its limitations for cardiac studies are due to its limited spatial resolution which decreases its accuracy in wall motion studies and virtually obviates its use for high resolution static imaging of such isotopes as ^{99m}Tc-PYP or ^{201}Tl.

A future application of multi-detector systems may be the cross-sectional imaging of dynamic cardiovascular studies. A group in Denmark has designed a system specifically to perform dynamic blood flow studies of the brain using radioactive xenon[5]. The system is constructed of 254 individual detectors arranged in multiple banks completely surrounding the head. Each detector is coupled to its own photomultiplier tube and associated electronics. This system has special digital logic circuits to derandomize incoming data and can function at count-rates of one million counts per second with a loss of only 1.5%. Conventional reconstruction methods produce cross sectional images of regional cerebral flow. The application of such a design to the heart has exciting possibilities.

POSITRON DETECTORS

Positron emitters are of interest for imaging studies of the cardiovascular system for several reasons. First, because of their unique method of localizing events, positron imaging systems do not require lead collimation. Since a typical collimator reduces the effective sensitivity of a conventional Anger camera by approximately 10^{-4}, the inherent sensitivity of a positron camera can be made higher. Therefore, these systems have relatively high detection efficiency as well as good spatial resolution. Second, since many metabolic markers contain oxygen, carbon, nitrogen, or potassium, it may be possible to find positron emitters for virtually any imaging problem. And third, tomographic capability is inherent in the detection scheme.

A variety of geometric arrangements for detectors have been introduced for positron imaging systems including: (1) positron cameras with opposed and specially modified Anger cameras, (2) opposed multi-crystal planar arrays, (3) opposed multi-wire proportional chamber detectors equipped with lead converters, (4) multi-bank hexagonal crystal arrays surrounding the patient, and (5) a ring of positron detectors.

The basic principles of positron detection are independent of detector type or geometry and are reviewed below. An isotope such as ^{11}C decays by the emission of a positively charged electron (positron) thereby converting an excess proton to a neutron. The positron travels a few millimeters after its ejection from the nucleus while undergoing a series of collisions with surrounding matter. At low or zero kinetic energy, the positron combines with a nearby electron in a matter-antimatter interaction. This annihilation reaction

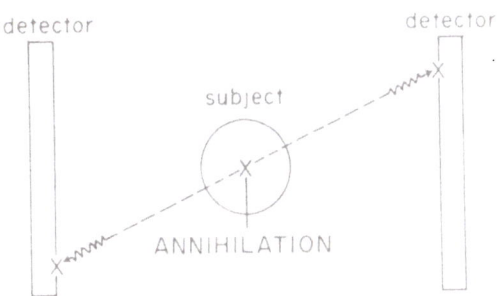

Figure 1-16. The position of the positron-electron interaction is along a line connecting the points of photon collision with the detectors.

results in the emission of two 511 keV photons which fly away at an angle of 180°. Annihilation events are recorded as coincident signals between two detectors. The position of the positron-electron interaction is along a line connecting the two detectors. This is illustrated in Figure 1-16. An image of the activity distribution of the source of radionuclide can be obtained by projecting the line connecting each set of recorded events through a given plane of the object. Annihilation events which originate within the plane will appear in focus while events originating elsewhere will be blurred. This is illustrated in Figure 1-17.

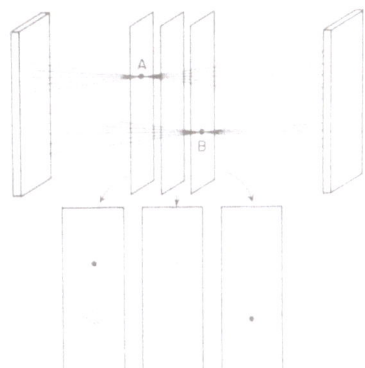

Figure 1-17. Concept of superposition tomography using parallel positron detectors.

The recording electronics of the positron imaging system are more complex than those of a simple Anger camera which produces a projection image of the object as a series of dots photographed from an oscilloscope screen. To record positron annihilation events, it is necessary to store the X-Y coordinates of the two photon detector interaction sites in digital form in the memory of a small computer. However, once these data are stored, it is advantageous and relatively simple to project them in various display modes.

THE SELECTION OF APPROPRIATE INSTRUMENTATION FOR CLINICAL
STUDIES

Present radioactive tracer techniques permit rapid, safe, noninvasive, and
repeatable measurements of cardiac performance. The parameter measured
with a cardiovascular nuclear medicine procedure will depend upon several
factors: (1) the type of radiopharmaceutical chosen (2) the method of administration, (3) the instrumentation utilized to make the measurement, and (4)
the time of observation. For example, the initial distribution of a labeled
albumin radiopharmaceutical as it traverses the central circulation is primarily
a function of blood flow. Sometime later, however, the distribution is a
function of regional blood volume and is unrelated to flow. If the first-transit
of such a tracer through the heart is recorded with a device of low frequency
response (on the order of 1-2 measurements per second) the resulting radio-
cardiogram curve can be used to determine cardiac output and to estimate
shunting. If, however, the recording is made with high temporal resolution
(greater than 20 measurements per second) the high frequency components of
the resulting curve can yield accurate determinations of both right and left
ventricular ejection fraction and a more precise measurement of shunting is
possible.

Four classes of instruments are currently available for cardiovascular nuclear medicine procedures: (1) the single detector system which includes the
scintillation probe and solid state detectors, (2) the Anger camera, (3) multi-
crystal camera, (4) positron detectors. Most single photon detection systems
employ a sodium iodide scintillation crystal to detect gamma photons and
convert incident kinetic energy to a flash of blue light. Photomultiplier tubes
then convert light energy to an electronic signal. Signals are passed through
appropriate amplification and discrimination steps to various readout or display devices. The instruments differ in the spatial resolution and sensitivity
they offer: single detector probe systems are often used with a flat-field
collimator resulting in very high sensitivity to gamma photons anywhere
within the field of view, while both Anger and multi-crystal cameras have
less sensitivity because of the necessity to collimate the detector with lead.
On the other hand, imaging systems can offer high spatial resolution and can
detect rapidly changing patterns of activity in a field of view because the
location of photons entering the crystal is determined electronically. Between
multi-crystal and single-crystal cameras, there are considerable differences.
Multi-crystal cameras are for better sensitivity (i.e. a greater number of
detectable events per second) at the cost of considerably reduced spatial
resolution. Spatial resolution is limited to the physical dimensions of each
crystal. Such designs are thus better suited to first-transit applications and
have limited utility for high resolution equilibrium studies. The spatial reso-

lution of single crystal cameras is far superior to that of multi-crystal designs and with newer generation cameras, sensitivity is more than adequate to obtain accurate first-transit studies. Single crystal cameras thus offer more versatility than multi-crystal designs.

DIGITAL RECORDING OF SCINTIGRAPHIC DATA

Computers have become increasingly important to clinical radionuclide cardiology. Quantitation of static images, the evaluation of changing radionuclide distribution with time, the acquisition of images synchronized with some physiologic trigger, and emission computed tomography are particularly dependent on computers for data acquisition and numerical analysis or reconstruction. Future clinical studies will become increasingly computer dependent.

Recall that gamma ray detectors count individual photons. Simple detectors convert the energy of an incident photon to a proportional electronic signal, or "Z" pulse, which is used for pulse height discrimination of primary photons from scattered and background radiation. Imaging devices produce an additional pair of signals for each detected photon. These X and Y signals are proportional to the X-Y location of the photon collision with the detector. Each detected photon thus constitutes a discrete electronic event with corresponding X, Y, and Z signals. These camera signals, being analog signals and characterized by voltage amplitudes which vary over some continuous range, are not compatible with the computer. The difference between analog and digital signals is illustrated in Figure 1-18. The computer requires input signals to be digital. Digital signals must meet certain stringent requirements: (1) the voltage must be equal to only one of two possible values at any given instant, and (2) the transition time between voltage levels must be short.

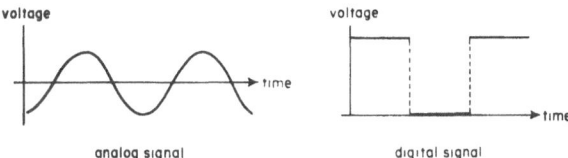

Figure 1-18. Analog signals may vary continuously over some range as a function of time. Digital signals may have only two possible values and the transition time between these two states must be very short.

Special electronic circuitry converts analog camera signals to digital form. These devices are termed appropriately analog-to-digital converters (ADCs). The most important characteristics of these analog-to-digital converters are their speed and accuracy. The maximum counting-rate of the imaging system determines the necessary conversion speed of the analog to digital converter. If a system is capable of detecting 100,000 events per second and we assume those events to be equally spaced in time, then the maximum time delay between events is 1 divided by the counting-rate, or 10 msec. After each photon is detected by the camera and subsesequently passed on to the analog-to-digital converter, 10 msec will pass before the next event arrives. The analog-to-digital converter circuit therefore has 10 msec to digitize the camera signal and prepare for the next event. If the detector system is capable of counting activity faster than the conversion rate of the analog-to-digital converter, then data will be lost between the camera and the computer. The interval during which data are lost is termed the dead time of the computer. A properly designed Nuclear Medicine computer system should never introduce computer dead time into the acquisition process.

The accuracy of an analog-to-digital converter is related to the number of binary digits (bits) used to digitize each camera signal. Ultimately, this figure determines the size of the acquisition matrix and therefore the digital spatial resolution of the system. Assume for example that 6 bit analog-to-digital converters are used to digitize the camera positioning signals X and Y. Six bits of information are capable of representing any integer number up to 2^6 or 64. The 12 bits of information used to code the digital image data are therefore capable of representing $64 \cdot 64$, or 4096, combinations. The analog-to-digital converter is therefore capable of resolving activity in one out of 4096 areas of detector surface. If 7 bits are used for each camera signal instead of 6, the resolution of the camera field is $2^7 \cdot 2^7$, or 1 in 16384. This conversion of analog signals to digital form should retain the specified resolution of the imaging system. Consider, for example, an Anger camera with a crystal of 25 cm diameter and a measured spatial resolution of 2.5 mm. Sampling theory requires the number of resolution elements to be twice the resolving power of the system. The number of required resolution elements across the diameter of the field of view is thus equal to $2 \cdot 250$ mm $\div 2.5$ mm $= 200$.

Nuclear Medicine computer systems are connected to imaging devices by feeding the X, Y and Z output signals to the analog-to-digital converters. The basic configuration for an analog-to-digital converter interfaced to a gamma camera is illustrated in Figure 1-19. Acquisition of digital images is accomplished by partitioning the camera field into discrete areas as shown in Figure 1-20. The physical dimensions of each area are determined by the size of the acquisition matrix and the gain setting of the analog to digital converters. This is shown in Figure 1-21.

Two modes of data acquisition are used with the digital computer. The frame mode acquisition builds a digital picture in computer memory as photons strike the face of the crystal. When acquisition is complete, images

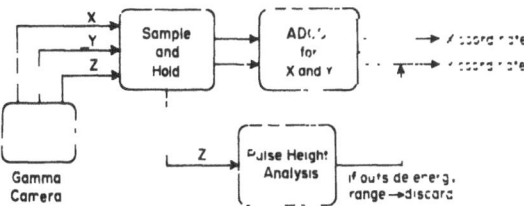

Figure 1-19. Basic configuration for ADC interface to Anger Camera.

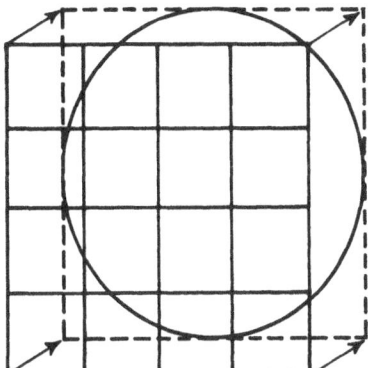

Figure 1-20. Digitizing the camera field. Imagine that a wire grid is placed over the crystal thus dividing the resultant images into discrete areas or picture elements (pixels).

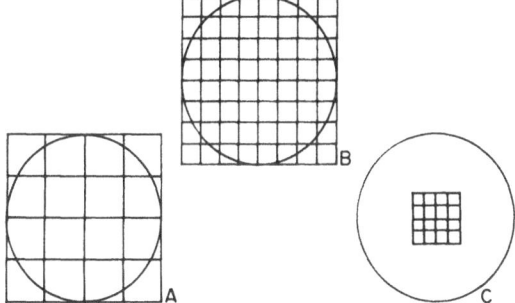

Figure 1-21. The physical dimensions of the crystal surface represented by each digital pixel is determined by the size of the acquisition matrix and the gain settings of the ADCs. In frame B the size of the acquisition matrix has been increased from 16 elements to 64 elements thus reducing the crystal surface represented by each digital pixel. In frame C the same digital resolution has been achieved by "zooming" the ADCs before digitizing the x, y positioning signals

are immediately available for processing or display. This is accomplished in the following manner. Suppose that three events, or photon–crystals interactions, occur on the face of the crystal in time sequence 1, 2 and 3, as shown in Figure 1-22. Each camera output is converted, one event at a time, to a digital number that represents the X, Y location or address of the event on

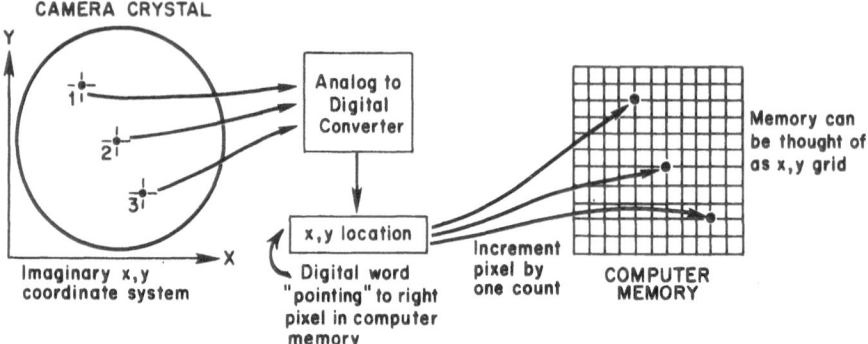

FRAME OR HISTOGRAM MODE

Figure 1-22. The frame mode acquisition of scintillation data.

the crystal face according to some imagined X, Y coordinate system. This digital address points to the proper element of the computer memory corresponding to that X, Y location. The computer memory has been organized into an X, Y grid of memory locations so that each memory location corresponds to a specific region of the crystal. As the analog-to-digital converter converts each X, Y pair. it calculates a digital number pointing to the corresponding location in computer memory and increments that location's value by exactly one count. Computer memory locations are thus utilized as simple counters with the count total in each location initially set to zero. The result is a one mapping of the total activity recorded by each discrete region on the crystal into a corresponding computer memory matrix. Thus, a digital picture is built up in computer memory during acquisition.

Alternatively, scintigraphic data may be acquired in list mode also known as serial mode. In list mode acquisition, images are not created as photons strike the crystal. Instead, as each event is converted into a digital address, the address is immediately inserted into a list, or number buffer. The computer memory is now organized as a long list of numbers. Periodically the elasped time is inserted into the buffer and coded in a special way so that it can later be distinguished from the adresses (Figure 1-23). When the buffer is full, it is transferred to some storage device such as magnetic tape or disk. At some later time after data collection is finished, the list mode data are retreived from the storage device and brought into some part of the computer memory. The computer user specifies the time intervals during which he would like to generate pictures. A program then takes all the address values from the list mode data buffer and generates a picture by incrementing locations in another area of computer memory set aside for this purpose. The digital picture is built up in exactly the same manner as in frame mode acquisition. The only difference is that the frames are formatted from data

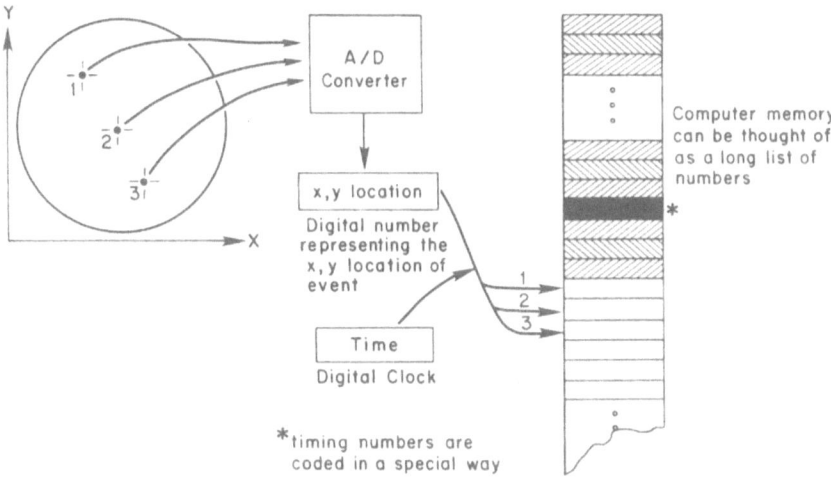

SERIAL OR LIST MODE

Figure 1-23. The serial or list mode acquisition of scintillation data.

coming from the storage device rather than from the camera. When the specified number of timing marks have been counted, the constructed picture is complete and can be viewed or stored for later recall. Usually, the timing marks are 10 msec apart. Thus, the smallest time interval for reconstructed pictures is 10 msec. List mode acquisition is designed to allow compact, rapid collection of high count-rate data. Unfortunately, most commercial nuclear medicine systems have severe limitations on the maximum allowable data rate during list mode acquisition. The importance of list mode acquisition is that other types of data, such as time markers and physiologic triggers, may be encoded in the list data stream. This formatting process offers flexible control over imaging parameters. For instance, following list mode acquisition of a first-transit cardiac study, viewing of the data for gross anatomic relation-ships may be accomplished by reformatting the data into frames of 2 sec duration. However, generation of ventricular time activity curves would require frames of 0.02 to 0.04 sec duration. List mode acquisition provides the necessary flexibility to accomplish these tasks. In addition, synchronized images of right ventricular or left ventricular performance may be accom-plished by reformatting data in specific time intervals following the occur-rence of the R-wave of the electrocardiogram. Unfortunately, the price of this versatility is bulky storage requirements and considerable time required to reformat the data.

An extremely important extension of frame mode acquisition is the tech-nique known as multiple-gated acquisition. In this mode, data from the camera are channeled to a series of matrices (or storage bins) in the comput-

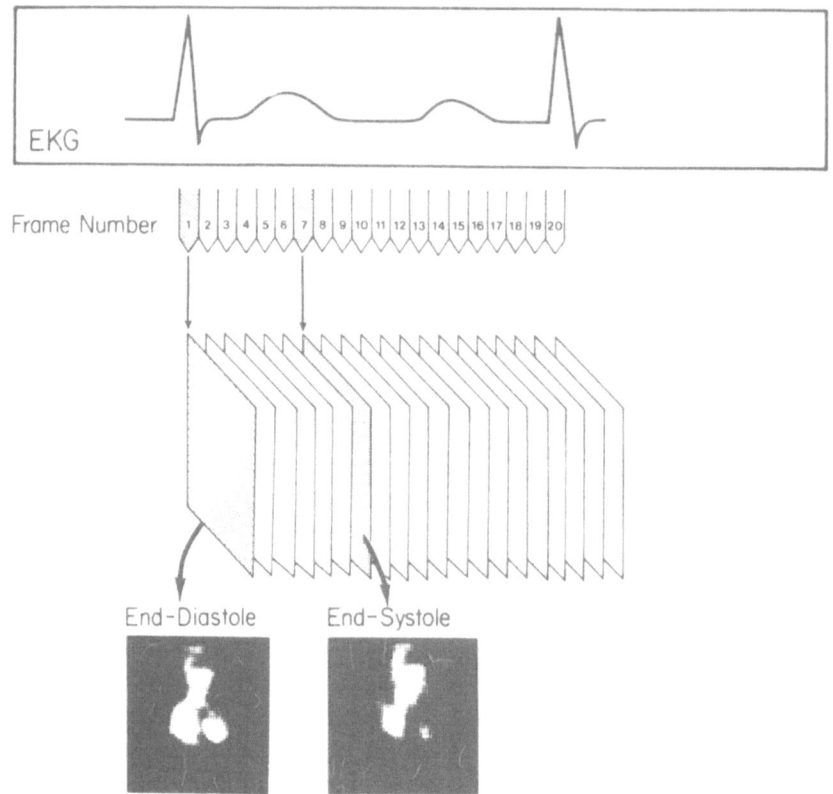

Figure 1-24. Basic concept of technique for multiple EKG gated image acquisition.

er's memory as shown in Figure 1-24. Each individual picture is still a one-to-one mapping of the crystal face in the computer memory. Individual matrices differ from one another in that they represent different time intervals following some physiologic event. A common application of this technique is the analysis of left ventricular blood pool activity for ejection fraction and wall motion. This form of acquisition is handled as follows. The computer will typically analyze some 10 heart beats from the input analog EKG signal and calculate the average R-R interval in milliseconds. The R-R interval is then divided into a fixed number of time intervals or frames following the R-wave. Following the initial occurrence of the R-wave, all camera data are directed into matrix 1. Acquisition continues in the matrix 1 for the previously calculated time interval per frame. When this time interval has elapsed, a special timing signal halts acquisition into matrix 1 and redirects camera data into matrix 2. This continues for each succeeding frame until the second occurrence of the R-wave. At this point, camera data are redirected to matrix 1 and are added to the data already resident. This sequence continues until acquisition is complete. Typically, acquisition occurs over many cardiac cycles building a series of images with increasing counting statistics representing a single, average, composite cardiac cycle.

DATA REPRESENTATION IN COMPUTER MEMORY

Just as digital signals may have only two possible voltage states, computer circuits may only have two states: ON or OFF. A useful comparison can be made to a string of light bulbs. Some of the bulbs in the string may be ON and some may be OFF, but no bulb can be somewhere between ON and OFF. For each bulb there are clearly only two distinguishable states. Computer circuits are also characterized by this ON and OFF state of operation. To make representation of these states more convenient, the number 1 is chosen to represent a circuit in the ON state, with 0 representing the OFF state. Following this line of reasoning, the computer data sequence: ON ON OFF OFF ON is represented by the sequence: 1 1 0 0 1. By attaching significance to their positions, the digits may be used to represent numeric quantities. Those quantities are generated using the binary (base 2) number system.

By definition, binary numbers are formed using two digits only: 1 and 0. Below are ten binary numbers and their decimal equivalents.

BINARY	DECIMAL
1	1
10	2
11	3
100	4
101	5
110	6
111	7
1000	8
1001	9
1010	10

Numeric operations in the binary system are representationally equivalent to the same operations in the decimal system. The only difference is a simple change of significance (or weighting value) of each digit position. For example, consider the decimal 173 also written and 173_{10}. The breakdown of this number is given by:

$$\begin{aligned} 173_{10} = 1 \cdot 10^2 &= 100 \\ 7 \cdot 10^1 &- 70 \\ 3 \cdot 10^0 &= 3 \\ \hline &170 \end{aligned}$$

The same breakdown technique applies to binary numbers. Consider the binary number 1011_2:

$$1011_2 = 1 \cdot 2^3 = 8$$
$$0 \cdot 2^2 = 0$$
$$1 \cdot 2^1 = 2$$
$$1 \cdot 2^0 = 1$$
$$\overline{\hphantom{11}}\,.$$
$$11$$

Binary numbers can be converted to their decimal equivalents.

Data are organized in computer memory according to a logical format. The individual circuits which represent individual digits are grouped sequentially into bytes (8 circuits) or word (16 circuits). A *byte* therefore contains 8 bits (or binary digits) or information while a *word* contains 16 bits of data. Image matrices are specified by their size (number of columns = X, number of rows = Y) and their depth (number of bits in each pixel). A typical example is 128×128 and each pixels contain up to 16 bits of information.

The number of bits per pixel is important in scintigraphic studies. Eight bits of data allows the number of counts per pixel to range from 0 to a maximum of 255 ($2^8 - 1$). Eight bits is entirely sufficient for routine dynamic studies but is usually insufficient for high resolution static images and may be inadequate for some multiple gated studies. Sixteen bits of data allow the representation of count values from 0 to 65, 536 (2^{16}). This is necessary for many static images but is wasteful for dynamic procedures. Some useful guidelines for comparing the acquisition capability of various nuclear medicine computer systems are given below:

STATIC IMAGING	RAPID DYNAMIC STUDIES	HIGH RESOLUTION, SLOW DYNAMICS
$128 \times 128 \times 6$	$64 \times 64 \times 8$	$64 \times 64 \times 16$
$256 \times 256 \times 8$	$128 \times 128 \times 8$	$128 \times 128 \times 16$
		$256 \times 256 \times 8$

THE EXTRACTION OF CLINICAL INFORMATION

We now have at least some understanding of how data are brought into a computer from a gamma camera and how those data are represented in numeric form in computer memory. Unfortunately, however, you cannot simply feed the computer data and have it eject an answer. The computer cannot mysteriously digest and assimilate all knowledge. If there is a method of doing something which can be broken down into simple steps requiring no human judgment, then it may be possible to program a computer to do it. The sequence of events is as follows: some one must first figure out how to solve the problem. He then instructs (programs) the computer how to perform that function. The computer then solves the problem in the same manner as the programmer. The only difference is that the computer does it many times faster.

COMPUTER OPERATIONS WHICH MAY HAVE CLINICAL SIGNIFICANCE MAY BE CATEGORIZED AS FOLLOWS:

1. Image display/data presentation
2. Numerical data extraction
3. Image processing
4. Tomographic reconstruction
5. General numerical and statistical calculations
6. File sorting/information retrieval (data base management)
7. Report generation

UNDERSTANDING EMISSION TOMOGRAPHY

Estimation of 3-dimensional form from projections

Although computer-assisted tomographic (CT or CAT) scanners which utilize X-rays as the imaging energy are now commonplace in large medical hospitals, emission tomographic systems have been disseminated much more slowly. The first tomographic imaging system used for medical studies was an emission scanner designed and built by Kuhl and his associates [5, 6] followed by Anger's tomoscanner [7, 8]. Many different methods for imaging a 3-dimensional radioactive source in tomographic cross section have been devised and tested over the past 20 years [9-13].

All tomographic systems whether transmission or emission, attempt to estimate one or more planar cross-sections of an object given a series of observations from several different view points. The observations are always in the form of *projections*, and in the case of emission tomography, a projection is the sum of all the radioactivity in the object as viewed from a particular point. Consider Figure 1-25 where an observer looks at a back-lighted pair of disk-shaped glass containers filled with a colored liquid. As the observer moves to observation points 1, 2 and 3, he begins to recognize the depth relationship of objects A and B because of their relative projected positions at the different view points. Figure 1-25 is in fact a good illustration of the data collection geometry for a multipinhole tomograph which will be discussed later. While the human perceptual ability is superior in many ways to the computer reconstruction algorithm used to estimate the structures in the two planes of this example, the principles are the same. If the observer had moved to point 4, he would have enormously improved his perception of the two structures. From the example of Figure 1-25, we can develop three basic intuitive tenants of tomography.

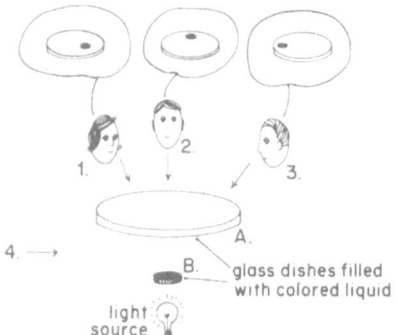

Figure 1-25. Schematic demonstration of the value of tomographic imaging.

First of all, the more views (projections) we have of the object, the better we can estimate its structure. Secondly, it is better to have widely spaced viewing points. For example, if the observer in Figure 1-25 is limited to only two views he will derive more perceptive input from view points 2 and 4 than, for example, from view points 1 and 2. Finally, in the example of Figure 1-25, any distortion of one or more views will hinder the perception of the 3-dimensional structure of the object. For emission tomography this means one needs good statistics, or many counts, from the source if the reconstructed image is to be noise free (although these counts can be spread over many views, or projections).

Multipinhole emission tomographs

The examples of Figure 1-25 can be readily extended to the multipinhole tomographic system (MTS) which is commercially available. The concept of the MTS is to produce n projections of the source object (n is the number of pinholes) using a scintillation camera fitted with a special collimator. The collimator is simply a thin sheet of lead placed 9–15 cm from the camera crystal, and the lead sheet has n small holes arranged in a regular pattern. Figure 1-26, Step 1 illustrates a 4-pinhole system ($n = 4$), showing the four projections of the source object which are produced on the crystal to form the *raw data image*. Special lead baffles are included to insure that the images do not overlap. The most recent version of the MTS was developed by Vogel, Kirch, and their colleagues [13] although the basic concept is not new.

Figure 1-26, Step II shows how the data are reconstructed to produce a 3-dimensional image. A computer program *backprojects* each image onto each of several planes, the number of planes being selectable by the operator. Notice that depth information is coded into the MTS image as a change in position of the n projections of this source were slowly moved nearer the collimator, the n projections of this source onto the crystal would appear as dots which moved outward toward the crystal edge. In attempting to determine where each of the n images came from, the computer program will apportion each image into each reconstructed plane, as shown in Figure 1-26, Step II. (In fact current back-projection programs are slightly more sophisticated in philosophy, but similar to that described here.) At the proper focal plane the contributions from the n images will summate; at other depths they do not add, but appear as noisy shapes. In Figure 1-26, three planes have been selected for reconstruction, with plane B as the correct focal plane. The image placed in places A and C by the backprojection program are incorrect, and they are called *blur-plane artifacts*. These are partially removed by another computer program which is usually called *iterative deblurring*. There are several ways to reduce the *blur-plane* artifacts, but the most common method is to use an iterative scheme based on the algebraic reconstruction technique (ART) developed by Gordon et al. [15, 16]. Briefly the algorithm works as follows. Following backprojection the iterative deblurring program develops a simulated raw data image containing the n small images by reversing the backprojection procedure.

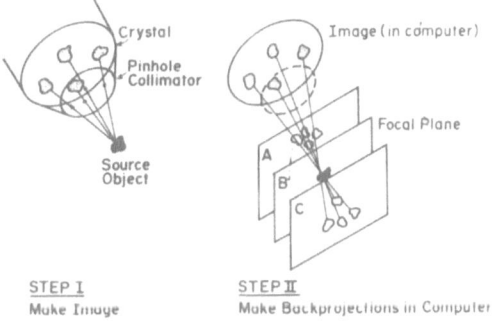

Figure 1-26. Basic concept of 4 pinhole tomographic imaging.

Data in each backprojected plane (planes A, B and C, Figure 1-26, Step II) are projected onto the crystal plane through each pinhole to form a simulated image. During this step, attenuation and other effects can be included. Keep in mind that the simulated image construction occurs in the computer memory and is accomplished mathematically using the known geometry of the

Make Image   Make Backprojections in Computer

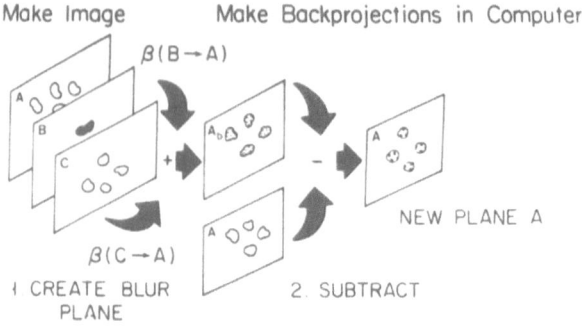

STEP Ⅲ

Deblur Image

Figure 1-27. Approach to deblurring of pinhole tomographic images.

MTS. Now if the backprojected reconstructions were perfect, this simulated image would be identical to the original raw data image. Unfortunately this is not the case, and an *error raw data image* can be formed by subtracting the simulated raw data image from the original raw data image. The completion of one iteration of the deblurring operation is accomplished by backprojecting the error raw data image onto each plane, as shown in Figure 1-27, Step III. This will tend to compensate the reconstructed images in each plane by removing some of the blur artifacts. The entire process can then be repeated several times, although computer processing speeds usually limit current MTSs to 1 or 2 iterations.

The multipinhole technique can enhance the visualization of objects which are obscured by overlying structures, and the technique can be applied by any nuclear imaging facility which has access to commonly-used low-energy radionuclides, a scintillation camera (preferably large field-of-view), and a small computer system. The major disadvantages of the method are incomplete removal of blur artifacts by the iterative deblurring software, poor focusing ability of the tomograph especially at depths greater than 15 cm from the collimator, and a limited field of view.

Slant-hole emission tomographs

One of the problems with the multipinhole tomographic method is the decrease in projection angle as depth increases moving away from the collimator. As discussed earlier, it is advantageous to take the projections of the object as far apart in angle as possible. The inherent geometry of the MTS prohibits this. To get around this problem another commercially-available system has been developed, the slant-hole emission tomograph (SET).

A special collimator is used on the SET consisting of a group of parallel holes which are slanted 20–30° with respect to a line perpendicular to the face of the crystal. Again a scintillation camera interfaced to a minicomputer system is employed. Figure 1-28 shows how the SET might collect data. The object to be imaged is placed approximately on the crystal center line and close enough to the collimator to ensure that the image falls on the crystal face. In Figure 1-28A an image is collected. Then the collimator, which is attached with a rotating collar, is rotated through some predetermined angle and another image is collected (Figure 1-28 B, C). This is repeated a number of times (usually 5-10 depending on data collection time) until a set of projections is obtained.

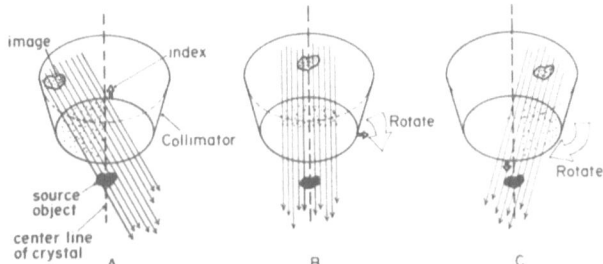

Figure 1-28. Slant-hole emission tomography – data collection sequence.

These projections are then reconstructed by a computer program, using methods similar to those discussed for the MTS. Blur artifacts are also a problem with the SET system. Computer programs to remove these are helpful but always leave some residue.

The obvious advantage of the SET over the MTS is the constant projection angle over the depth of the object being imaged. This characteristic implies that the SET reconstructed planes would have less variation in quality, as a function of their distance away from the collimator, than similar MTS planes would have. The relative disadvantages of the SET method are a limited field of view in depth, and the inability to image dynamic processes in tomographic section (all projections are not taken simultaneously). The relative merits of the two techniques for clinical imaging are still being evaluated.

Coded aperture methods

Since coded-aperture methods have not been applied clinically to a wide extent, they will be discussed only briefly. It was previously mentioned that lead baffles are used with the multipinhole system to prevent overlap of the images. If these are omitted and the images are allowed to overlap, the raw data image is referred to as being *coded,* or scrambled, in such a way that not only is the depth information coded into a position displacement, but also which image «belongs" to a given pinhole can no longer be distinguished. Reconstruction of several planes is accomplished with methods which simultaneously decode the raw data image in depth while resolving the overlap of images from the various pinholes[9–11, 17–19].

Figure 1-29 demonstrates the data collection and optical reconstruction with a multipinhole coded aperture tomographic system. Only two pinholes are included for the sake of clarity, although 10–50 pinholes are often used in actual systems. In Figure 1-29, Step I, the raw data image from an X-shaped source shows the characteristic overlap of images from each pinhole. In Step II an optical method of reconstructing the data is illustrated. In this example two planes of reconstruction are selected – one at the focal plane of the source object, and another plane further away. A diffuse light source is used to illuminate a sheet of film which contains the raw data image. Another opaque film containing the pinhole patterns is placed between the raw data film and a translucent viewing screen. Each pinhole works like a lens to form an image on the viewing screen as shown. At the correct point in the focal plane the crosses summate to form the desired reconstruction of the source object, but note that two unwanted crosses are reproduced on each side of the source object. These unwanted crosses are an example of the *in plane blurring* effect characteristic of coxed aperture systems. Blur artifacts occur in the focal plane as well as other planes, whereas the MTS and SET methods must contend with only one of these blurring problems. To summarize, the coded aperture techniques have more apparent sensitivity because each pinhole can use all of the crystal detector, but the price which is paid for this increase in efficiency is difficulty in decoding and reconstructing the images. The net effect is that the source strength-to-background noise ratio does not increase even though the sensitivity rises.

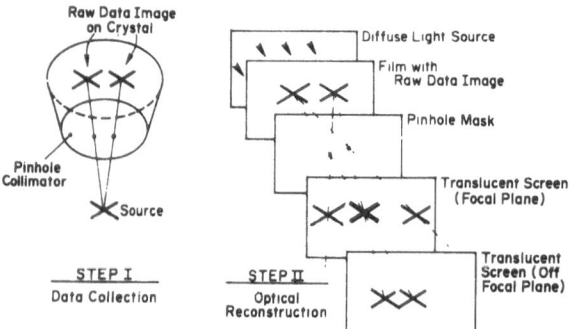

Figure 1-29. Multipinhole coded aperture tomography – data collection and optical reconstruction.

The operation in Figure 1-29, Step II can also be carried out on digital computer by an operation called cross correlation, or "matched filtering". Suffice it to say that the final outcome is the same as that illustrated in Figure 1-29, except computer processing offers some advantages in flexibility of the reconstruction and in viewing the reconstructed images.

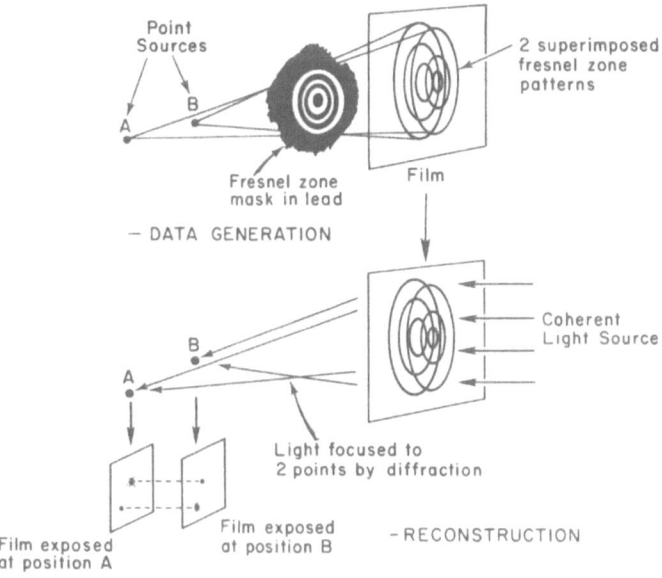

Figure 1-30. Demonstration of how two point sources are coded on film with a Fresnel zone and then reconstructed.

Another type of coded-aparture tomographic method is the Fresnel zone technique shown in Figure 1-30. The technique is exactly analogous to the coded aperture multipinhole method just described, except the focusing ability of the Fresnel zone pattern is used to focus the raw data and produce the reconstructed images. Fresnel zone data can also be reconstructed using a digital computer, and the same comments given above for the coded aperture multipinhole technique apply to Fresnel zone systems. Other types of coded aperture systems using moving arrays of holes have been developed and show promise [10] but will not be discussed here.

Transverse section imaging

All of the techniques previously described can be categorized loosely as off-plane blurring techniques because they use a blurring effect to reduce the contrast of objects which are not in the reconstructed focal plane. As previously discussed, the blurring is never complete with these methods, and blur artifacts always remain to reduce the contrast of the desired focal plane object. To get around this problem Kuhl's[5, 6] transverse section scanning method is often used as the method for collecting data. In Figure 1-31, a schematic depiction of the transverse section approach is illustrated. Again one is gathering projections around the source object (the heart in this case) at many different viewing angles, and reconstructing the activity in a plane from these projections. In Figure 1-6 the apparatus illustrated uses many different detectors to generate several projections simultaneously while the entire detector gantry rotates slowly about the patient. This particular geometry was introduced by Kuhl and is used in other machines[12, 13] although other geometries are appropriate and will be discussed.

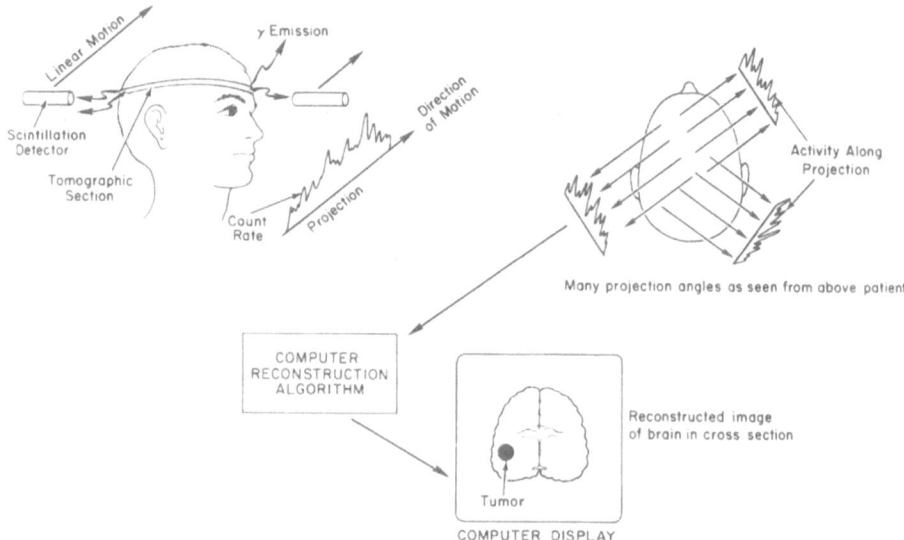

Figure 1-31. Schematic of tomographic brain section made by viewing many projections of the activity, storing these projections in digital form, and reconstructing the section with a numerical algorithm.

The differentiation between the off-plane blurring systems previously discussed and the transverse section systems is that in general the transverse section systems only consider projections from a single plane during data collection. Activity in other planes parallel to the plane (slice) of interest is not recorded; therefore, there is no blurring artifact from activity outside the focal plane as with the off-plane blurring methods. This fact is evidenced by the greatly improved images which are produced by the transverse section machines.

Figure 1-31 schematically illustrates emission transverse section scanning (ETSS) of the brain. In ETSS terminology the *projection* takes on the particular meaning of a one-dimensional function of count-rate recorded while scanning past the source as shown in Figure 1-31. Many of these projections of the activity within the slice, or section, are collected over different angles (usually 30–80). A computer program reconstructs the activity distribution within the section by one of two methods: a) filtered backprojection (which will include for the discussion given here Fourier methods, convolution methods, or linear superposition), or b) iterative reconstruction.

Filtered backprojection (FBP) has been described elsewhere [16, 20–23] and will be summarized here. Consider the image formed by backprojecting many projections of a point source infinitely as shown in Figure 1-32. As previously discussed, the backprojection operation apportions the activity at each point in the projection equally into the area of reconstructed image which could have contributed to that point on the projection. This portion of the image lies along a line, called a *raysum*, perpendicular to the projection. Broadening of the reconstructed object is caused by improper summation of all the raysum contributions about the center of the object. The backprojected image could be resharpened by applying a 2-dimensional filter, called a "deconvolution filter", as shown in Figure 1-32B. Note that the filter does not provide perfect compensation – some undershoot and ringing effects about the main peak occur. The same effect can be achieved much faster by applying the same filter to each projection before the backprojection operation. This is illustrated by Figures 1-32C and 1-32D. Filtered backprojection methods are fast, rela-

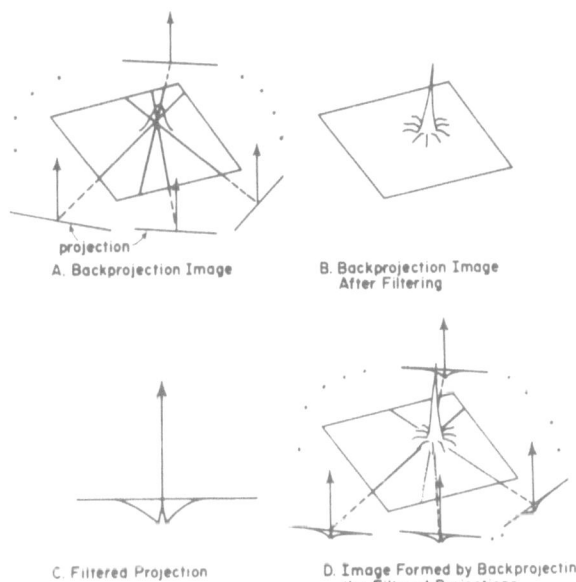

A. Backprojection Image

B. Backprojection Image
After Filtering

C. Filtered Projection

D. Image Formed by Backprojecting
the Filtered Projections

Figure 1-32. Development of the concept of reconstruction by filtered backprojection.

tively accurate, and can be modified to work for most emission tomographic applications. They are also one-step methods that do not require repetitive operations to succeed. For these reasons FBP msthods are the most widely used.

The concept of iterative reconstruction has been previously discussed under the Multipinhole Emission Tomographs section. The ART algorithm as applied to ETSS will be briefly discussed. The first step of ART is simple backprojection shown in Figure 1-32. A set of simulated projections is then calculated by reversing the backprojection procedure using the reconstructed image. This will give a set of simulated projections which have a smeared point source in each. A set of error projections is produced by subtracting the simulated projections from the actual raw data projections. This error projection is then backprojected into the current reconstruction. The procedure is repeated for 3-8 iterations to complete the reconstruction. Attenuation effects are usually inserted during the simulated projection procedure. ART is much slower than FBP, but provides better attenuation correction and better reconstructions than FBP when the projections are noisy (low count rates)[23]. An excellent discussion of reconstruction algorithms for emission tomography is given in reference [24].

The projections around the source can also be collected using a rotating scintillation camera[25-27]. By digitizing strips of the camera image, the computer can reconstruct multiple slices of an object. Cameras usually have 0.1, or less, the sensitivity of a rotating multidetector transverse scanner when compared on a per-slice basis; however, the rotating cameras gather data for many slices during one slow rotation.

More recently, coincidence detection systems have been constructed to detect the annihilation of β^+ particles emitted by certain special radionuclides[28-34]. These radionuclides, which are positron emitters, generally have short half-lives ranging from 2 hr to a few seconds. This means they must be produced by a cyclotron at or near the site of the imaging system, an obvious disadvantage. The radiation dose to the patient is also higher, since the tissue receives radiation not only from the β^+ particle, but also from the two back-to-back 511 keV gammas which are released during the annihilation process. On the other hand, the annihilation coincidence detection (ACD) systems have some distinct advantages when compared to more commonly used lead-collimated single photon (or "singles counting") systems. The first is the ability to collimate the detector response electronically. Only back-to-back gammas emitted within the cylindrical space between the detector crystals of an ACD pair will be recorded, since the coincidence circuit requires essentially simultaneous registration of a photon at both crystals (see Figure 1-33). Event A in Figure 1-33A will be recorded, whereas event B will not. The second big advantage of ACD systems is the insensitivity of the recorded

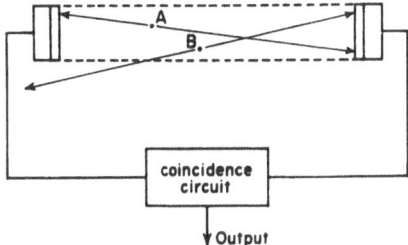

A. Electronic Collimation

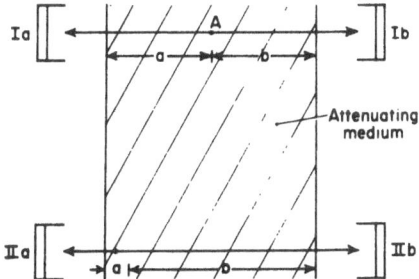

B. Insensitivity to Position of Source

Figure 1-33. Advantages of annihilation coincidence detection.

count rate to the position of a source within an attenuating medium. Figure 1-33B shows two positron-emitting point sources within an attenuating medium. Both ACDs will record equal count rates for source strengths that are the same. This property of the ACD systems makes attenuation correction simplier than single-photon systems when performing tomographic imaging. Another advantage of ACD systems is the ability to form many pairs of detectors in an array, increasing the sensitivity of the system. In Figure 1-33B, for example, one can form four detector pairs by adding coincidence circuitry (Ia-Ib, IIa-IIb, IIa-Ib, and Ia-IIb). It turns out, however, that very small doses must be used in multipaired ACD systems to avoid overloading the system with accidental random events called " singles ". Ring geometries of detectors are often used for ACD systems to get the densest arrangement of dctector crystals – hence, the most sensitivity. Finally, some of the positron emitters such as ^{11}C, ^{13}N, and ^{15}O can be incorporated into natural compounds, analogs, or synthesized drugs for the study of *in-vivo* metabolic processes. This ability to label a metabolic agent with a positron emitter without altering its chemical nature has opened a new frontier in imaging physiologic function.

Although single-photon tomography cannot match the technical advantages of ACD systems listed above, the widespread availability of inexpensive radionuclides makes the single photon techniques attractive when clinical studies are considered. A number of single-photon tomographs are commercially available of the multidetector and rotating camera types. One single-photon tomograph has recently been designed to study brain blood flow in tomographic cross-section [13].

Practical myocardial imaging with ^{201}Tl and ^{99m}Tc-pyrophosphate

The technique and instrumentation for myocardial imaging with ^{201}Tl and ^{99m}Tc-pyrophosphate, as described in this book, is summarized in Table 1-2. Quality control of instrumentation, radiopharmaceuticals and imaging technique are important aspects of reliable myocardial imaging and will be discussed in the following chapters.

Table 1-2. Practical myocardial imaging with ^{201}Tl and ^{99m}Tc-pyrophosphate

	^{201}Tl	^{99m}Tc-pyrophosphate
Dose	2 mCi	15 mCi
Injection	i.v.	i.v.
Time between injection and imaging	5-10 min	1½-2 hr
Gamma camera	Single crystal, 37 PMT	Single crystal, 37 PMT
Collimator	Parallel-hole, high-resolution (or general purpose)	Parallel-hole, high-resolution (or general purpose)
Energy peak	80 keV	140 keV
Window	20%	20%
Counts/view	300,000	300,000-500,000
Views	Anterior, 45° left-anterior-oblique, left-lateral	Anterior, 45° left-anterior-oblique, left-lateral
Computer matrix selection	128×128	128×128
Sequence when dual imaging is performed	#1	#2

REFERENCES

1. Blumgart HL, Weiss S: Studies on the velocity of blood flow. J Clin Invest 4:15, 1927.
2. Hevesy G: The absorption and translocation of lead by plants: A contribution to the application of the method of radioactive indicators in the investigation in the change of substance in plants. Biochem J 17:439, 1923.
3. Prinzmetal M, Corday E, Bergman HC, Schwartz L, Spritzler RJ: Radiocardiography: a new method for studying the blood flow through the chambers of the heart in human beings. Science 108:340, 1948.
4. Bender MA, Blau M: The autofluoroscope. Nucleonics 21:52, 1963.
5. Kuhl DE, Edwards RQ: Image separation radioisotope scanning. Radiology 80:653, 1963.

6. Kuhl DE, Edwards RQ, Ricci AR, et al.: The Mark IV system for radionuclide computed tomography of the brain. Radiology 121:405, 1976.

7. Anger HO: Multiplane tomographic gamma-ray scanner. In: Medical radioisotope scintigraphy, Vol I, p 203. Vienna: Int. Atomic Energy Agency, 1969.

8. Anger HO: Multiplane tomographic scanner. In: Tomographic imaging in nuclear medicine, p 2, Freedman GS, ed. New York: Soc. Nucl. Med., 1973.

9. Chang LT, Kaplan SN, MacDonald B, et al.: A method of tomographic imaging using a multiple pinhole coded aperture. J Nucl Med 15:1063, 1974.

10. Chang LT, MacDonald B, Perez-Mendez V: Coded aperture imaging of gamma rays using multiple pinhole arrays and multiwire proportional chamber detector. IEEE Trans Nucl Sci 5-22:374, 1975.

11. Koral RF, Rogers WL, Knoll GF: Digital tomographic imaging with time-modulated and pseudo random coded aperture. J Nucl Med 16:402, 1975.

12. Bowley AR, Taylor CG, Causer DA, Barber DC, et al.: A radioisotope scanner for rectilinear, transverse section and longitudinal section scanning: (ASS-the Aberdeero Section Scanner). Br J Radiol 46:262, 1973.

13. Stokely EM, Sveinsdottir, Lassen NA, Rommer P: A single photon dynamic computer assisted tomograph for imaging brain function in multiple cross sections. J Comput Assist Tomogr 4:230, 1980.

14. Vogel RA, Kirch D, LeFree M, et al.: A new method of multiplane tomography using a seven pinhole collimator and an Anger scintillation camera. J Nucl Med 19:648, 1978.

15. Gordon R: A tutorial on ART (algebraic reconstruction techniques). IEEE Trans Nucl Sci 5-21:78, 1974.

16. Gordon R, Herman GT: Three dimensional reconstruction from projections: a review of algorithms. Int Rev Cytol 38:111, 1974.

17. Mertz L, Young NO: Fresnel transformation of images. In: Proc. Int Conf on Optical Instrumentation, p 305. London: Chapman & Hall, 1961.

18. Barret HN: Fresnel zone plate imaging in nuclear medicine. J Nucl Med 13:382, 1972.

19. Rogers WL, Han KS, Jones LW, et al.: Applications of a fresnel zone plate to gamma ray imaging. J Nucl Med 13:612, 1972.

20. Shepp LA, Logan BF: The Fourier reconstruction of a head section. IEEE Trans Nucl Sci 5-21:21-43, 1974.

21. Bracewell RN: Strip integration in radioastronomy. Aust J Phys 9:198, 1956.

22. Cho ZH: General views on 3-d image reconstruction and computerized transverse axial tomography. IEEE Trans Nucl Sci 5-21:44, 1974.

23. Herman GT, Rowland SW: Three methods for reconstructing objects from X rays: a comparative study. Com Graphics and Image Processing 2:151, 1973.

24. Budinger TF, Gullberg GT, Huesman RH: Emission computed tomography. In: Image reconstruction from projections; implementation and applications, Herman GT, ed. Vol. 32 of Topics in Applied Physics, p 147. New York: Springer-Verlag, 1979.

25. Anger HO, Price DC, Yost PE: Transverse-section scanning with the scintillation camera. J Nucl Med 8:314, 1967.

26. Keyes JW, Orlandea N, Heetderks WJ, et al.: The humongotron – a scintillation camera transaxial tomograph. J Nucl Med 18:381, 1977.

27. Jasyczak RJ, Murphy PH, Huard D, Burdine JA: Radionuclide emission computed tomography of the head with ^{99m}Tc and a scintillation camera. J Nucl Med 18:373, 1977.

28. Chesler DA: Positron tomography and three-dimensional reconstruction technique. In: Tomographic imaging in nuclear medicine, p 176, Freedman GS, ed. New York: Soc. Nucl Med, 1973.

29. Phelps ME, Hoffman EJ, Mullani NA, et al.: Application of annihilation coincidence detection to transaxial reconstruction tomography. J Nucl Med 16:210, 1975.

30. Phelps ME, Hoffman EJ, Highfill R, Kuhl DE: A new emission computed axial tomography for positron emitters. J Nucl Med 18:603, 1975.

31. Bohm C, Eriksson L. Bergtrom, et al.: A computer assisted ring detector positron camera system for reconstruction tomography of the brain. IEEE Trans Nucl Sci 5-25:624, 1978.

32. Cho ZH, Chan JK, Eriksson L: Circular ring transverse axial positron camera for 3-dimensional reconstruction of radionuclides distribution. IEEE Trans Nucl Sci 5-23:613, 1976.
33. Robertson JS, Marr RB, Rosenblum M, et al.: 32-crystal positron transverse section detector. In: Tomographic imaging in nuclear medicine, p 142, Freedman GS, ed. New York: Soc. Nucl. Med., 1973.
34. Ter-Pogossian MM, Mullani NA, Hood JT, et al.: Design considerations for a positron emission transverse tomography (PETTV) for imaging of the brain. J Comput Assist Tomog 2:539, 1978.

ACCUMULATION OF
RADIOPHARMACEUTICALS

2. MECHANISMS OF THALLIUM-201 MYOCARDIAL ACCUMULATION

FRANS J. TH. WACKERS and GERARD SAMSON

Thallium is a metallic element of group IIIA of the periodic table with biological similarities to potassium. Thallium was first used successfully for external imaging of the human heart by Kawana et al.[1]. In 1970 these investigators reported on the use of a mixture of short-lived thallium isotopes, mainly ^{199}Tl, for myocardial imaging. Lebowitz et al.[2] reported in 1975 the production of ^{201}Tl and suggested that this might be a more favorable isotope for clinical imaging with the Anger scintillation camera. Scintiscans obtained in the goat, indicated that the relative myocardial concentration was sufficient to allow external imaging[3]. In the same year we reported the feasibility of myocardial imaging in patients with and without acute myocardial infarction[4].

The practical advantages of ^{201}Tl over other suitable myocardial imaging agents such as potassium-43 (^{43}K), rubidium-81 (^{81}Rb), and cesium-129 (^{129}Cs), are its relatively low energy photons which makes it possible to employ high-resolution low-energy collimators and its physical half-life of 73 hr which provides sufficiently long shelf-life for practical clinical imaging.

Toxicological considerations do not play a role using ^{201}Tl as thallous chloride. The concentration of thallous chloride in a dose of 2 mCi of ^{201}Tl is less than 4 µg. The LD_{50} of thallous chloride is a factor 10^4 more. The minimal lethal dose in man is reported to be 12 mg/kg[5].

TISSUE DISTRIBUTION AND RADIATION DOSE

Usually, estimations of radiation dose to patients are based on extrapolation of data derived from animal experiments. We assessed the effective half-life, tissue distribution and radiation dose of ^{201}Tl from analysis of tissue samples obtained at post mortem in six patients[6].

From sequential whole-body measurements we determined the effective half-life of ^{201}Tl to be 57 ± 4.32 hr (mean $\pm$ SD). Figure 2-1 shows an example of sequential images obtained in a patient. The biological half-life of thallous chloride was estimated to be 10.3 ± 3.4 days. The daily excretion of thallium

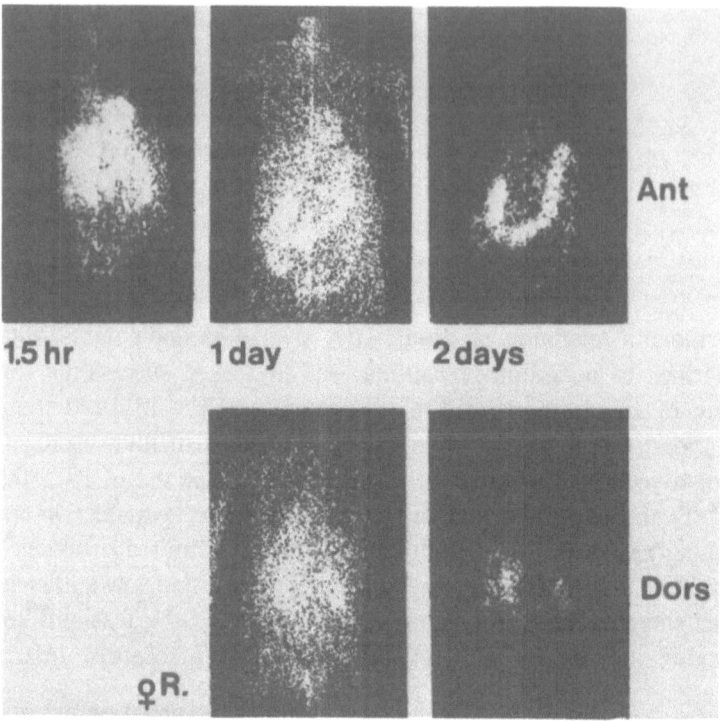

Figure 2-1. Sequential imaging with ^{201}Tl at 1.5 h, 1 day and 2 days after injection. It can be appreciated that redistribution of ^{201}Tl throughout the body occurs. Initially most of the activity is concentrated in heart, liver and spleen. One day after injection, the concentration in the heart has relatively decreased and most of the activity is located in skeletal muscle, kidneys and intestines. On the second day after injection most of the ^{201}Tl activity is in the large bowel (and feces) and kidneys. Abbreviations: Ant = anterior view; Dors = dorsal view. Reproduced with permission from Ref. [49].

in the urine and stools amounts to 3.5% and 2% respectively. Table 2-1 shows the relative accumulation of ^{201}Tl in various organs. The organ distribution of ^{201}Tl at the time of death in seven patients is expressed as mean percentages of administered activity. As shown in Table 2-1, the total myocardium accumulates approximately 4% of the administered dose, whereas this is 9% for the liver and 4% for the kidney. The major portion of injected ^{201}Tl is accumulated in skeletal muscle. These values are in general agreement with the distribution pattern observed in animals [3, 7, 8]. The tissue radiation doses in various organs were calculated using the MIRD model [9] (Table 2-2). The greatest radiation dose is absorbed by the kidneys (1.34 rad/mCi). We found a relatively high radiation dose for the heart. For this calculation, radiation from adjacent organs (liver, spleen, kidneys) was also taken into account. The whole-body radiation dose was calculated to be 0.21 rad/mCi. Although the reported radiation dose to various organs differs

Table 2-1. Distribution of ^{201}Tl in various organs (mean percentage ($\pm$SD) of injected dose). Data are derived from post mortem tissue analysis in six patients (two males, four females)

Myocardium	3.6%	$\pm$ 0.7
Lungs	4.0	$\pm$ 1.3
Liver	8.7	$\pm$ 2.1
Spleen	0.65	$\pm$ 0.21
Kidney	4.1	$\pm$ 1.5
Thyroid	0.1	$\pm$ 0.02
Testis	0.18	$\pm$ 0.03
Ovaries	0.031	$\pm$ 0.011
Skeletal muscle	41.3	$\pm$ 5.5
Skeleton, red marrow	13.0	$\pm$ 4.6
Blood	2.2	$\pm$ 0.3
Pancreas	0.25	$\pm$ 0.08
Adrenals	0.039	$\pm$ 0.004
Prostate	0.04	$\pm$ 0.01
Stomach wall	0.56	$\pm$ 0.10
Intestines	3.0	$\pm$ 0.5
Bladder contents	0.7	$\pm$ 0.2
Feces	2.0	$\pm$ 0.5
Connective tissue, lymphatic system, central nervous system, etc.	15.6	$\pm$ 7.8

Table 2-2. Radiation dose (rad/mCi) of ^{201}Tl for various organs and whole body

	Samson et al. [6] *	Philips Duphar [46] *	New England Nuclear [47]	Feller et al. [48]
Myocardium	1.30 ± 0.36 (SD)		0.34	0.17
Lungs	0.45 ± 0.15	0.33		0.12
Liver	0.63 ± 0.17	0.50	0.62	0.15
Spleen	0.45 ± 0.14			
Kidney	1.34 ± 0.55	0.85	1.5	0.39
Thyroid	0.48 ± 0.12	0.43	0.74	
Testis	0.49 ± 0.11	0.43	0.54	0.30
Ovaries	0.37 ± 0.10	0.49	0.57	
Skeletal muscle	0.23 ± 0.05	0.28		
Skeletal bone	0.16 ± 0.05			
Red marrow	0.35 ± 0.10	0.50	0.34	
Blood	0.15 ± 0.04			
Pancreas	0.39 ± 0.10			
Adrenals	0.36 ± 0.05			
Prostate	0.29 ± 0.08			
Intestines	0.73 ± 0.14		0.65	
Bladder	0.24 ± 0.06			
Whole body	0.21 ± 0.03	0.22	0.24	0.24

* Data based on post mortem human tissue analysis

considerably, there is a general agreement concerning the whole-body dose. These differences may be explained by errors introduced by extrapolation from animal data and whether or not redistribution of ^{201}Tl over the body is taken into account. The skeletal muscle mass which is the most important pool for ^{201}Tl accumulation is relatively larger in man than in small animals

THALLIUM-201 KINETICS

Following an intravenous injection, ^{201}Tl disappears very rapidly from the blood: 91.5% is removed with a half-life of 5 min. The remaining activity disappears with a half-life of 40 hr. More than 50% of the latter activity is concentrated in the erythrocytes. Myocardial activity increases rapidly immediately following intravenous injection, reaching a plateau at approximately 20 min and remaining relatively constant for 60 min. Following the plateau myocardial activity decreases slowly owing to physical decay and slow egress of ^{201}Tl from the myocardium (see below)[10]. Significant redistribution of ^{201}Tl occurs over an interval of 24 hr following administration. The relative concentration in the heart and kidneys is initially significantly higher than after 24 hr. At this time the relative activity in the limbs has increased[11]. Initial myocardial/background (lung) ratio may differ considerably in individual patients but generally averages 1.97:1 (range 1.5 to 2.8:1)[10]. Markedly increased pulmonary uptake is seen in heavy smokers and in patients with pulmonary congestion. Boucher et al.[12] reported increased pulmonary uptake of ^{201}Tl following exercise as an indicator of abnormal left ventricular function in patients with coronary artery disease.

The accumulation of ^{201}Tl in the myocardial cells very likely involves both passive and active membrane transport systems. Mullins and Moore[13] demonstrated that the muscle fiber membrane of a frog was unable to distinguish between potassium (K^+) and thallium (Tl^+) ions. An explanation for this is the close similarity of the radius of the hydrated ions of thallium (1.44 Å) and potassium (1.33 Å), which is an important determinant of passive lipid-layered membrane penetration.

Gehring and Hammond[14] reported that at low concentration Tl^+ activates the $Na^+ K^+$ ATPase system, the active transport system for maintaining the high intracellular concentration of K^+. Britten and Blank[15] demonstrated that Tl^+ had a $10\times$ higher affinity for the $Na^+ K^+$ ATPase system than K^+. Gelbart et al.[16] reported preliminary findings in the intact animal suggesting an active role of the $Na^+ K^+$ ATPase system in ^{201}Tl cellular uptake. Following occlusion of the left anterior descending artery in dogs, they obtained serial myocardial biopsies. It appeared that myocardial ^{201}Tl concentration was dependent on flow *and* the regional ATPase concentration.

Adolph et al.[17] produced regional myocardial hypoxia in dogs by perfusing the left anterior descending artery with jugular venous blood. Thus, normal coronary perfusion ensured adequate delivery of ^{201}Tl. Nevertheless, definite deficits in myocardial accumulation of ^{201}Tl occurred in the anterior wall. After reperfusion of the left anterior descending artery with arterial blood and an additional intravenous injection of ^{201}Tl, these anterior wall defects disappeared.

Thus, myocardial intracellular accumulation appears to occur both by a passive and an active oxygen dependent transport mechanism.

Strauss et al.[18] demonstrated in dogs an excellent relationship ($r = 0.97$) between regional myocardial distribution of ^{201}Tl and radioactive microspheres determined myocardial blood flow. This correlation was excellent over a wide range of values for myocardial blood flow. However, under conditions of reactive hypermia ^{201}Tl accumulation was not increased to the same extent in the high flow regions as myocardial blood flow. Mueller et al.[19] confirmed this excellent correlation between ^{201}Tl tissue accumulation and regional myocardial blood flow in a series of closed-chest anesthetized dogs with normal and abnormal myocardial perfusion. DiCola et al.[20] investigated the pathophysiologic correlates of ^{201}Tl myocardial uptake in a 24-hr-old closed-chest canine infarct model. Reduction in regional ^{201}Tl uptake correlated well with the magnitude of tissue creatine phosphokinase depletion (Figure 2-2) and microsphere estimates of regional transmural blood flow

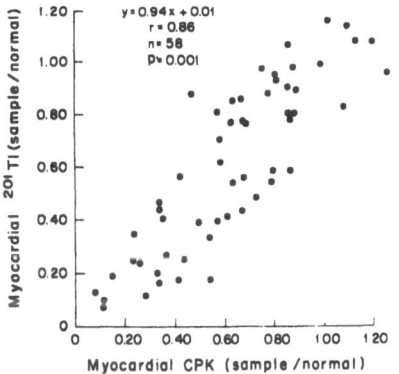

Figure 2-2. Relationship between myocardial ^{201}Tl and creatine phosphokinase (CPK) activities in 58 biopsy samples obtained from dogs 24 h following embolic infarction. Activities are expressed as ratios between infarct sample and the mean of normal samples obtained in each individual study. The magnitude of local tissue enzyme decrease correlates well with regional decrease in ^{201}Tl myocardial accumulation. Reproduced with permission from DiCola et al.[20].

(Figure 2-3). It is of note that evidence of myocardial necrosis was present histologically, whenever ^{201}Tl uptake was reduced to less than 0.86 (ratio sample/normal) of normal concentration.

For accumulation of ^{201}Tl in the myocardium, myocardial *blood flow* is the most important determinant. However for clinical use, it is extremely important to know, in addition, the time course of myocardial *extraction* after an intravenous injection, since regional myocardial blood flow in the clinical situation may change rapidly (e.g., exercise induced ischemia or spontaneous angina). This aspect has been studied by Weich et al. [21] and L'Abbate et al. [22]. Weich et al. [21] demonstrated in dogs that myocardial extraction of ^{201}Tl is highly efficient. During the first transit of a bolus of ^{201}Tl through the coronary circulation 88% of the total amount is extracted. This fraction remained constant with pacing or propanolol administration. However, during hypoxia and acidosis, the extraction fraction decreased significantly to 78% and 79% respectively. The effect of hypoxia persisted after normalization of oxygen level in blood.

L'Abbate et al. [22] studied myocardial kinetics of ^{201}Tl and ^{42}K in man by continuous sampling from the aortic root and coronary sinus. They found that the values for the initial extraction fraction of ^{201}Tl was similar to those obtained in animals. For ^{201}Tl this value was 87% and for ^{42}K 85%. The net maximal myocardial uptake of ^{201}Tl per 100 g of tissue measured by this

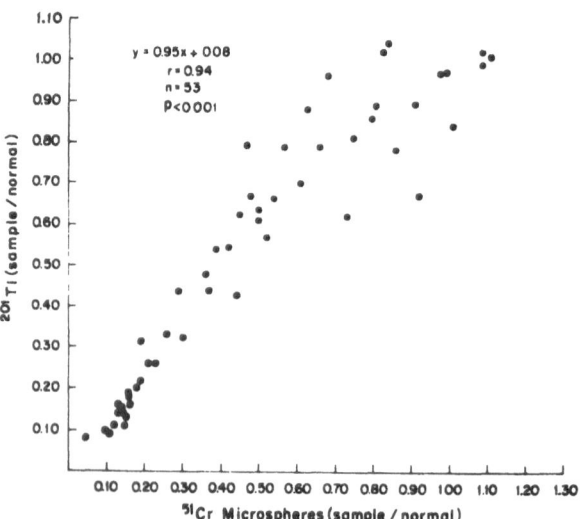

Figure 2-3. Relationship between transmural myocardial ^{201}Tl uptake and relative regional myocardial blood flow as estimated by the microspheres (^{51}Cr) technique. Activities are expressed as ratios between infarct sample and the mean of normal samples obtained in each individual study. The microsphere estimates of transmural regional myocardial blood flow correlate well with transmural ^{201}Tl uptake. Reproduced with permission from DiCola et al. [20].

method ranged in these patients from 1.0 to 2.7% of the injected dose and was positively related to myocardial blood flow. The net uptake of ^{42}K ranged from 1.4 to 2.4%, but was not correlated with myocardial blood flow.

This detailed study indicated another important difference between ^{42}K and ^{201}Tl. The myocardial washout of ^{42}K was considerably faster than for ^{201}Tl, expecially at higher heart rates and myocardial blood flow. This is in agreement with experimental data obtained by Gehring and Hammond[14]. From the relative characteristics and kinetics of both ^{42}K and ^{201}Tl, these investigators concluded that perfusion defects frequently seen on post-exercise scintiscans in patients with coronary artery disease, are more likely to be the result of an actual severe *reduction* of perfusion to ischemic areas, rather than an inadequate increase of regional myocardial perfusion [22].

The rapid extraction from the blood, its relatively lower concentration in surrounding organs and its relatively slower clearance from the heart (compared to potassium and rubidium) are important characteristics that account for the superiority of ^{201}Tl over other presently available myocardial imaging agents [23]. According to the fractionation principle defined by Sapirstein [24],

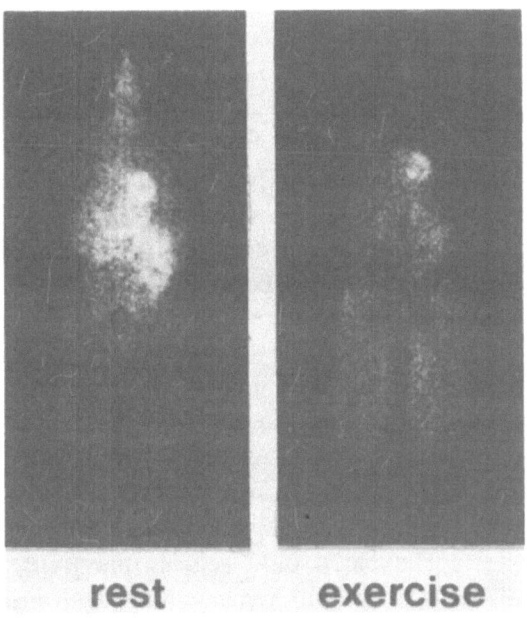

rest   exercise

Figure 2-4. Whole-body imaging of a patient at rest and exercise. At rest ^{201}Tl accumulates in the heart, but also in the liver, spleen, kidneys and gastrointestinal tract. Following exercise ^{201}Tl activity is most prominent in the heart. Most of the remaining activity is located in the exercising muscles of the thighs. Note the almost absent activity in the splanchnic region. These images illustrate that ^{201}Tl is accumulated according to the distribution of cardiac output. Reproduced with permission from Ref. [49].

an indicator that is totally or nearly totally extracted during the first pass can be used to estimate regional perfusion as a fraction of the cardiac output. Figure 2-3 demonstrates the change in distribution of cardiac output as visualized by ^{201}Tl accumulation following exercise as compared to the resting state. Strauss et al. [25] confirmed that the concentration of ^{201}Tl and microspheres were similar ($r = 0.93$) in the heart, kidney, thyroid and skeletal muscle in both control and norepinephrine-treated animals. This was however not the case in organs with a dual circulation: that is the liver and lungs.

The close relationship between regional myocardial perfusion and regional myocardial ^{201}Tl concentration explains the clinical results in identifying (acute or prior) myocardial infarction . Additionally, the rapid extraction of ^{201}Tl during the first transit, the rapid clearance from the blood, the dependence on normal oxygenated conditions and the relatively slow washout from the myocardial cells, are factors that account for the success of ^{201}Tl stress scintigraphy. For clinical practice, exercise induced ischemia maintained for only 30–60 sec appears to be sufficient time for ^{201}Tl to accumulate in the myocardium, in proportion to the regional blood flow at the end of exercise. On the other hand, approximately 30% false negative results are obtained by ^{201}Tl stress scintigraphy [26]. Patterson et al. [27] and Wharton et al. [28] demonstrated in a canine model that the duration of ischemia maintained after injection of ^{201}Tl is of critical importance to visualize regional perfusion defects. An ischemic "steady state" of at least 2–3 min af⁺ r injection was required in order to visualize perfusion defects.

Originally it was assumed that ^{201}Tl would remain fixed in the myocardium for several hours since the net clearance rate of ^{201}Tl was in the range of 7 hr. However, clinical studies demonstrated that exercise induced perfusion defects filled in and disappeared, apparently by redistribution of the radionuclide within 2-4 hr after injection [29]. Pohost and Beller [28-39] have extensively investigated this phenomenon of redistribution in animal experiments and in clinical studies.

The disappearance of ^{201}Tl defects over a 4-hr period of reperfusion after transient coronary occlusion in anesthetized dogs, results from further accumulation of ^{201}Tl in the previously ischemic zone, as well as from washout from the normal myocardium [35, 40]. Since only approximately 4% of the injected ^{201}Tl is accumulated in the heart, a very large systemic reservoir of ^{201}Tl is present outside the heart. The blood only acts as the transport vehicle [36]. As long as myocardial cellular integrity remains intact with maintenance of the electrochemical gradient for ^{201}Tl, the initial concentration of ^{201}Tl is proportional to the product of perfusion and extraction fraction. Subsequently, a continuous exchange of ^{201}Tl will take place: [201]Tl enters the cells (uptake) and ^{201}Tl leaves the cells (washout). Thus, in the presence of an imbalance between rate of uptake and rate of washout, the net concentration of ^{201}Tl will change. In the following, this is illustrated when ^{201}Tl is given during exercise. Immediately following exercise in a patient with significant coronary artery disease, an imbalance may be present: the normal myocardium contains a relatively high concentration due to absolute increase of blood flow during the exercise, whereas the transiently ischemic myocardium will have a relatively lower concentration of ^{201}Tl. The local concentration of ^{201}Tl will continue to change until a static equilibrium condition is achieved. In the post-exercise resting phase the blood flow, and thus the *uptake* of ^{201}Tl, for both myocardial regions will be *similar*, thus disappearance of local differences in ^{201}Tl concentration must be achieved by a *difference* in the *washout* rate of the previously ischemic region and that of the normal region.

The intrinsic washout rate of myocardial cells was studied experimentally by Beller et al. [34, 35] and Okada et al. [37] by serial measurements of ^{201}Tl myocardial activity. Thallium-201 (30 µCi) was injected directly into the coronary arteries. Since 88% of the injected dose is extracted, recirculation back to the heart from the systemic pool becomes insignificant. The intrinsic washout curve was monoexpenential over a time range of 5 min to 2 hr after injection. The average half-life ($t^{1/2}$) for ^{201}Tl in the myocardium was 75 min. This is in marked contrast to the $t^{1/2}$ for net washout (difference between import and export of ^{201}Tl), which is 7-8 hr. In this situation, ^{201}Tl is continuously replaced by new ^{201}Tl from the systemic pool. Grunwald et al. [39] demonstrated that the intrinsic washout of ^{201}Tl may be significantly altered by severe hypoperfusion. In dogs that underwent varying degrees of partial occlusion of the left anterior descending coronary artery, intrinsic washout could be prolonged as much as 300 min ($t^{1/2}$). Thus, the dynamic exchange of ^{201}Tl and differences in intrinsic washout are responsible for normalization of ^{201}Tl scintiscans at delayed imaging after exercise.

In patients with (acute or old) myocardial infarction the regional difference in uptake of ^{201}Tl will be constant at all times, as is the washout rate. Therefore, persistent defects can be noted in these patients. In patients with acute episodes of myocardial ischemia (unstable angina) one has to assume that changes occur both in the rate of uptake (impaired active extraction) and the rate of washout of ^{201}Tl.

EFFECT OF CARDIAC DRUGS ON THALLIUM-201 UPTAKE

Since many patients with cardiac disease are using one or more cardiac drugs, the effects of these drugs on ^{201}Tl myocardial accumulation is potentially important. *Digoxin,* a known inhibitor of the Na^+ K^+ ATPase system, appears to decrease ^{201}Tl accumulation. Costin and Zaret [41] could demonstrate a 22% net decrease in ^{201}Tl uptake in anesthetized dogs following administration of digoxin. However, Weich et al. [21] found no effect of intravenous acetylstrophantidin on the extraction fraction of ^{201}Tl. Similarly, Hamilton et al. [7] could not demonstrate in dogs an effect of digoxin in myocardial to background ratio by external imaging. Schelbert et al. [42] studied the effect of ouabain in fetal mice hearts and found a decrease of 31.1% in ^{201}Tl uptake. Zimmer et al. [43] reported a 60% inhibition of ^{204}Tl uptake in monolayer cultured Girardi cells. Recently Krivokapich et al. [44] described the exchange characteristics of ^{201}Tl and ^{42}K in an arterially perfused isolated rabbit interventricular septum. Paradoxically, these investigators noted that acetylstrophanthidin resulted in an increase in both the influx and efflux of ^{201}Tl in contrast to the decrease in influx and increase of efflux seen with ^{42}K. These contradictory findings may be explained by the observation by Britten and Blank [15] that thallous ions have a higher affinity than potassium ions for the Na$^+$ K$^+$ ATPase and therefore more ouabain is required to displace thallium than an equivalent amount of potassium. *Propanolol* also inhibits the Na$^+$ K$^+$ ATPase system. Costin and Zaret [41] noted a 32% decrease in ^{201}Tl uptake, whereas Hamilton et al. [7] found a decrease of only 11%, and the decreased myocardial uptake was not identifiable by clinical inspection of the image or analysis of myocardium/background ratio. Schelbert et al. [42] found a decrease of 35.5% for ^{201}Tl uptake in fetal mouse hearts when exposed to propanolol. *Furosemide* [7] and *procainamide* [42] produced no significant change in ^{201}Tl uptake.

Of all drugs, the images appeared to be most affected by *dipyridamole* [7], a potent coronary vasodilator. This drug increased left ventricular myocardial uptake of ^{201}Tl by 60%. Gould et al. [45] further investigated the potential value of *dipyridamole* as an alternative mode to produce marked heterogeneity in regional myocardial blood flow in the presence of coronary artery disease. They demonstrated that pharmacologic coronary vasodilatation by *dipyridamole* is as effective (sensitivity 67%) as maximal treadmill exercise in creating myocardial perfusion abnormalities detectable with ^{201}Tl myocardial imaging.

In conclusion, the accumulation of ^{201}Tl in the myocardium probably involves both passive and active membrane transport systems. The most important determinants for the initial distribution after injection are regional myocardial blood flow and unimpaired myocardial extraction. Subsequently, a continuous exchange of ^{201}Tl takes place, such that half of all the intracellular ^{201}Tl is replaced within 75 min. The balance between the rate of uptake and the washout rate of ^{201}Tl determines the ultimate myocardial distribution of ^{201}Tl.

Various cardiac drugs may alter cardiac uptake of ^{201}Tl. The changes produced by *digoxin* and *propanolol* are not of sufficient magnitude to impair the diagnostic potentials of practical cardiac imaging with ^{201}Tl. Only *dipryidamole* increases ^{201}Tl myocardial accumulation significantly and improves visual contrast and myocardial/background ratios in images.

REFERENCES

1. Kawana M, Krizek H, Porter J, Lathrop KA, Charleston D, Harper PV: Use of [199]Tl as a potassium analog in scanning. J Nucl Med 11:333, 1970 (abstract).
2. Lebowitz E, Greene MW, Fairchild R, Bradley-Moore PR, Atkins HL, Ansari AN, Richards P, Belgrave E: Thallium-201 for medical use. I. J Nucl Med 16:151-155, 1975.
3. Bradley-Moore PR, Lebowitz E, Greene MW, Atkins HL, Ansari AN: Thallium-201 for medical use. II: Biologic behavior. J Nucl Med 16:156-160, 1975.
4. Wackers FJTh, van der Schoot JB, Busemann Sokole E, Samson G, van Niftrik GJC, Lie KI, Durrer D, Wellens HJJ: Noninvasive visualization of acute myocardial infarction in man with thallium-201. British Heart J 37:741-744, 1975.
5. Negherbon WO: Handbook of toxicology, Vol III, p 750. Philadelphia: W.B. Saunders 1959.
6. Samson G, Wackers FJTh, Becker AE, Busemann Sokole E, van der Schoot JB: Distribution of thallium-201 in man. Verhandlungsbericht der 14. Internationalen Jahrtagung der Gesellschaft für Nuclear Medizin, Berlin: Band I, 15-18 Sept., 1976.
7. Hamilton GW, Narahara KA, Yee H, Ritchie JL, Williams DL, Gould KL: Myocardial imaging with thallium-201: effect of cardiac drugs on myocardial images and absolute tissue distribution. J Nucl Med 19:10-16, 1978.
8. Lie R, Thomas RG, Scott JK: The distribution and excretion of Tl-204 in the rat with suggested MPC's and a bio-assay procedure. Health Phys 2:334, 1960.
9. Snyder WS, Ford MR, Warner GG, Watson SB: "S" absorbed dose per unit cumulated activity for selected radionuclides and organs. NM/MIRD pamphlet #11. New York: Society of Nuclear Medicine, 1975.
10. Ritchie JL, Hamilton GW: Biologic properties of thallium. In: Thallium-201 myocardial imaging, pp 9-28, Ritchie JL, Hamilton GW, Wackers FJTh, eds. New York: Raven Press, 1978.
11. Atkins HL, Budinger TF, Lebowitz E, Ansari AN, Greene MW, Fairchild RG, Ellis KJ: Thallium-201 for medical use. III: Human distribution and physical imaging properties. J Nucl Med 18:133-140, 1977.
12. Boucher CA, Zir LM, Beer GA, et al.: Increased lung uptake of thallium-201 during exercise myocardial imaging: clinical, hemodynamic and angiographic implications in patients with coronary artery disease. Am J Cardiol 46:189, 1980.
13. Mullins LJ, Moore RD: The movement of thallium ions in muscle. J. Gen Phys 43:759-773, 1960.
14. Gehring PJ, Hammond PB: The interrelationship between thallium and potassium in animals. J Pharmacol Exp Ther 155:187-201, 1967.
15. Britten JS, Blank M: Thallium activation of the (Na^+-K^+)-activated ATPase of rabbit kidney. Biochim Biophys Acta 159:160-166, 1968.
16. Gelbart A, Doherty PW, McLaughlin PR, Harrison DC: Na^+, K^+-ATPase and coronary blood flow as determinants of thallium-201 uptake by ischemic myocardium. Circulation 54, suppl II, II:70, 1976.
17. Adolph R, Romhilt, D, Hishiyama H, Sodd V, Blue J, Gabel M: Use of positive and negative imaging agents to visualize myocardial ischemia. Circulation 54, suppl II, II:220, 1976.
18. Strauss HW, Harrison K, Langan JK, Lebowitz E, Pitt B: Thallium-201 for myocardial imaging: relation of thallium-201 to regional myocardial perfusion. Circulation 51:641-645, 1975.
19. Mueller TM, Marcus ML, Ehrhardt JC, Chaudhuri T, Abboud FM: Limitations of thallium-201 myocardial perfusion scintigrams. Circulation 54:640-646, 1976.
20. DiCola VC, Downing SE, Donabedian RK, Zaret BL: Pathophysiological correlates of thallium-201 myocardial uptake in experimental infarction. Cardiol Res XI:141-146, 1977.
21. Welch HF, Strauss HW, Pitt B: The extraction of thallium-201 by the myocardium. Circulation 56:188-191, 1977.
22. L'Abbate A, Biagini A, Michelassi C, Maseri A: Myocardial kinetics of thallium and potassium in man. Circulation 60:776-785, 1979.

23. Nishiyama H, Sodd VJ, Adolph RJ, Saenger EL, Lewis JT, Gabel M: Intercomparison of myocardial imaging agents: ^{201}Tl, ^{129}Cs, ^{43}K, and ^{81}Rb. J Nucl Med 17:880-889, 1976.
24. Sapirstein LA: Regional blood flow by fractional distribution of indicators. Am. J. Physiol 193:161-168, 1958.
25. Strauss HW, Harrison K, Pitt B: Thallium-201: non-invasive determination of the regional distribution of cardiac output. J Nucl Med 18:1167-1170, 1977.
26. Ritchie JL, Zaret BL, Strauss HW, Pitt B, Berman DS, Schelbert HR, Ashburn WL, Berger HJ, Hamilton GW: Myocardial imaging with thallium-201: a multicenter study in patients with angina pectoris or acute myocardial infarction. Am J Cardiol 42:345-350, 1978.
27. Patterson R, Halgash D, Micelli K, Miao J, Rogers J, Eng C, Horowitz S, Goldsmith S: "Steady state" problems in myocardial perfusion imaging to detect transient ischemia: critical role of the duration of the ischemic state after thallium-201 injection. Am J Cardiol 43:357, 1979.
28. Wharton TP, Neill WA, Oxendine JM, Painter LN: Duration of regional ischemia and degree of reactiva hyperemia following ischemia affect magnitude of initial thallium-201 defect. Circulation 60: suppl II, II:173, 1979.
29. Pohost GM, Zir LM, Moore RH, McKusick KA, Guiney TE, Beller GA: Differentiation of transiently ischemic from infarcted myocardium by serial imaging after a single dose of thallium-201. Circulation 55:294-302, 1077.
30. Gewirtz H, O'Keefe DD, Pohost GM, Strauss HW, McIlduff JB, Daggett WH: The effect of ischemia on thallium-201 clearance from the myocardium. Circulation 58:215-219, 1978.
31. Pohost GM, O'Keefe DD, Gewirtz H, Strauss HW, Beller GA, Newell JB, Chaffin JS, Daggett WM: Thallium redistribution in the presence of severe fixed coronary stenosis. J Nucl Med 19:680, 1978.
32. Berger BC, Watson DD, Sipes JN, Pohost GM, Teates CD, Beller GA: Redistribution of thallium at rest in patients with coronary artery disease. J Nucl Med 19:680, 1978.
33. Watson DD, Beller GA, Berger BC: The mechanism of thallium-201 redistribution. Am. J. Cardiol 43:357, 1979.
34. Watson DD, Beller GA, Irving JF, Teates CD: A kinetic model for thallium myocardial redistribution. J Nucl Med 19:680, 1978.
35. Beller GA, Pohost GM: Time course and mechanism of resolution of thallium-201 defects after transient myocardial ischemia. Am J Cardiol 41:379, 1978.
36. Beller GA, Watson DD, Pohost GM: Kinetics of thallium distribution and redistribution: clinical applications in sequential myocardial imaging. In: Cardiovascular nuclear medicine, 2nd edition, pp 225-242, Strauss HW, Pitt B, eds. St. Louis: Mosby, 1070.
37. Pohost GM, Alpert NM, Ingwall JS, Strauss HW: Thallium redistribution: mechanisms and clinical utility. Semin Nucl Med 10:70, 1980.
38. Okada RD, Jacobs ML, Newell JB, Strauss HW, Daggett WM, O'Keefe DD, Pohost GM: Thallium-201 kinetics in nonischemic canine myocardium. Circulation 60 suppl II, II-172, 1979.
39. Grunwald AM, Holzgrefe HH, Teates CD, Watson DD, Beller GA: Altered thallium-201 transport in ischemic myocardium. Circulation 60, suppl II, II:172, 1979.
40. Schelbert H, Schuler G, Ashburn W, Covell J: Time course of redistribution of Tl-201 after transient ischemia. J Nucl Med 18:598, 1977.
41. Costin JC, Zaret BL: Effect of propanolol and digitalis upon radioactive thallium and potassium uptake in myocardial and skeletal muscle. J. Nucl Med 17:535, 1976.
42. Schelbert H, Inwall J, Watson R, Askburn W: Factors influencing the myocardial uptake of thallium-201. J Nucl Med 18:598, 1977.
43. Zimmer L, McCall D, D'Addabbo L, Whitney K: Kinetics and characteristics of thallium Exchange in cultured cells. Circulation 60, suppl II, II:138, 1979.
44. Krivokapich J, Shine KI: The effects of hyperkalemia and glycoside on ^{201}thallium exchange in rabbit myocardium. Circulation 60, suppl II, II:173, 1979.
45. Gould KL, Westcott RJ, Albro PC, Hamilton GW: Noninvasive assessment of coronary stenoses by myocardial imaging during pharmacologic coronary vasodilatation. Am. J. Cardiol 41:279-287, 1978.

46. Huising WB, DeJong RBJ: Calculation of radiation dose in humans from i.v. injected thallous chloride (Tl-201) based on human distribution data. Internal report Philips-Duphar, BV, Petten, The Netherlands, 1978.
47. New England Nuclear. Package Insert: Catalog #NRP-427, 1978.
48. Feller PA, Sodd VJ: Dosimetry of four heart-imaging radionuclides: ^{43}K, ^{81}Rb, ^{129}Cs, and ^{201}Tl. J Nucl Med 16:1070-1075, 1975.
49. Wackers FJTh, Busemann Sokole E, Samson G, van der Schoot JB: Atlas of ^{201}Tl myocardial scintigraphy. Clin Nucl Med, 2:64-74, 1977.

3. MECHANISMS OF TECHNETIUM-99m-PYROPHOSPHATE ACCUMULATION IN DAMAGED MYOCARDIUM

L. Maximilian Buja, Robert W. Parkey, Ernest Stokely, Frederick J. Bonte and James T. Willerson

The purpose of this chapter is to summarize the available information concerning the pathophysiological basis for the use of the "hot spot" myocardial imaging technique, ^{99m}Tc stannous pyrophosphate in the detection of irreversibly damaged myocardial tissue, including acute myocardial infarcts. ^{99m}Tc-pyrophosphate is classified as a "hot spot" imaging technique since it concentrates in acutely infarcted myocardium. Table 3-1 identifies other "hot spot" imaging techniques that also allow the recognition of acute myocardial necrosis. This chapter will concentrate on the use of ^{99m}Tc-pyrophosphate as an "infarct avid" or "hot spot" agent to detect acute myocardial infarcts.

Table 3-1. "Hot spot" radionuclide imaging techniques for detecting acute myocardial infarcts

A. Nonimmunologic mechanisms of accumulation in damaged myocardium
 1. Technetium-99m-phosphates
 2. Technetium-99m-tetracycline
 3. Technetium-99m-glucoheptonate
 4. Technetium-99m-heparin
 5. Mercury-203-mercurials

B. Immunologic mechanisms for radionuclide uptake in the identification of damaged cellular constituents
 1. Iodine-131-antibody to myosin
 2. Iodine-131-antibody to mitochondria

C. Labeling of inflammatory infiltrate
 1. Gallium-67 citrate
 2. Indium-111 leukocytes·

EXPERIMENTAL STUDIES

Following experimental canine coronary occlusion, myocardial necrosis initially develops in maximally ischemic subendocardial regions followed by a progressive spread of irreversible injury into less severely ischemic zones located in the subepicardium[1, 2]. Prolonged coronary artery occlusion is accompanied by a progressive increase in collateral blood flow into the ischemic region[3-5]. The presence, location and size of collateral perfusion and related border zone phenomena within the ischemic region have been the subject of debate and active evaluation [1, 6-8]. Histologic study has demonstrated that the established transmural infarct in the dog has histopathologically distinct zones which appear to correlate with differences in regional perfusion (Figure 3-1). Experimental canine and human infarcts share many similar histologic features [9, 10]. Human infarcts do, however, have more irregular and complicated zonal development which may itself be a manifestation of even more complex patterns of collateral perfusion.

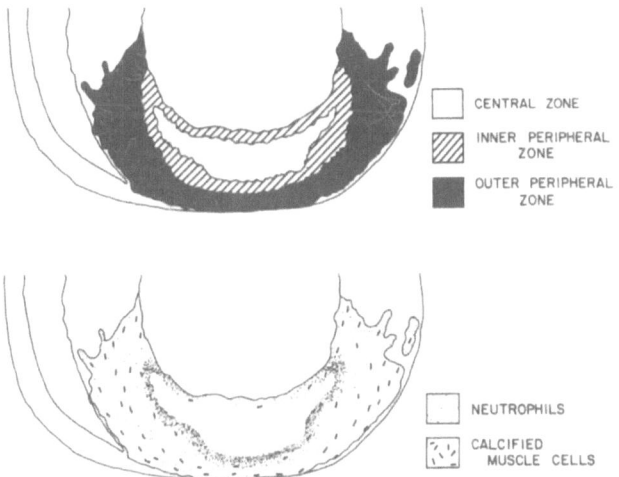

Figure 3-1. Histological zones of the typical transmural myocardial infarct produced by permanent ligation of a proximal coronary artery in the dog. (From Ref. [13] by permission.)

Acute myocardial infarcts typically have subendocardially located central zones which contain necrotic myocardium without neutrophilic infiltrate [2, 9, 10]. Necrotic muscle cells in this region do not exhibit calcification; however, calcification may be observed in necrotic blood vessels. Lack of muscle cell calcification and sparcity of neutrophils in this region appear best explained by the virtual absence of blood flow to this zone initially and the subsequent lack of collateral perfusion of this zone.

Bounding the central infarct region is a peripheral zone of myocardium where coronary blood flow is 10–40% of control values after several hours of coronary occlusion [2]. Calcium accumulation in this zone is associated with widespread hypercontraction damage and heavy neutrophil accumulation [2]. Mitochondrial calcification occurs when at least partial mitochondrial function is retained during the initial stages of calcium influx thus allowing the formation of calcium phosphate precipitates which serve as foci for progressive calcification after mitochondrial function ceases (Figure 3-1) [2, 11]. Pathological calcium accumulation in this setting results from calcium complexing with organic macromolecules and the formation of soluble amorphous calcium phosphate precipitates[2]. There is progressive growth of insoluble hydroxy apatite-like deposits as well. It should be emphasized that the infarct zones shown in Figure 3-1 often have irregular margins and interdigitate with one another. The relative size of the various regions varies for different infarcts and a central infarct zone may not be found with small, patchy and/or subendocardial infarcts.

PATHOPHYSIOLOGY OF ^{99m}Tc-PYROPHOSPHATE SCINTIGRAPHY

The pathophysiological basis for an abnormal ^{99m}Tc-pyrophosphate myocardial scintigram is the selective accumulation of this radiopharmaceutical in severely damaged and necrotic myocardium with calcium accumulation and residual blood flow (Figures 3-2 to 3-4)[2, 12–20].

NORMALIZED LEVELS OF ^{201}TI AND OF ^{125}I (15μ) MICROSPHERES
IN DIFFERENT REGIONS OF
CANINE TRANSMURAL ACUTE MYOCARDIAL INFARCTS

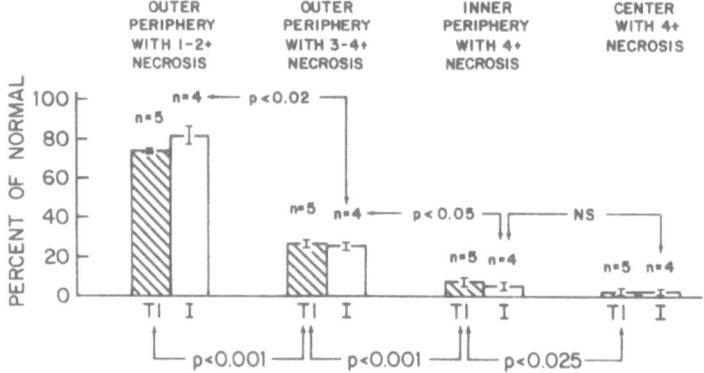

Figure 3-2. Regional blood flow measured by ^{201}Tl and ^{125}I microspheres in established canine myocardial infarcts. (From Ref. [13] by permission.)

In experimental animals, ^{99m}Tc-pyrophosphate uptake has a predictable time course following permanent coronary occlusion. Technetium-99m-pyrophosphate scintigrams become abnormal within 12 hr after coronary occlusion and increase in intensity over the next 48 to 72 hr. They decrease in intensity thereafter and are usually negative by 1 to 2 weeks after experimental coronary occlusion[2, 12-14]. A similar time course has been observed in most patients with myocardial infarcts[18, 21, 22]. Available evidence suggests that the timing of ^{99m}Tc-pyrophosphate uptake depends on the rate of evolution of infarction and on variations in the degree of perfusion in the ischemic region.

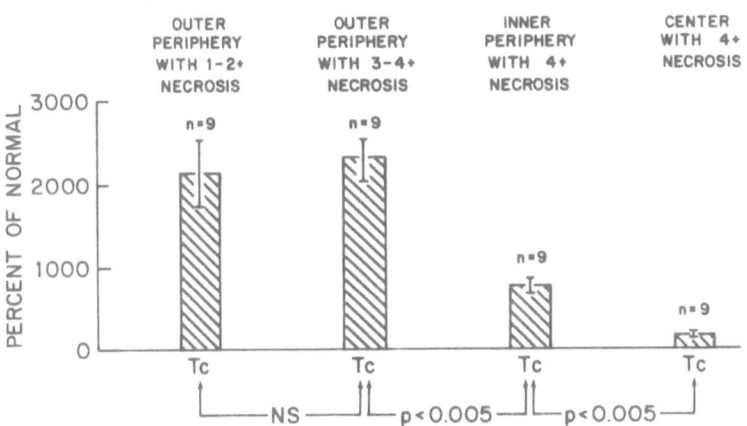

NORMALIZED LEVELS OF ^{99m}Tc–PYP
IN DIFFERENT REGIONS OF
CANINE TRANSMURAL ACUTE MYOCARDIAL INFARCTS

Figure 3-3. Regional levels of ^{99m}Tc-pyrophosphate in canine myocardial infarcts. Major concentration of ^{99m}Tc-pyrophosphate is in regions of extensive necrosis in the outer periphery of the infarcts. The edges of the infarcts also exhibit high ^{99m}Tc-pyrophosphate uptake in zones of focal necrosis with relatively abundant blood flow. (From Ref. [13] by permission.)

Thus, severe temporary ischemia followed by reflow may result in an abnormal scintigram within hours after the onset of myocardial damage [23, 24]. In contrast, ordinarily 12 hr or longer appears necessary for development of abnormal ^{99m}Tc-pyrophosphate scintigrams with permanent coronary occlusion. This is probably best explained by slower evolution of phenomena important in ^{99m}Tc-pyrophosphate concentration such as calcium accumulation and collateral perfusion [12-14].

Analytical studies have demonstrated that the selective *in vivo* concentration of ^{99m}Tc-pyrophosphate in altered soft tissues is ordinarily associated with elevated tissue calcium content, but that a linear relationship between ^{99m}Tc-pyrophosphate accumulation and calcium levels does not occur [2, 14]. Lack of a linear relationship can be adequately explained by noting that there are different affinities of ^{99m}Tc-pyrophosphate for various types of tissue calcium stores as well as regional differences in the delivery of ^{99m}Tc-pyrophosphate attributed to local vascularity and blood flow variations [12-14].

We have obtained data that suggest that the concentration of ^{99m}Tc-pyrophosphate may result from complexing to soluble and insoluble inorganic calcium deposits [2, 12–14]. Dewanjee has suggested that ^{99m}Tc-pyrophosphate uptake in myocardial infarcts results primarily from polynuclear complexing with denatured macromolecules [25]. It has also been shown that partial complexing of ^{99m}Tc-pyrophosphate with serum proteins is associated with only minimal reduction in its affinity for binding to hydroxyapatite or amor-

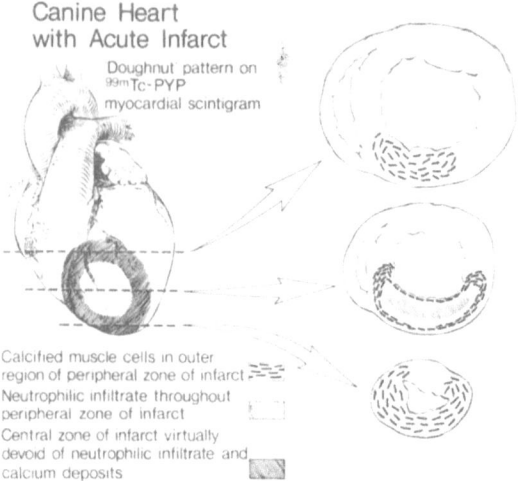

Canine Heart
with Acute Infarct

Doughnut pattern on
⁹⁹ᵐTc-PYP
myocardial scintigram

Calcified muscle cells in outer
region of peripheral zone of infarct
Neutrophilic infiltrate throughout
peripheral zone of infarct
Central zone of infarct virtually
devoid of neutrophilic infiltrate and
calcium deposits

Figure 3-4. Typical localization of ⁹⁹ᵐTc-pyrophosphate in a large anterior myocardial infarct results in a "doughnut" scintigraphic pattern. This pattern is characterized by a peripheral region of intense uptake surrounding a central region of considerably lower activity. (From Ref. [12] by permission.)

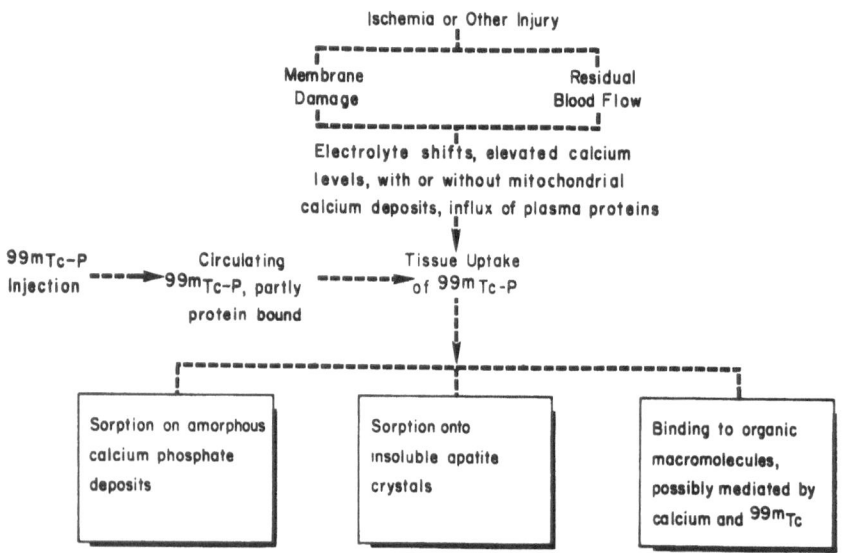

Figure 3-5. Pathophysiological mechanisms of ⁹⁹ᵐTc-pyrophosphate uptake. (From Ref. [14] by permission.)

phous calcium phosphate *in vitro* [14]. Thus, available data suggest multiple mechanisms for *in vivo* concentration of ⁹⁹ᵐTc-pyrophosphate, including complexing with soluble and insoluble inorganic calcium deposits as well as organic macromolecules (Figure 3-5) [2].

Studies done in our institution have also suggested that the abnormal concentration of ^{99m}Tc-pyrophosphate in the myocardium depends upon the presence of irreversible myocardial damage [2, 12–14]. Evidence has been provided by autoradiographic studies which have shown extensive ^{99m}Tc-pyrophosphate uptake in frankly necrotic muscle cells as well as significant uptake in a small population of damaged, lipid-laden muscle cells mixed with frankly necrotic myocardium [2, 14]. These experimental findings have been supported by clinical pathologic studies in more than 50 patients [20, 26]. These studies in patients have shown that ^{99m}Tc-pyrophosphate myocardial scintigraphy accurately detects subendocardial as well as transmural myocardial infarcts. Abnormal ^{99m}Tc-pyrophosphate scintigrams in patients with unstable angina pectoris and chronic ischemic heart disease have been associated with the presence of multifocal, irreversible myocardial damage in the form of coagulation necrosis, myocytolysis and/or fibrosis, and the histologic age of the lesions was consistent with acute injury at the time of the ^{99m}Tc-pyrophosphate myocardial scintigrams in the patients studied [19, 20]. Abnormal ^{99m}Tc-pyrophosphate myocardial scintigrams may also be found with myocardial necrosis of varying etiology, including necrosis resulting from cardioversion [15, 27–29], heat injury [30, 31], contusion [32], metastatic cardiac tumor and metastatic myocardial calcification [21, 33,34]. Approximately 3 g of necrotic muscle is required for consistent detection of lesions with ^{99m}Tc-pyrophosphate scintigraphy [35].

Thus, extensive evidence suggests that an abnormal ^{99m}Tc-pyrophosphate myocardial scintigram is a sensitive indicator of myocardial necrosis and that an abnormal ^{99m}Tc-pyrophosphate myocardial scintigram does not occur when the severity of myocardial damage is limited to reversible injury unassociated with myocardial necrosis. It should be stressed, however, that an abnormal ^{99m}Tc myocardial scintigram can be due to any etiology responsible for myocardial necrosis consisting of 3 g or more of irreversible damage when the scintigram is performed within the correct time frame.

REFERENCES

1. Reimer KA. Lowe JE, Rasmussen MM, et al.: The wavefront phenomenon of ischemic cell death. I. Myocardial infarct size vs duration of coronary occlusion in dogs. Circulation 56:786, 1977.
2. Buja LM, Parkey RW, Bonte FJ, et al.: Pathophysiology of "cold spot" and "hot spot" myocardial imaging agents used to detect ischemia or infarction. In Nuclear cardiology, p 105, Willerson JT, ed. Philadelphia: F.A. Davis, 1979.
3. Gregg DE: The natural history of coronary collateral development. Circ Res 35:335, 1974.
4. Bishop SP, White FC, Bloor CM: Regional myocardial blood flow during acute myocardial infarction in the conscious dog. Circ Res 38:429, 1976.
5. Rivas F, Cobb FR, Bache RJ, et al.: Relationship between blood flow to ischemic regions and extent of myocardial infarction. Serial measurement of blood flow to ischemic regions in dogs. Circ Res 38:439, 1976.

6. Hirzel HO, Nelsen GR, Sonnenblick EH, et al.: Redistribution of collateral blood flow from necrotic to surviving myocardium following coronary occlusion in the dog. Circ Res 39:214, 1976.

7. Hirzel HO, Sonnenblick EH, Kirk ES: Absence of a lateral border zone of intermediate creatine phosphokinase depletion surrounding a central infarct 24 hours after acute coronary occlusion in the dog. Circ Res 41:673, 1977.

8. Hearse DJ, Opie LH, Katzeff IE, et al.: Characterization of the "border zone" in acute regional ischemia in the dog. Am J Cardiol 40:716, 1977.

9. Mallory GK, White PD, Salcedo-Salgar J: The speed of healing of myocardial infarction. A study of the pathologic anatomy in seventy-two cases. Am Heart J 18:647, 1939.

10. Baroldi G: Different types of myocardial necrosis in coronary heart disease: a pathophysiologic review of their functional significance. Am Heart J 89:742, 1975.

11. Buja LM, Dees JH, Harling DF, et al.: Analytical electron microscopic study of mitochondrial inclusions in canine myocardial infarcts. J Histochem Cytochem 24:508, 1976.

12. Buja LM, Parkey RW, Dees JH, et al.: Morphologic correlates of technetium-99m stannous pyrophosphate imaging of acute myocardial infarcts in dogs. Circulation 52:596, 1975.

13. Buja LM, Parkey RW, Stokely EM, et al.: Pathophysiology of technetium-99m stannous pyrophosphate and thallium-201 scintigraphy of acute anterior myocardial infarcts in dogs. J Clin Invest 57:1508, 1976.

14. Buja LM, Tofe AJ. Kulkarni PV, et al.: sites and mechanisms of localization of technetium-99m phosphorus radiopharmaceuticals in acute myocardial infarcts and other tissues. J Clin Invest 60:724, 1977.

15. Pugh BR, Buja LM, Parkey RW, et al.: Cardioversion and "false positive" technetium-99m stannous pyrophosphate myocardial scintigrams. Circulation 54:399, 1976.

16. Bonte FJ, Parkey RW, Graham KD, et al.: A new method of radionuclide imaging of myocardial infarcts. Radiology 110:473, 1974.

17. Bonte FJ, Parkey RW, Graham KD, et al.: Distribution of several agents useful in imaging myocardial infarcts. J Nucl Med 16:132, 1975.

18. Parkey RW, Bonte FJ, Buja LM, et al.: Myocardial infarct imaging with technetium-99m phosphates. Semin Nucl Med 7:15, 1977.

19. Buja LM, Poliner LR, Parkey RW, et al.: Clinicopathologic study of persistently positive technetium-99m stannous pyrophosphate myocardial scintigrams and myocytolytic degeneration after acute myocardial infarction. Circulation 56:1016, 1977.

20. Poliner LR, Buja LM, Parkey RW, et al.: Clinicopathologic correlations in 52 patients studied by technetium-99m stannous pyrophosphate myocardial scintigraphy. Circulation 59:257, 1979.

21. Willerson JT, Parkey RW, Buja LM, et al.: Are ^{99m}Tc-stannous pyrophosphate myocardial scintigrams clinically useful? Clin Nucl Med 2:137, 1977.

22. Willerson JT, Parkey RW, Bonte FJ, et al.: Technetium stannous pyrophosphate myocardial scintigrams in patients with chest pain of varying etiology. Circulation 51:1046, 1975.

23. Bruno FP, Cobb FR, Rivas F, et al.: Evaluation of technetium stannous pyrophosphate as imaging agent in acute myocardial infarction. Circulation 54:71, 1976.

24. Reimer KA, Martonffy K, Schumacher BL, et al.: Localization of ^{99m}Tc labeled pyrophosphate and calcium in myocardial infarcts after temporary coronary occlusion in dogs. Proc Soc Exp Biol Med 156:272, 1977.

25. Dewanjee MK, Kahn PC: Mechanisms of localization of ^{99m}Tc-labeled pyrophosphate and tetracycline in infarcted myocardium. J Nucl Med 17:639, 1976.

26. Holman BL, Ehrie M, Lesch M: Correlation of acute myocardial infarct scintigraphy with postmortem studies. Am J Cardiol 37:311, 1976.

27. DiCola VC, Freedman GS, Downing SE, et al.: Myocardial uptake of technetium-99m stannous pyrophosphate following direct current transthoracic countershock. Circulation 54:980, 1976.

28. Schneider RM, Hayslett JP, Downing SE, et al.: Effect of methylprednisolone upon technetium-99m pyrophosphate assessment of myocardial necrosis in the canine countershock model. Circulation 56:1029, 1977.

29. McDaniel MM, Morton ME: ^{99m}Tc-pyrophosphate imaging demonstrating skeletal muscle and myocardial activity following cardioversion. Clin Nucl Med 2:57, 1977.
30. Adler N, Camin LL, Schulkin P: Rat model for acute myocardial infarction. Application to technetium-labeled glucoheptonate, tetracycline and polyphosphate. J Nucl Med 17:203, 1976.
31. Davis MA, Holman BL, Carmel AN: Evaluation of radiopharmaceuticals sequestered by acutely damaged myocardium. J Nucl Med 17:911, 1976.
32. Go RT, Chiu CL, Doty DB, et al.: Radionuclide imaging of experimental myocardial contusion. J Nucl Med 15:1174, 1974.
33. Epstein DA, Solar M, Levin EJ: Demonstration of long-standing metastic soft tissue calcification by ^{99m}Tc-diphosphonate. Am J Roentgenol 128:145, 1977.
34. Janowitz WR, Serafini AN: Intense myocardial uptake of ^{99m}Tc-diphosphonate in a uremic patient with secondary hyperparathyroidism and pericarditis: case report. J Nucl Med 17:896, 1976.
35. Poliner LR, Buja LM, Parkey RW, et al.: Comparative evaluation of several different noninvasive methods of infarct sizing during experimental myocardial infarction. J Nucl Med 18:517, 1977.

NORMAL SCINTIGRAPHIC IMAGES

4. THALLIUM-201 MYOCARDIAL IMAGING

FRANS J. TH. WACKERS

Three views are routinely obtained for ^{201}Tl scintigraphy: 0° anterior, 45° left-anterior-oblique, both views with the patient supine and a left-lateral view, with the patient lying on his right side.

Following intravenous injection of ^{201}Tl, the scintiscans of a normal subject only demonstrate the left ventricle [1–3]. In patients with normal myocardial perfusion, the left ventricle appears horseshoe or ovoid in shape (Figure 4-1). The central area of decreased activity represents the left ventricular cavity and is normal. The accumulation of ^{201}Tl in the normal left ventricle is usually homogeneous. However, some areas with apparent diminished uptake may occur in the normal subject. These variations of the normal image will be discussed more extensively below.

The right ventricle, because of its smaller myocardial mass and relatively less ^{201}Tl accumulation per gram of tissue, is usually on a resting study not, or only faintly, visualized. However, following exercise, the right ventricle is clearly visualized (Figure 4-2).

ANALOGUE OR COMPUTER PROCESSED IMAGES?

The interpretation of ^{201}Tl scintiscans should preferably be done from analogue unprocessed images. When digitized images are used, the analogue unprocessed images should be at hand for comparison. In our experience, computer processing, contrast enhancement, smoothing, various methods for background correction and especially color display, possess the potential danger of exaggerating and distorting the slight variations in ^{201}Tl accumulation that may be seen in normals. Without any doubt, computer processing may greatly enhance the readability of the images. However, initially subtle areas of diminished ^{201}Tl activity on the analogue images may, after computer processing, appear as definite defects and lead to misinterpretation. One should be very cautions to read perfusion defects present *only* on processed images. Although the *sensitivity* of ^{201}Tl scintigraphy can be increased by these methods, the painful trade-off is that of decreased *specificity* [4]. When black and white display is used, a continuous gray scale should be applied. For

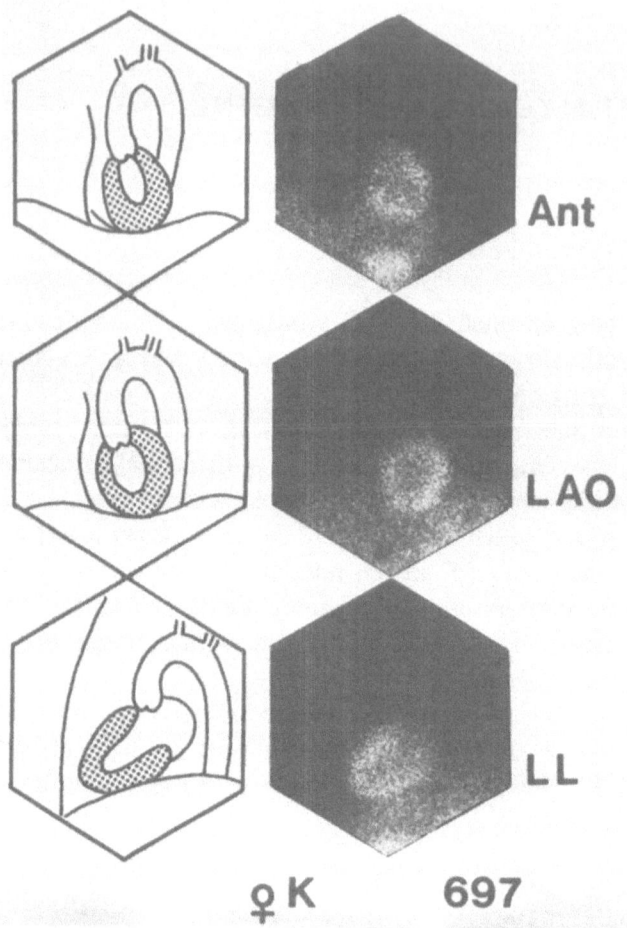

Figure 4-1. Thallium-201 scintiscans in three projections of a normal subject. On the left are representations of the anatomy. Only the left ventricle is visualized. The accumulation of ^{201}Tl is almost homogenous. The central area of decreased activity is the left ventricular cavity. Abbreviations: ANT = anterior; LAO = 45° left-anterior-oblique; LL = left-lateral. Reproduced with permission from Ref. [1].

color display (which we do not favor) it is of utmost importance that this is well standardized. On heavily processed images it will be difficult to differentiate between subtle variations of normal and actual perfusion abnormalities. "Dial a lesion" is the name of this dangerous game. All ^{201}Tl imaging data presented in this volume are based upon the interpretation of analogue unprocessed images.

exercise

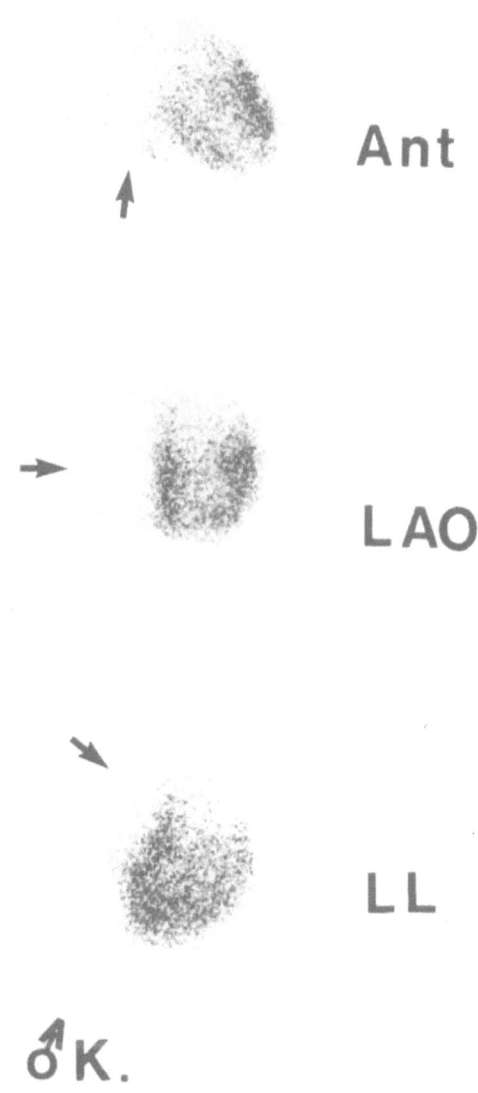

Ant

LAO

LL

♂ K.

Figure 4-2. Thallium-201 scintiscans following exercise of a normal subject. The right heart, especially the right ventricle, is also visualized (arrows). Reproduced with permission from Ref. [1].

PROJECTION OF ACTIVITY ONTO THE PLANE OF VIEW

Correct interpretation of ^{201}Tl studies depends on a thorough understanding of the anatomy of the heart as projected on the different scintigraphic views. These images are not directly comparable to those obtained by dye ventriculography which silhouettes a small segment of the ventricular wall (Figure 4-3). In contrast, in ^{201}Tl myocardial perfusion scintigraphy the configuration of the heart is related to the total amount of myocardial mass perpendicular to the crystal face of the gamma camera at any given location. Figure 4-4 illustrates this for the left-anterior-oblique view. A transverse section through

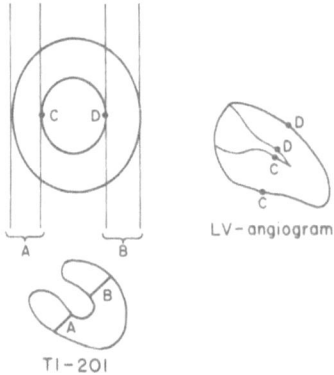

Figure 4-3. Generation of ^{201}Tl scintiscans. In contrast to dye left ventriculography, which visualizes the silhouette (C, D) of the left ventricle, ^{201}Tl scintiscans represent the projection of the total amount of myocardial mass (A, B) perpendicular to the plane of view.

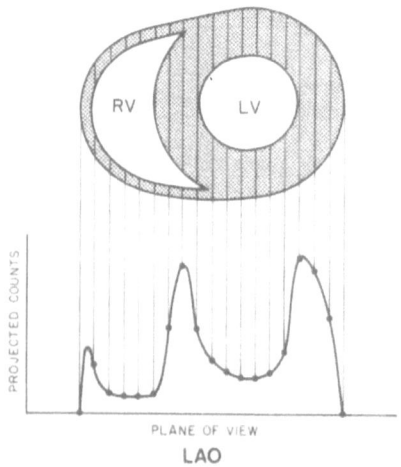

Figure 4-4. Generation of ^{201}Tl scintiscans. The projection of ^{201}Tl activity on the plane of view is demonstrated for the left-anterior-oblique position. See text. Abbreviations: A = anterior wall; L = lateral wall; S = interventricular septum; LV = left ventricle; RV = right ventricle.

the heart is schematically shown and its projection onto the plane of view. This plane is almost parallel to the anterior wall and at an angle with the interventricular septum and the lateral wall. The shaded profile represents the approximate summation of the projected myocardial mass. Assuming that the distribution of ^{201}Tl in the myocardium is homogeneous, the septum and the lateral wall will register more ^{201}Tl activity per unit region due to their greater mass than will the anterior wall. Additionally, radiation emanating from myocardium distant to the crystal face (the posterior wall) contributes less to the total image, because of high absorption of the low energy (80 keV) photons by tissue and the cardiac blood pool, which itself contains only a minimal amount of ^{201}Tl (<0.001% of injected dose/gram). Thus, the gamma camera appears to look «through» the ventricular wall parallel to the plane of view into the ventricular cavity, which results in a horseshoe or ovoid image. The same effect causes perfusion defects to be seen more clearly in a tangential view (Figure 4-5).

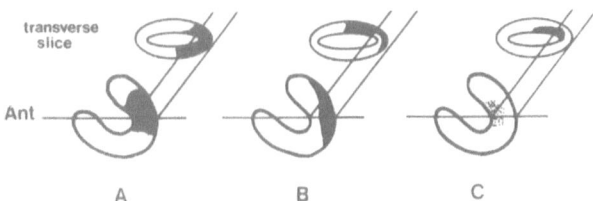

A   B   C

Figure 4-5. The projection of areas of diminished ^{201}Tl accumulation depends on its location and extent. The schematic drawings illustrate this for the anterior view. Three situations are depicted: transmural lateral infarct (A); posterior wall infarct with epicardial extension to the lateral wall (B), and small subendocardial area of infarction (C). *A:* Defects are best seen tangentially when they generate a discontinuation of activity originating from the myocardial wall perpendicular to the plane of view. The amount of normal overlying myocardium determines the amount of residual activity present in the defect. *B:* The posterior wall infarction will not produce a defect on the image since it is seen *en face* and more importantly, due to the distance, the posterior wall contributes little to the image in the anterior view because of radiation attenuation. The lateral extension may only be recognized as an abnormal configuration of the anterolateral wall. *C:* A subendocardial lesion may produce an abnormal image depending on the extent of the lesion and the amount of normal overlying myocardium. Even if the extent is large enough to produce a defect it may be difficult to recognize this abnormality with certainty. The local thinning of the anterolateral may be too subtle to be appreciated on the scintiscans. Moreover, if the area of subendocardial infarction is extensive it may be impossible to differentiate this condition from dilated left ventricle with thin myocardium.

CARDIAC ANATOMY ON THALLIUM-201 SCINTISCANS

To visualize all segments of the left ventricle at least once, it is mandatory to obtain multiple views. We routinely take three views (0° anterior, 45° left-anterior-oblique, and the 90° left-lateral view), although in an individual patient additional views may be necessary.

The projection of the heart in the three standard views is illustrated by sections through a normal human heart obtained at post mortem and positioned as *in situ*.

Anterior view

In Figure 4-6 the plane of section is parallel to the surface of the crystal of the gamma camera in the anterior position. The plane of section is through the anterior wall, with a thin layer still present, rather than through the center of the heart to represent the greater contribution of myocardium closest to the detector. The interventricular septum is at an angle to the plane of section and contributes importantly to the caudal part of the horsehoe in this view. Since activity from the inferoposterior wall is also projected in this area and

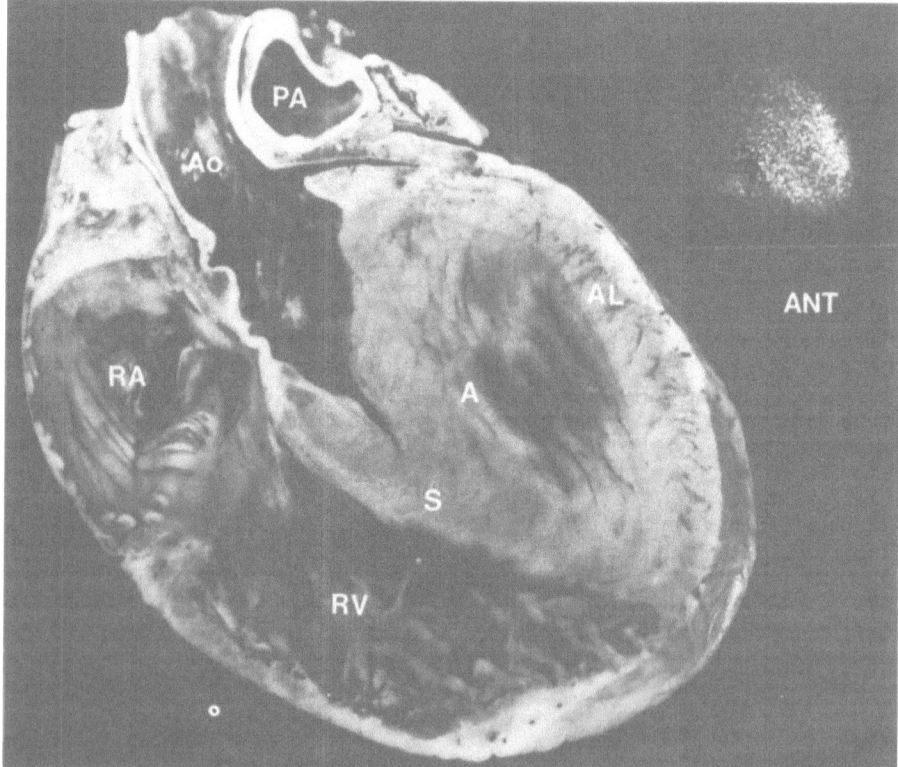

Figure 4-6. Section through a normal human heart parallel to the crystal surface of the gamma camera in the 0° anterior position. The heart is positioned as *in situ*. See text. An anterior view ^{201}Tl scan is shown for comparison. Abbreviations: RA = right atrium; RV = right ventricle; S = interventricular septum; A = anterior wall; AL = anterolateral wall; Ao = aorta; PA = pulmonary artery. Reproced with permission from Ref. [1].

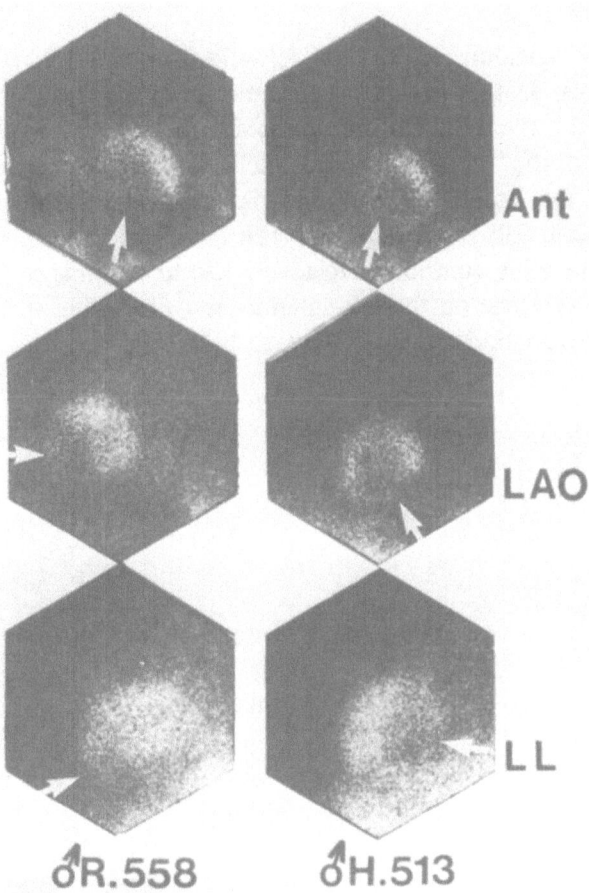

Figure 4-7. Thallium-201 scintiscans in a patient with an apicalseptal infarction (left) and a patient with an inferoposterior infarction (right). Note that on the anterior view in both patients a similar image is obtained. On the left-anterior-oblique images the location of the defect is clearly shown to be septal (left) in one patient, and posterior (right) in the other patient. Reproduced with permission from Ref. [1].

thus superimposed on that of the septum, the caudal part of the horseshoe is composed of radioactivity from these three anatomic areas of the left ventricular wall. The superimposed activity from septum and inferoposterior wall is illustrated in Figure 4-7, which demonstrates the scintiscans of a patient with an apical-septal and a patient with an inferoposterior wall infarction. The anterior view is essentially similar in both patients, but on the 45° left-anterior-oblique and left-lateral views, the difference in anatomic location of the perfusion defects becomes evident. This demonstrates that multiple views are necessary for precise anatomic localization of a myocardial infarction.

Left-anterior-oblique view

In figure 4-8 the cardiac anatomy for the 45° left-anterior-oblique view is shown. The interventricular septum is almost perpendicular to the crystal face and free of superimposed structures. On the scintiscans this activity is projected as the medial part of the "doughnut". The lateral part of the doughnut represents activity from the lateral free wall and partly from the posterior wall. The pure anteroapical wall is viewed upon "en face", in front of the cardiac blood pool and therefore contributes relatively less to the image. The configuration of the left ventricle on the left-anterior-view may differ in the individual patient. These variations will be discussed below.

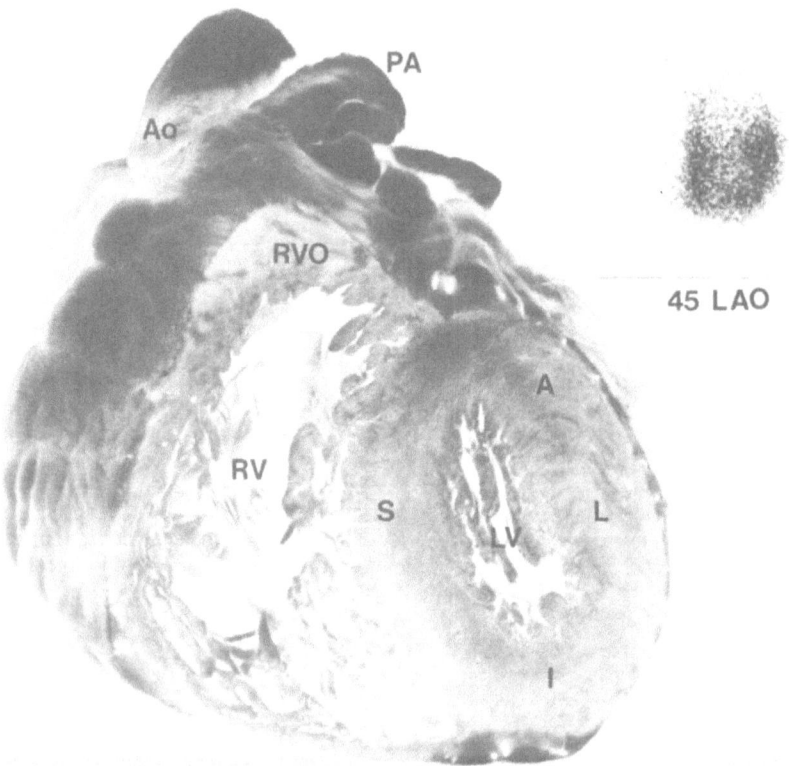

Figure 4-8. Section through a normal human heart parallel to the crystal surface of the gamma camera in the 45° left-anterior-oblique position. The heart is positioned as *in situ*. See text. A left-anterior-oblique ^{201}Tl scan is shown for comparison. Abbreviations: RV = right ventricle; RVO = right ventricular outflow tract; S = interventricular septum; A = anterior wall; L = lateral wall; I = inferior wall; Ao = aorta; PA = pulmonary artery. Reproduced with permission from Ref. [1].

Left-lateral view

Figure 4-9 illustrates the cardiac anatomy of the left-lateral view. The right ventricular outflow tract is anterior to the left ventricle. The anterior wall, perpendicular to the plane of section, has been cut off. From Figure 4-9, it is obvious that the anterior wall is super-imposed on activity of the septum. However, owing to tissue absorption, the contribution of the septum to the image may be less important. The inferoposterior wall is projected on the caudal part of the horseshoe.

The anatomy of the left ventricle, as projected onto the various scintigraphic views, is schematically shown in Figure 4-10. In the left-anterior-oblique view the (postero)lateral wall is not always visualized in the same way. Usually the symmetrical image shown in A can be seen, but sometimes an asymmetrical image is obtained as shown in B, in which the posterolateral wall seems considerably thicker than the septum. Configuration B can be explained by a slight deviation of the longitudinal axis of the heart towards the medial line. The apparent thickness of the lateral wall is an effect of "blurring" by cardiac motion on ungated static images (see below and Figure 4-14).

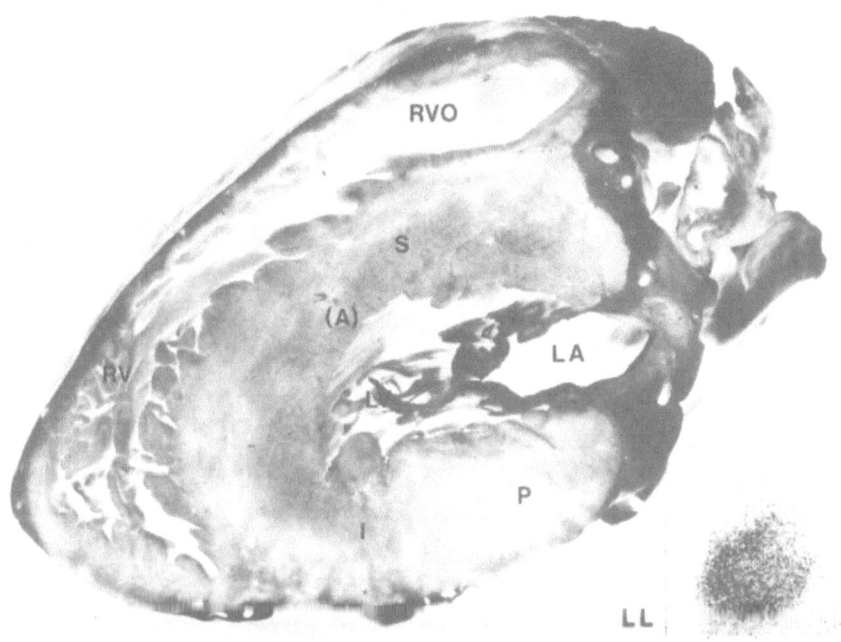

Figure 4-9. Section through a normal human heart parallel to the crystal surface of the gamma camera in the 90° left-lateral position. The heart is positioned as *in situ*. See text. The scintiscan displays a left-lateral view for comparison. Reproduced with permission from Ref. [1].

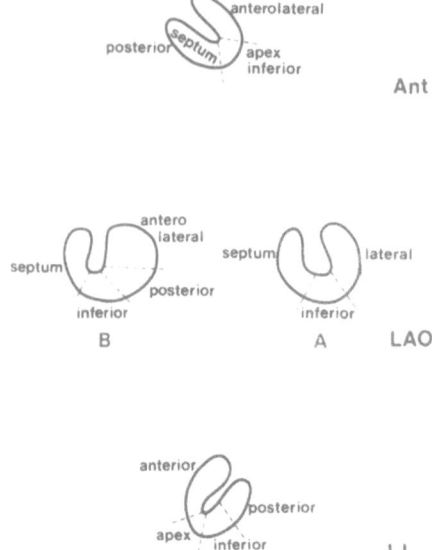

Figure 4-10. Schematic representation of the anatomy of the left ventricle as projected on different views. See text. Reproduced with permission from Ref. [1].

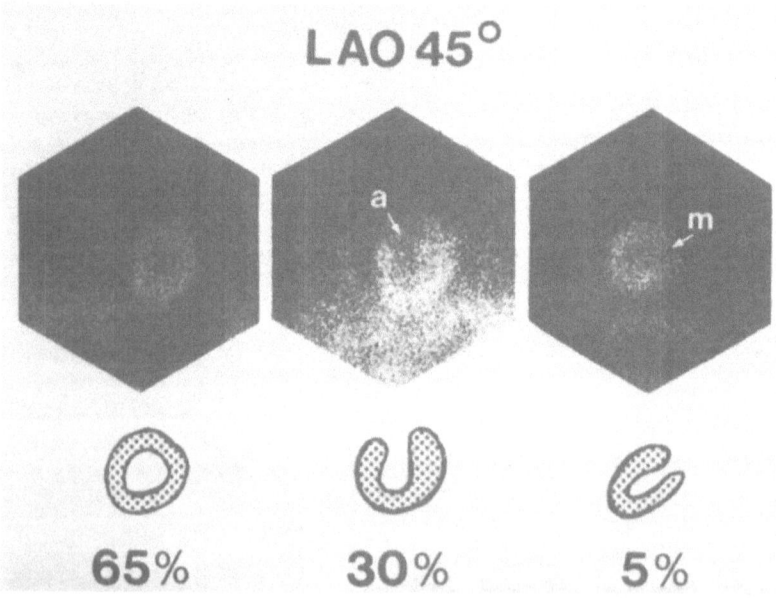

Figure 4-11. Variation in the configuration of the normal left ventricle on the 45° left-anterior-·oblique view (LAO). The percentages indicate the prevalence in a random group of 500 ^{201}Tl studies. Arrows indicate the area of diminished activity due to the aortic (a) and mitral orifice (m). Reproduced with permission from Ref. [1].

The 45° left-anterior-oblique view may also display important individual variation in configuration due to the position of the heart (Figure 4-11). In our series, the « typical » doughnut pattern is seen in 65% of the patients. In

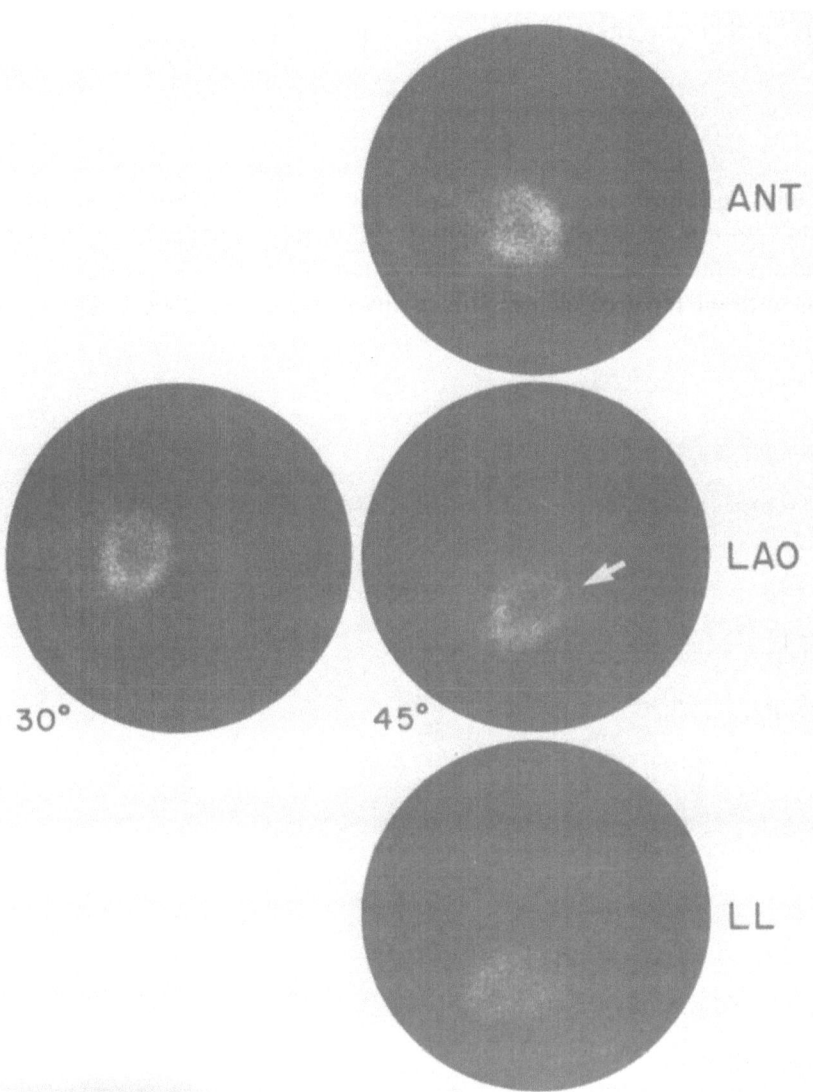

Figure 4-12. Example of a post-exercise ^{201}Tl study in a patient with a slightly medially rotated heart. The standard 45° left-anterior-oblique (LAO) view shows an apparent lateral wall defect (arrow). However, it can be appreciated that the septum is curved instead of straight. This indicates that the lateral aspect of the heart is viewed (compare to left-lateral (LL) view). By rotating the position of the camera head to 30° a normal left-anterior-oblique view is obtained. The septum is straight and maximal separation of right and left ventricle is obtained. The "defect" with 45° obliquity is due to the mitral orifice.

30% of the patients, the aortic orifice can be seen as a definite area of absent activity. In 5% of the patients, the 45° left-anterior-oblique view displays a horseshoe shape, the lateral area of diminished activity representing the mitral orifice. Because this horseshoe image is the result of a more medially directed long axis of the left ventricle, it can be converted into a normal dougnut pattern by changing the angle of obliquity to 30° (Figure 4-12).

EFFECT OF MOTION ARTIFACT ON THALLIUM-201 IMAGES

Numerous investigations have shown that ^{201}Tl myocardial imaging in patients with chronic or acute coronary insufficiently provides highly satisfactory results and important clinical information. This may be considered surprising since all reported clinical studies involve ungated static ^{201}Tl studies.

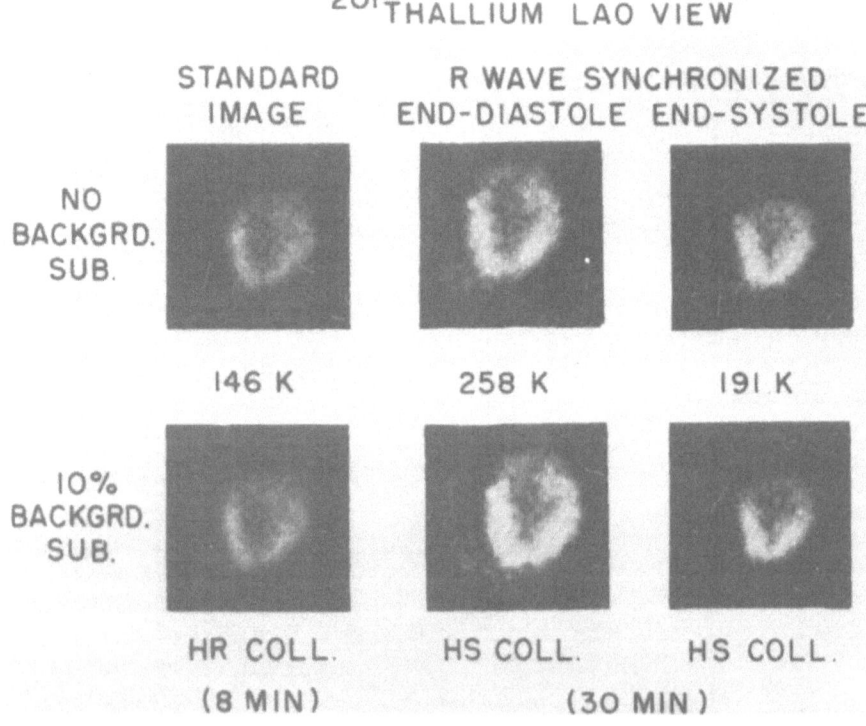

Figure 4-13. Comparison of a standard non-synchronized ^{201}Tl study (left) and a R-wave synchronized study (middle and right) in the same normal subject. Blurring in all areas due to motion artifact is readily apparent in the standard image. The loss of resolution is especially prominent at the outer margin of the ventricular cavity and the outer edge of the ventricular myocardium. Overall, the configuration or pattern of the unsynchronized image corresponds most closely to the end-diastolic R-wave synchronized image. Reproduced with permission from Hamilton et al.[5]

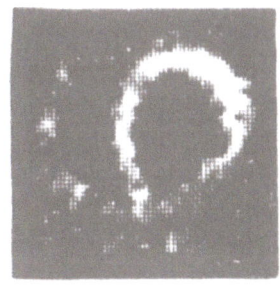

201 THALLIUM

WALL MOTION
STUDY
LAO
INF. HYPOKINESIS   ED—ES

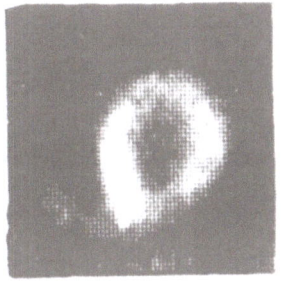

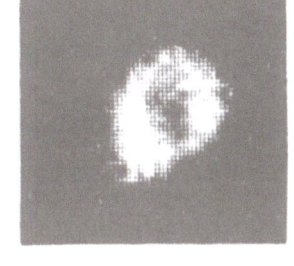

END—DIASTOLE   END—SYSTOLE

Figure 4-14. Wall motion study by R-wave synchronized ^{201}Tl images in a normal subject. The end-systolic image is subtracted from the end-diastolic image. The difference image (top) shows regions of myocardial motion. Much greater motion is noted in the posterolateral wall than in the septum due to movement of the whole left ventricle anteriorly during systole. This accounts for the asymmetrical image often seen as the 45° left-anterior-oblique view. Reproduced with permission from Hamilton et al. [5].

These static images represent the integrated radioactivity of the beating heart over a given time period. Hamilton et al. [5] and Alderson et al. [6] demonstrated the feasibility of R-wave synchronized ^{201}Tl imaging (Figures 4-13 and 4-14). The synchronized motion free images appeared to resolve the myocardium more clearly and defects were more radily apparent than with standard nonsynchronized images (Figures 4-15 and 4-16). In addition, left ventricular wall motion could also be analyzed. Systolic myocardial thickening and wall motion could be appreciated by visual inspection or by computer analysis. One of the motion artifacts, a lateral wall that appears significantly thicker than the septum, is visible on the left-anterior-oblique view (Figure 4-10). The R-wave synchronized ^{210}Tl images demonstrate that this is partially due to the cardiac contraction. As the myocardium contracts inwards, the geom-

^{201}THALLIUM LAO VIEW

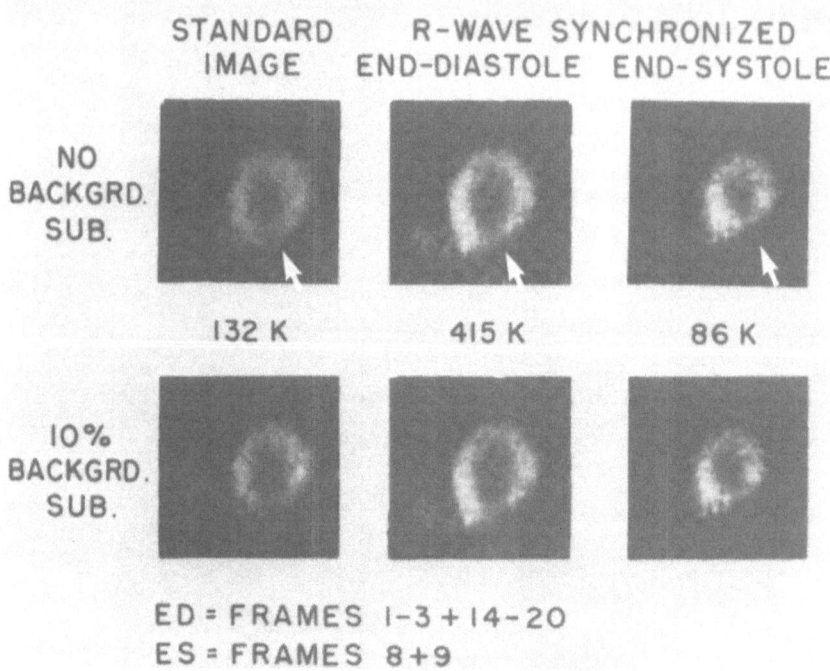

STANDARD   R-WAVE SYNCHRONIZED
IMAGE   END-DIASTOLE END-SYSTOLE

NO BACKGRD. SUB.

132 K   415 K   86 K

10% BACKGRD. SUB.

ED = FRAMES 1-3 + 14-20
ES = FRAMES 8 + 9

Figure 4-15. Comparison of standard non-synchronized and R-wave synchronized ^{201}Tl studies in the same patient with previous inferior myocardial infarction. The standard image shows only a small apical defect. The synchronized images (particularly end-systole) show this to be due to thinning of the inferior wall. Reproduced with permission from Hamilton et al.[5].

etric center of the ventricle moves forward, with the effect that lateral wall motion is maximized and the septum appears akinetic relative to a fixed reference point. as a result, the summed image over time appears to have a thicker lateral wall, while images gated for end-diastole usually demonstrate equal thickness in the septum and lateral wall (Figures 4-13 and 4-14). Overall, the configuration of the unsynchronized image corresponds most closely to the end-diastolic image of the synchronized study.

It is not yet established that R-wave synchronized ^{201}Tl imaging yields better detection of perfusion abnormalities than conventional static imaging[7]. Since the clinical results in patients with coronary artery disease, although not perfect are quite satisfactory, many patients would have to be studied to demonstrate a statistically significant difference. Strauss et al.[8] reported that gated ^{201}Tl imaging may be useful for better recognition of asymmetrical septal hypertrophy. The disproportional upper septal thickesing during systole can better be appreciated on the gated images.

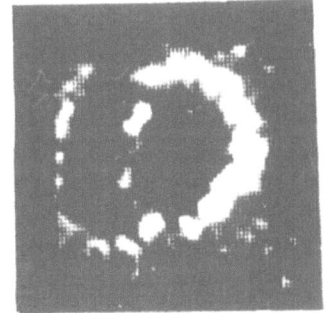

^{201}THALLIUM
WALL MOTION
STUDY
LAO

NORMAL PATTERN   ED—ES

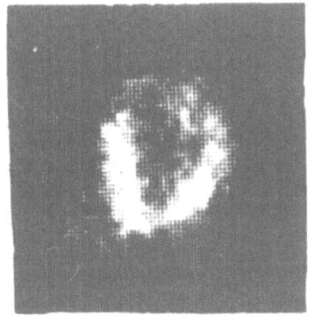 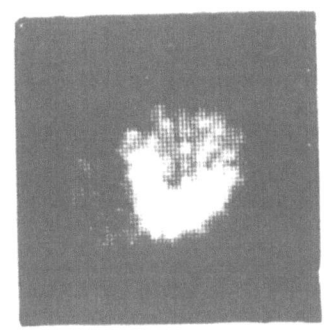

END—DIASTOLE   END—SYSTOLE

Figure 4-16. Wall motion study by R-wave synchronized ^{201}Tl images in a patient with previous inferior myocardial infarction. The inferior wall demonstrates clearly decreased motion. Reproduced with permission from Hamilton et al. [5].

An important potential advantage of cinematic display of ^{201}Tl studies is that subtle abnormalities may be more readily recognized when the blurring effect is reduced. In addition, the analysis of both regional myocardial perfusion and regional wall motion may be helpful for an improved overall image interpretation.

At present, a major disadvantage of gated ^{201}Tl imaging is the much longer time required to obtain a single view (20–30 min). Such lengthly studies are particularly undesirable not only for studies after exercise in which redistribution of ^{201}Tl is known to occur, but also in patients with acute myocardial infarction or ischemia where long imaging times are often too uncomfortable for the patient, or may interfere with patient management. New and more flexible computer software presently offers an alternative mode: a 300,000 counts ^{201}Tl study is acquired with R-wave synchronization. Subsequently, the data can be displayed either as a static study or as a 4–8 frame movie. In our experience, the movie display provides little additional information since the total counts in each frame is relatively low.

NORMAL VARIATIONS AND EFFECT OF HEART POSITION

The occurrence of slight regional differences in myocardial ^{201}Tl activity as normal variants and the appearance of artifactual defects due to variations in cardiac position render interpretation of ^{201}Tl scintiscans a difficult task. Familiarity with the spectrum of normal patterns will help avoid the pitfalls of reading ^{201}Tl scintiscans (Figure 4-17).

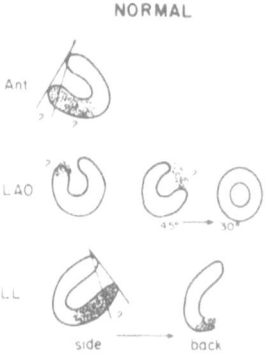

Figure 4-17. Schematic representation of the various anatomic areas on ^{201}Tl scintiscans in which apparent defects may be present that not necessarily represent true myocardial perfusion abnormalities. See text

Apex

A well-known and recognized area of normally decreased ^{201}Tl activity on the scintiscans is the apex of the left ventricle. This is due to normal thinning of the myocardium and is usually noted in patients whose heart is in a vertical position. A typical "normal" apical defect appears as a narrow slit-like area, aligned with the long axis of the ventricle and usually is present on all three views (Figure 4-18). In patients with an abnormally dilated left ventricule (Figure 4-19), this apical defect may be larger and at times difficult to distinguish from an apical infarction. A helpful guideline is that the decreased uptake of a true myocardial infarct is almost always asymmetrically located on one or more views, because the area of decreased uptake extends into the anterior or inferior wall. In contrast, the marked apical thinning that can be

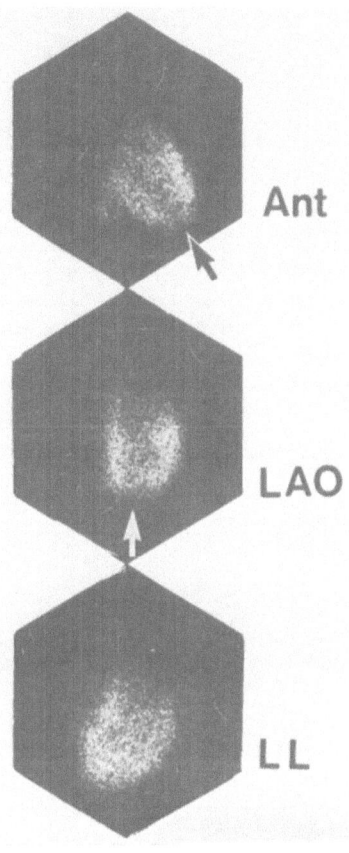

Figure 4-18. Thallium-201 scintiscans in a normal subject following exercise. An area of diminished activity at apex can be appreciated especially in the anterior and left-anterior-oblique views.

encountered in a dilated ventricle always is symmetrical along the long axis of the left ventricle.

Aortic orifice

Although most patients will display a "doughnut" pattern on the 45° left-anterior-oblique view, a horseshoe pattern or a high septal area with decreased activity is seen often. This normal defect represents the aortic valve area (Figure 4-11). This pattern is consistent enough to be reliably appreciated and will seldom pose a problem. In patients with a horizontal heart and/or a tortuous ascending aorta, the cardiac base may be almost vertical, possibly leading to the conclusion that the area of decreased activity representing the

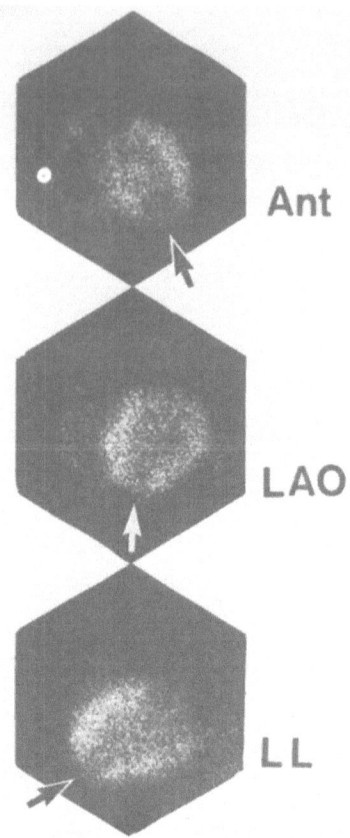

Figure 4-19. Thallium-201 scintiscans in a patient with long standing hypertension. In addition the patient had severe chronic obstructive lung disease. The right ventricle is visualized. The left ventricle is enlarged and dilated. The apical defect is due to the enlargement and dilation of the left ventricle and does *not* represent an apical infarct.

aortic orifice is a perfusion defect of the interventricular septum. However, the anterior view will readily demonstrate the actual horizontal position of the heart (Figure 4-20), providing clues to the proper interpretation of the left-anterior-oblique view.

Base of the heart

On the anterior or left-lateral view, the high posterobasal part of the horse-shoe occasionally demonstrates diminished ^{201}Tl activity (Figures 4-17 and 4-21). One should be extremely cautious not to overread such apparent "single view" basal perfusion defects. It is impossible to determine with certainty from the ^{201}Tl scintiscans the actual plane of the atrioventricular

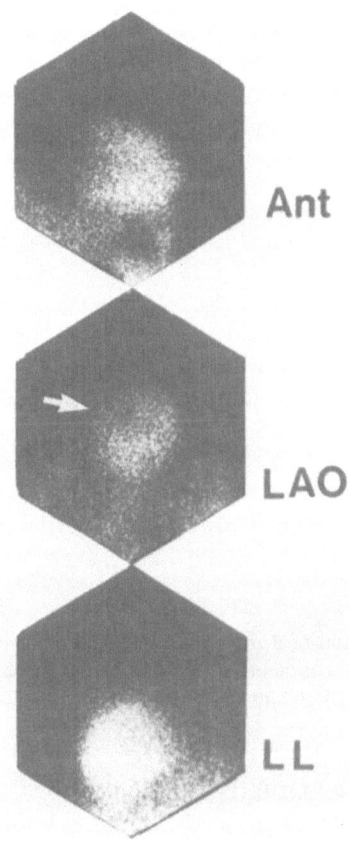

Figure 4-20. Normal ²⁰¹Tl scintiscans of a patient with a horizontal position of the heart and a tortuous ascending aorta. The cardiac base is almost vertical (anterior view). The left-anterior-oblique view demonstrates an apparent perfusion defect high in the septum (arrow), which represents the aortic orifice.

valve ring, i.e., the open end of the horsehoe. Therefore, it is difficult to differentiate between the absence of a small part at the end of the horseshoe and a more vertical than usual heart base. The latter will occur when the heart is in a horizontal position. Foreshortening of the inferior wall may then lead to apparent high posterobasal defects.

TYPICAL ARTIFACTS

Defects on ²⁰¹Tl scintiscans, that appear on only one view, probably are artifacts. In our experience, a true infarct rarely presents as a "single view" defect. These "one view" artifacts can be unmasked by repositioning the

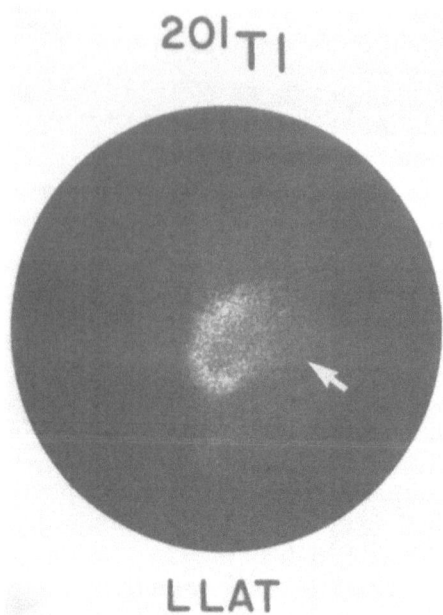

Figure 4-21. Thallium-201 scintiscan in left-lateral position of a normal subject. The other two views (anterior and left-anterior-oblique) were normal. A posterobasal perfusion defect seems to be present. In this patient the heart is in a horizontal position and the apparent defect is caused by foreshortening of the inferoposterior wall.

patient or by obtaining additional views. Typical artifacts can be described for each view.

Anterior view: inferior wall

In normal subjects the horseshoe image on the anterior view displays ^{201}Tl activity in the anterolateral wall approximately equal to that in the inferoseptal region. Sometimes the anterolateral wall has slightly more activity, but the inferoseptal region is well visualized. Figure 4-22 shows a ^{201}Tl study of a patient with chronic obstructive lung disease. The views obtained routinely are the anterior supine, left-anterior-oblique supine and the left-lateral view with the patient on the right side. The images demonstrate visualization of the right ventricle on the left-anterior-oblique view, as can be expected in patients with lung disease, but surprisingly there is an apparent inferior wall defect on the anterior view. Yet this patient had no history of coronary artery disease and no electrocardiographic evidence of previous myocardial infarction. The anterior view was repeated with the patient *sitting upright* in front of the gamma camera. The anterior erect image clearly visualizes the inferoseptal region: a normal anterior image. This artifactual defect conceivably is due to

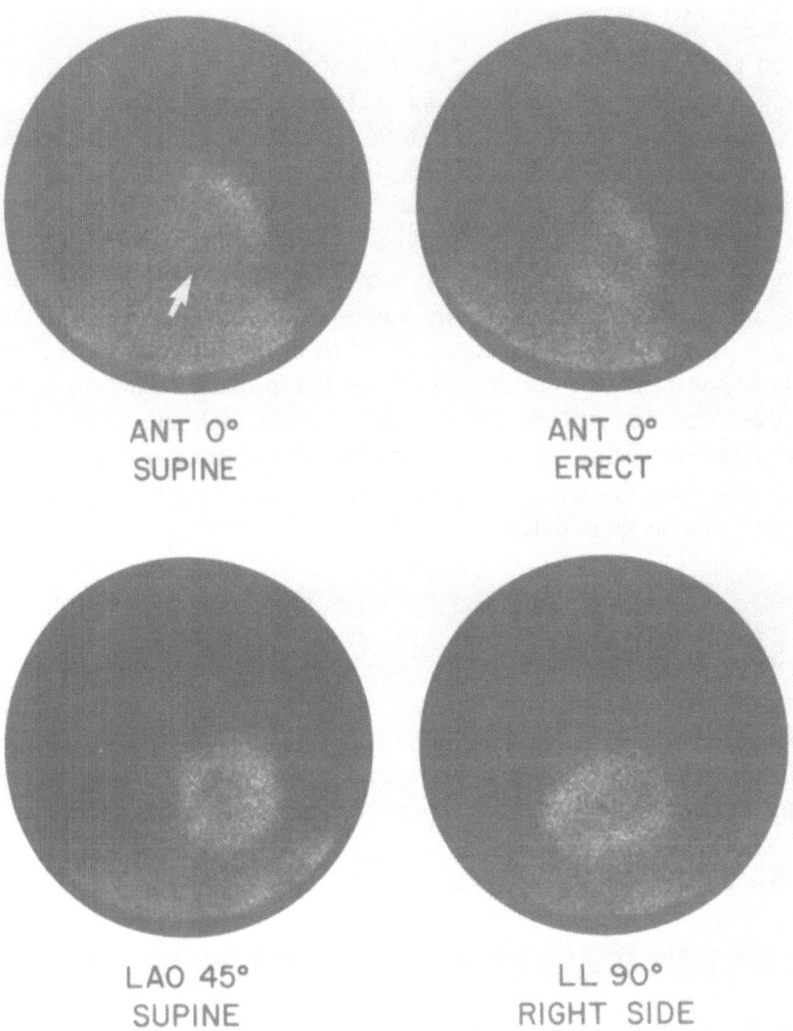

ANT 0°
SUPINE

ANT 0°
ERECT

LAO 45°
SUPINE

LL 90°
RIGHT SIDE

Figure 4-22. Thallium-201 scintiscans at rest in patient with chronic obstructive lung disease. In supine position the anterior view shows an apparent defect at the inferior wall (arrow). The same view obtained with the patient sitting upright shows normal perfusion of the inferior wall. This artifactual defect is likely to be caused by radiation attenuation by the diaphragm.

attenuation of myocardial radiation by adjacent structures, and since it was abolished by moving the patient from supine to erect position, it is likely that the left hemidiaphragm is responsible. This finding is rare and we have observed it in only 10 or 15 patients among the approximately 3000 patients we have studied with ^{201}Tl. The phenomenon may be encountered especially in patients who are obese or have lung disease.

Left-anterior-oblique view: lateral wall and septum

On the left-anterior-oblique view the position of the heart rather than that of the patient is more often responsible for artifactual solitary defects.

Lateral wall

The effect of a heart more medially rotated than normal has already been discussed on p. 82 (Figure 4-12). In this situation, the 45° left-anterior-oblique view is not perpendicular to the long axis of the left ventricle, and the projection of the heart is more comparable to the left-lateral view. A horse-shoe image is obtained and the apparent defect at the high lateral wall is the open end of the horseshoe, which represents the atrioventricular ring. In these patients, a view that displays the septum vertically and the left-ventricle as a "doughnut" should be obtained.

Septum

We discussed above the apparent high septal defect caused by the horizontally positioned heart on the left-anterior-oblique view (Figure 4-20).

In patients with a dilated and enlarged left ventricle, the long axis is frequently deviated to the left. A routine 45° left-anterior-oblique view in these cases displays an image similar to that of an anterior view and demonstrates an apparent septal defect, caused by the normally open end of the horseshoe (Figure 4-23). A steeper (60°) left-anterior-oblique angle is more likely to project the ventricle along its long axis and will visualize the true image of the septum and the typical doughnut pattern. This phenomenon may explain previous reports of septal defects in patients with left bundle branch block [9]. In our study of 40 patients with left bundle branch block without evidence of previous myocardial infarction [10], the septum was always well visualized although it appeared thinner than usual in one-third of the patients. In these patients, frequently the obliquity of the left-anterior-oblique view had to be adjusted because of enlargement and dilation of the left ventricle.

Left-lateral view: inferior wall

A common artifactual defect similar to that described for the anterior view may be obtained with greater frequency in the left-lateral view. We studied

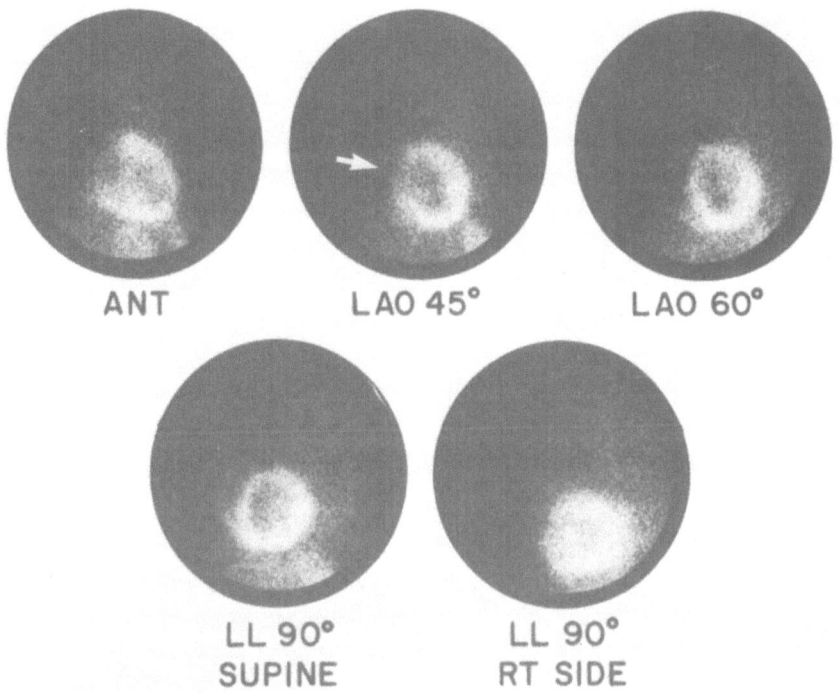

ANT   LAO 45°   LAO 60°

LL 90°   LL 90°
SUPINE   RT SIDE

Figure 4-23. Thallium-201 scintiscans in a patient with left bundle branch block pattern on the electrocardiogram. The left ventricle is dilated and rotated clockwise. On the standard 45° left-anterior-oblique view a septal perfusion defect appears to be present. However, the configuration of the left ventricle in this view is very similar to that in the anterior view, indicating clockwise rotation. The left-anterior-oblique 60° and 90° views clearly visualize the septum. Although the septum is thinner than usual, no perfusion defect is present.

the effect of patient positioning on left-lateral ^{201}Tl images in 28 patients[11]. The left-lateral image was performed with the patient *supine* and with the patient *lying on his right side*. False-positive inferoposterior defects (Figure 4-24) were obtained in five patients (18%) in the left-lateral supine view, but not in the left-lateral view with the patient lying on his right side.

The left-lateral supine images were more often technically inadequate than those obtained with the patient lying on his right side (6/28 vs 3/28). When the image obtained with the patient on the right side was technically inadequate, the companion supine image was equally inadequate. Possible explanations for the apparent false-positive defects include (a) geometric considerations and (b) radiation attenuation by adjacent structures. Figure 4-25 demonstrates the change in alignment of the heart as the patient moves from supine position to the right side down position: the long axis of the heart shifts from horizontal toward vertical. When the patient is on his right side, the inferoposterior segments are parallel to the detector, providing an *en face*

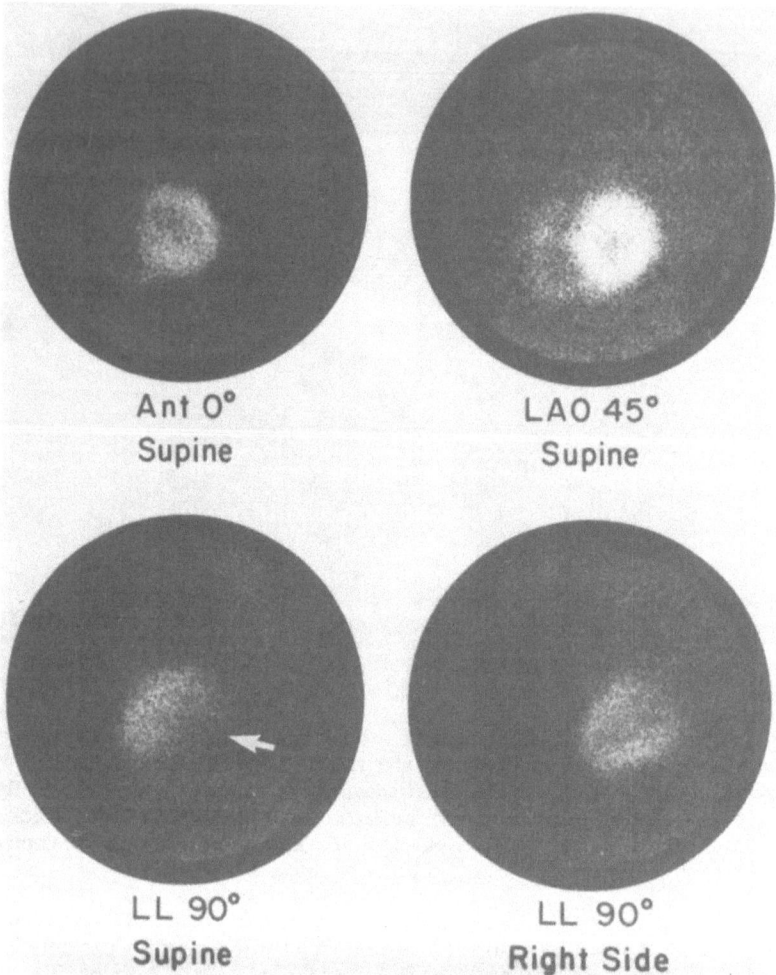

Ant 0°
Supine

LAO 45°
Supine

LL 90°
Supine

LL 90°
Right Side

Figure 4-24. Thallium-201 scintiscans following exercise in a patient with normal coronary arteries. A definite inferoposterior wall defect is seen on the left-lateral supine view. The anterior and left-anterior-oblique views are normal. A left-lateral view obtained with the patient lying on his right side demonstrates a normal inferoposterior wall. The two left-lateral images were obtained immediately after each other. Reproduced with permission from Ref. [11].

image of this region. However, with the patient supine, the inferoposterior wall is more perpendicular to the detector, which may lead to foreshortening of the inferoposterior segments. While false-positive defects in the left-lateral supine position could result from distortion of these segments, the most likely explanation for false-positive defects in the supine image is attenuation by the left hemidiaphragm (Figure 4-26). The left-lateral view is an important projection for visualization of the inferoposterior wall without overlying radioactivity. Unfortunately, in many laboratories the left-lateral view is obtained with

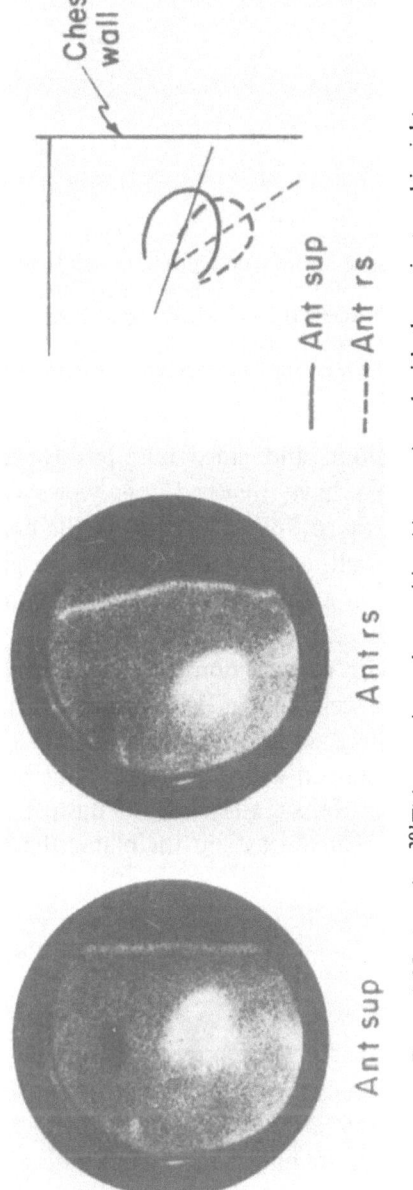

Figure 4-25. Anterior ^{201}Tl images in supine position (Ant sup), and with the patient on his right side (Ant rs). When turned from supine to right side, the long axis of the heart becomes more "vertical" as schematically illustrated. Lead marker and left mid-axillary line served as fixed external reference. Reproduced with permission from Ref. [11].

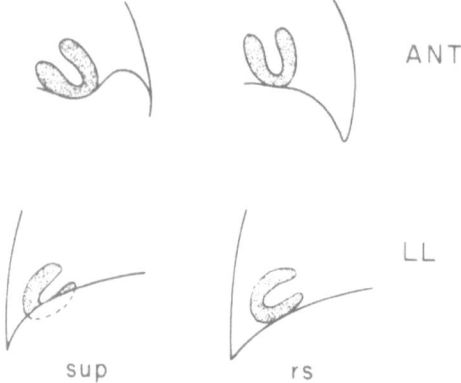

ANT

LL

sup   rs

Figure 4-26. Schematic illustrations of interrelationship between left hemi-diaphragm and heart in supine (sup) position and with the patient on his right side (rs). Top panel shows anterior (Ant) view and lower panel shows left-lateral (LL) view. In supine position, excursion of the left hemidiaphragm above the inferior border of the heart may result in attenuation of ^{201}Tl radiation from the inferoposterior myocardial segments. Reproduced with permission from Ref. [11].

the patient in supine position and since false-positive defects have been obtained some investigators have replaced this view with a steeper left-anterior-oblique projection. Since this angle displays the projection of a different part of the ventricular wall, it does not visualize the posterior wall at all, expecially in patients with an enlarged left ventricle (Figure 4-23). For accurate interpretation of ^{201}Tl scans "complete imaging" is mandatory. The reported decreased sensitivity of detection for inferior wall abnormalities by ^{201}Tl imaging [9, 10] may be well be related to incomplete myocardial imaging. We believe that the left-lateral images are an important component of ^{201}Tl imaging. They should be obtained with the patient lying on his right side and the detector head parallel to the sagittal plane of the patient above the table top. Care should be taken that the patient maintains the correction position, to ensure good quality images.

Obese patients

In extremely obese patients attenuation of radiation by breast tissue may cause artifactual areas of diminished activity. Such areas usually will appear as anteroapical defects on the anterior and left-lateral view, while the location may vary on the left-anterior-oblique view. Figure 4-27 displays examples of [201]Tl "defects", that were created by breast tissue.

Solitary "one view" defects are unusual in ^{201}Tl imaging and when they appear a technical explanation should be sought, such as abnormal position or size of the heart, or attenuation of radiation by structure adjacent to the heart.

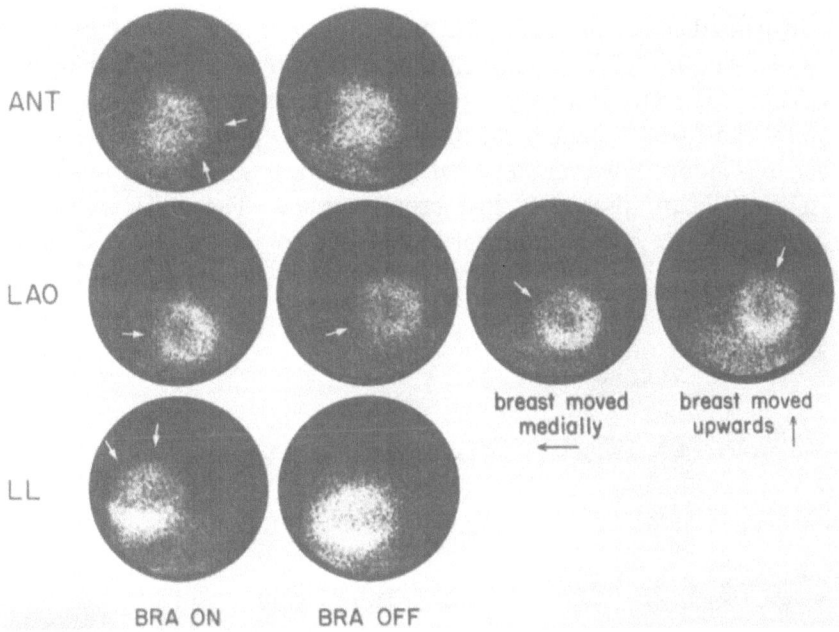

ANT

LAO

LL

breast moved
medially

breast moved
upwards ↑

BRA ON   BRA OFF

Figure 4-27. Thallium-201 scintiscans in a patient with heavy breasts. Left images with bra on. Apparent perfusion defects (arrows) are present in all views. With bra off the defects change in location due to different position of the left breast. On the left-anterior-oblique view defects can be created by moving the breast in different directions.

There is one exception: an isolated defect at the anterior wall on the left-lateral view (see chapter 6, Figure 6-2) is usually a true defect representing perfusion abnormality restricted to the anterior wall. Occasionally solitary defects cannot be explained by one of the above described factors. In a resting study this is a problem and the study should be considered as "questionable". In post-exercise studies the disappearance of solitary defects at delayed imaging indicates presence of transient ischemia.

For the application of multiple pinhole or coded aperture ^{201}Tl tomography it is extremely important to be familiar with the pseudodefects described above. Since they are primarily due to radiation attenuation and position of the heart, similar artifacts can be expected on the reconstructed images.

Relative accumulation of thallium-201

Thallium-201 scintiscans usually are analyzed to detect a difference in radio-nuclide accumulation: in patients with ischemic heart disease the area with diminished activity is considered abnormal since it reflects diminished myo-

cardial blood flow. However, the images only demonstrate *relative uptake* of
^{201}Tl. In particular circumstances the area with *more* uptake may be abnormal, while the area with diminished uptake may represent normal myocardium. The ^{201}Tl scans of a patient referred to the coronary care unit because of atypical chest pain (Figure 4-28) show less activity in the anterolateral wall. Further evaluation, however, revealed asymmetrical septal hypertrophy and not ischemic heart disease as had been expected. The ^{201}Tl scans show *increased* uptake in the inferoseptal region due to increased septal muscle mass.

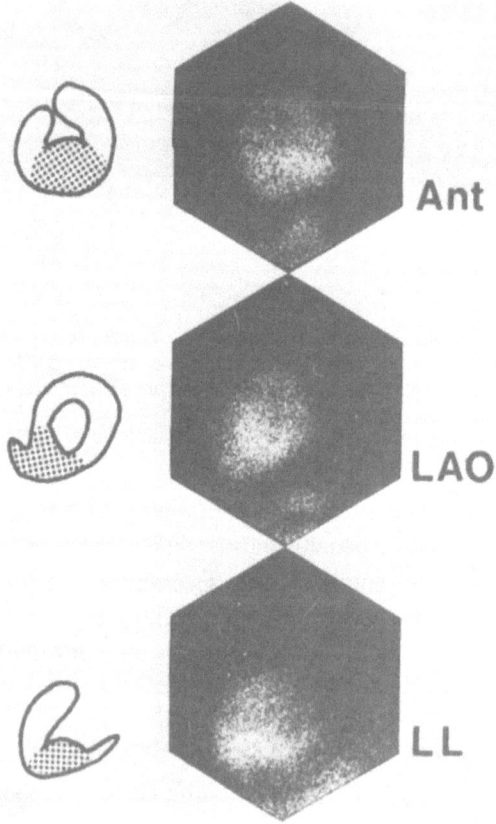

Figure 4-28. Thallium-201 scintiscans in a patient with asymmetrical septal hypertrophy. Accumulation of ^{201}Tl is inhomogeneous. Increased uptake in the inferoseptal region reflects increased muscle mass. Left a schematic illustration.

Figure 4-29 shows the ^{201}Tl scans of a patient with coronary spasm, shortly after relief of the pain sublingual nitroglycerin. Again, the abnormal region seems to be the anterolateral wall. However, these scintiscans demonstrate *increased* uptake of ^{201}Tl in the inferior wall as the result of reactive hyper-

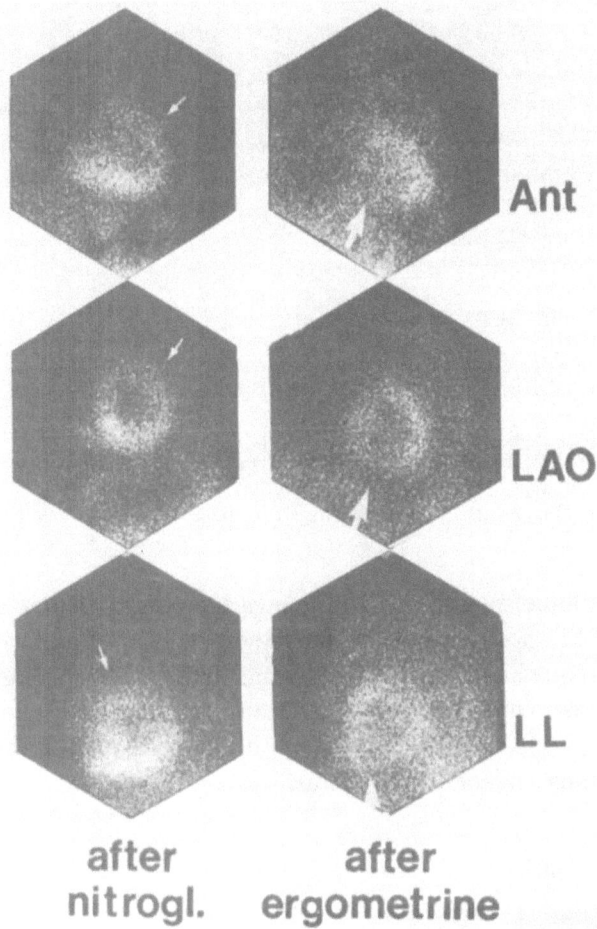

Ant

LAO

LL

after
nitrogl.

after
ergometrine

Figure 4-29. Thallium-201 scintiscans in a patient with angiographically normal coronary arteries and vasospasm of the right coronary artery. Left. scintiscans shortly after relief of pain by nitroglycerin. An area of diminished activity seems to be present at the anterolateral wall. Right, scintiscans after provocation of vasospasm by i.v. ergometrine. Perfusion defect is present at the inferior wall (arrows). After nitroglycerin reperfusion hyperemia in the inferior wall caused relatively increased ^{201}Tl uptake.

emia after relief of vasospasm in the right coronary artery (also see chapter 10, p. 212).

The display of relative activity of ^{201}Tl may lead to distortion of the images. Figure 4-30 shows three left-lateral views. A normal horseshoe pattern is present in the normal subject and this pattern is still recognizable in the patient with a small anterior wall defect.

In contrast, the image is distorted in the patient with a large anterior wall defect; the base of the heart and the lateral wall (parallel to the crystal face),

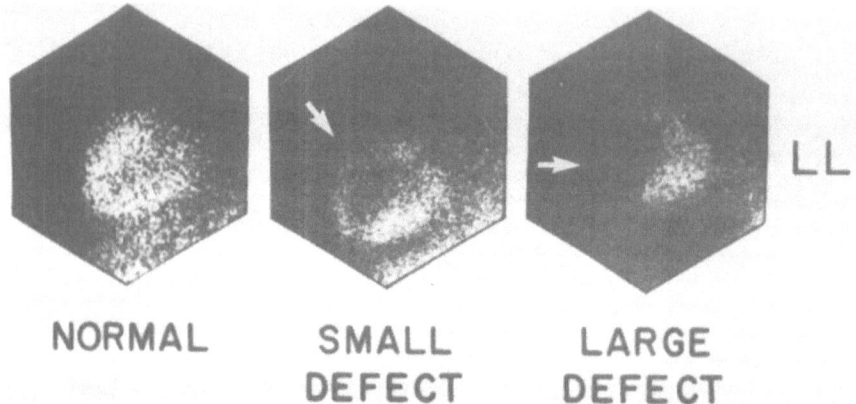

Figure 4-30. Three left-lateral views. Left, normal images displaying the usual horseshoe pattern. Middle, small anterolateral defect. The horseshoe pattern is preserved. Right, large anterior wall defect. Relative contribution of radiation of the base of the left ventricle is greater due to loss of contribution of the anterior wall. This results in distorted image and "closure" of the open end of the horseshoe.

which usually do not contribute significantly to the image, are now visualized resulting in "closure" of the open end of the horseshoe.

In summary, correct interpretation of ^{201}Tl scintiscans depends (1) on thorough knowledge of the variability of normal ^{201}Tl scans, (2) familiarity with the effects on the images of abnormal position or size or the heart and (3) the effects of patients positioning and/or body habitus.

Visualization of the right ventricle

In normal subjects the right ventricle is not visualized at rest [1-3]. Visualization of the right ventricle on ^{201}Tl images is determined by right ventricular myocardial blood flow and right ventricular myocardial mass. Under normal conditions the left ventricle has approximately 25% more myocardial mass and correspondingly higher myocardial blood flow than the right ventricle. Consequently, only the left ventricle is well visualized.

Visualization of the right ventricle at rest is always abnormal, indicating increased right ventricular workload. This may be pressure overload or volume overload [15, 16]. Thus, patients with a variety of congential heart disease, acquired heart disease or pulmonary disease may demonstrate visualization of the right ventricle at rest [17-19]. Additionally, resting tachycardia may cause visualization of the right ventricle. In the latter condition there is also increased uptake of ^{201}Tl in the left ventricle.

In patients with acute myocardial infarction often the right ventricle may be visualized. This may be due to tachycardia, relative low contribution of

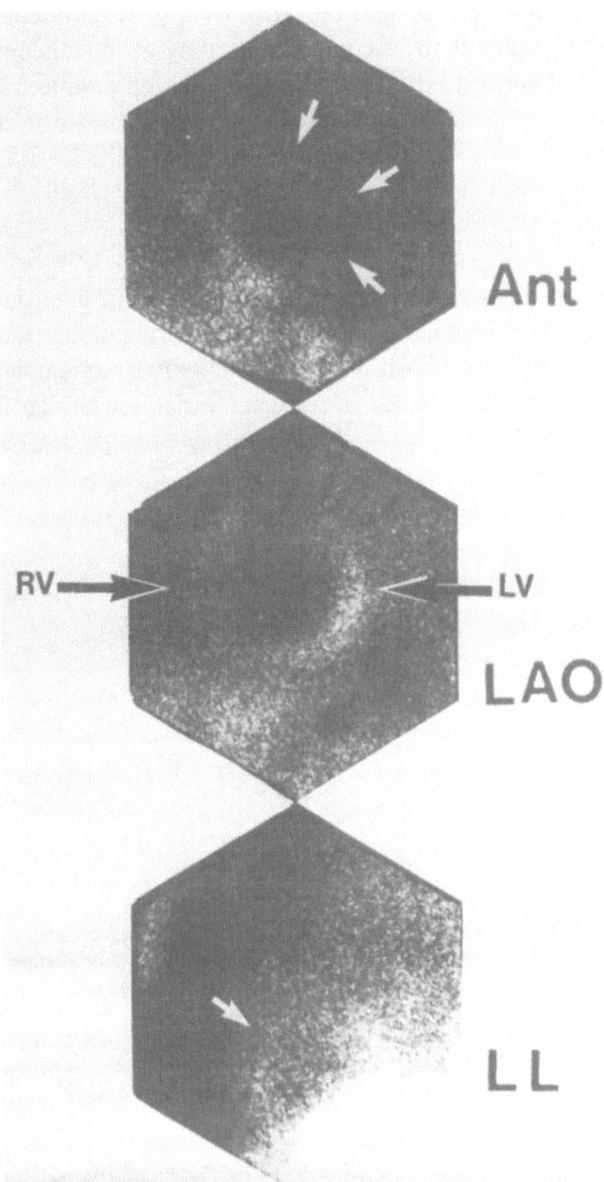

Figure 4-31. Patient with massive anteroseptal infarct. The left ventricle (LV) is almost not visualized. On the left-anterior-oblique view (LAO) the septum is completely absent. The right ventricle (RV) is clearly visualized. See Figure 6-9 in chapter 6.

radiation by the left ventricle due to an extensive perfusion defect (Figure 4-31), increased right ventricular workload due to increased pulmonary (wedge) pressure, or a combination of these factors.

Occasionally, in patients with visualization of the right ventricle, the inferior wall of the right ventricle seems to be thin or to display a perfusion defect (Figure 4-19). It is probably incorrect to interpret this finding as evidence of right ventricular infarction. However, the significance of this observation as yet has to be determined.

Interobserver variability

In addition to experience, an important subjective aspect affects the interpretation of ^{201}Tl scintiscans. We compared observer variability among four experienced investigators from two institutions [20]. Observer agreement occurred in 79% of the studies (Figure 4-32), a degree of variability similar to

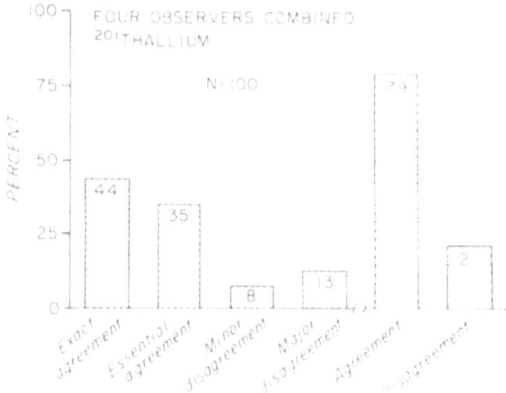

Figure 4-32. Variability among four observers in reading 100 ^{201}Tl scintiscans. Scintiscans could be read as normal (N), abnormal (AB) or borderline (B). N N N N = all four observers read the same study as "normal", B B B AB = three observers read the same study as "borderline", one observer disagreed and read as "abnormal". The graph shows percentages of exact agreement (N N N N, B B B B, or AB AB AB AB), essential agreement (N N N B, AB, AB, AB, B, B B B N, B B B AB), minor disagreement (N N B B, AB AB B B), and major disagreement (N/AB). Agreement is sum of exact and essential agreements. Disagreement is sum of minor and major disagreements. Reproduced with permission from Trobaugh et al. [19].

that previously found for coronary angiography [21]. The relative degree of interobserver variability was dependent on whether the studies were read as normal, abnormal or borderline. Greater interobserver agreement occurred for studies read as normal or abnormal than for those read as borderline (Figure 4-33). Improved observer agreement was also noted when observers read studies from their own institution, suggesting an unintentional bias. From this study it was also apparent that there was disagreement not so much in the description of the images as well as in the final interpretation.

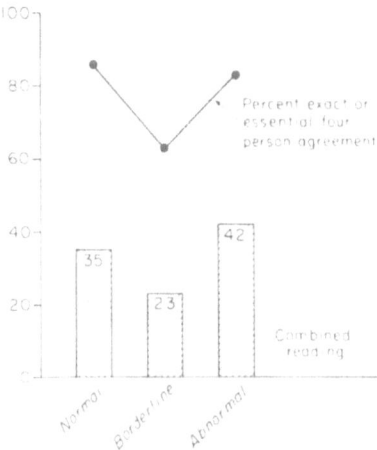

Figure 4-33. Variability among four observers in reading 100 ^{201}Tl scintiscans. Agreement among various observers was greater for studies read as normal or abnormal than for those read as borderline. The graph shows the average percentage of cases read as normal, borderline or abnormal for the four observers. Above, average percentage of exact or essential (see Figure 4-32) agreement is indicated: of the average number of 35 scans read as normal there was exact or essential agreement in 86% of the cases. This occurred in only 63% of the scans read as borderline and in 83% of the scans read as abnormal. Reproduced with permission from Trobaugh et al. [19].

CONCLUSION

Thallium-201 scintiscans may sometimes be difficult to interpret. Valuable clinical information can be obtained when the study is properly performed and analyzed by a careful and experienced observer.

REFERENCES

1. Wackers FJTh, Busemann Sokole E, Samson G, van der Schoot JB: Atlas of ^{201}Tl myocardial scintigraphy. Clin Nucl Med 2:64-74, 1977.
2. Cook DJ, Bailey I, Strauss HW, Rouleau J, Wagner Jr, HN, Pitt B: Thallium-201 for myocardial imaging: appearance of the normal heart. J Nucl Med 17:583-589, 1976.
3. Wackers FJTh, Sokole EB, Samson G, van der Schoot JB: Anatomy of the normal myocardial image. In: Thallium-201 myocardial imaging, pp 41-53, Ritchie SL, Hamilton GW, Wackers FJ, eds. New York: Raven Press, 1978.
4. Massie B, Botvinick E, Arnold S, Shames D, Brundage B, Sheldon K: Effect of contrast enhancement on the sensitivity and specificity of Tl-201 scintigraphy. Am J Cardiol 43:357, 1979.
5. Hamilton GW, Narahara KA, Trobaugh GB, Ritchie JL, Williams DL: Thallium-201 myocardial imaging: characterization of the ECG-synchronized images. J Nucl Med 19:1103-1110, 1978.
6. Alderson PO, Wagner JR, HN, Gomez-Moeiras JJ, Rehn TG, Becker LC, Douglas KH, Manspeaker HF, Schindledecker GR: Simultaneous detection of myocardial perfusion and wall motion abnormalities by cinematic ^{201}Tl imaging. Radiology 127:531-533, 1978.

7. McKusick KA, Bingham J, Pohost G, Strauss HW: Comparison of Defect detection on ungated vs Gated thallium-201 cardiac images. J. Nucl Med 19:725, 1978.

8. Pohost GM, Fallon JT, Strauss HW: Radionuclide techniques in cardiomyopathy. In: Cardiovascular nuclear medicine. 2nd edition, pp 326-340, Strauss HW, Pitt B, eds. St. Louis: Mosby, 1979.

9. McGowan RL, Welch TG, Zaret BL, Bryson AL, Martin ND, Flamm MD: Noninvasive myocardial imaging with potassium-43 and rubidium-81 in patients with left bundle branch block. Am J Cardiol 38:422-428, 1976.

10. Wackers FJTh, Busemann Sokole E, Samson G, Van der Schoot JB, Lie KI, Durrer D, Wellens HJJ: Thallium-201 for visualization of acute myocardial infarction in the presence of left bundle branch block. Herz 2:163-166, 1977.

11. Johnstone DE, Wackers FJTh, Berger HJ, Hoffer PB, Kelley MJ, Gottschalk A, Zaret BL: Effect of patient positioning on left lateral thallium-201 myocardial images. J Nucl Med 20:183-188, 1979.

12. Berger HJ, Gottschalk A, Zaret BL: Dual Radionuclide study of acute myocardial infarction: comparison of thallium-201 and technetium-99m stannous pyrophosphate imaging in man. Ann Intern Med 88:145-154, 1978.

13. Blood DK, McCarthy DM, Sciacca RR, Cannon PJ: Comparison of single dose and double-dose thallium-201 myocardial perfusion scintigraphy for the detection of coronary artery disease and prior myocardial infarction. Circulation 58:777-788, 1978.

14. Bulkley BH, Rouleau J, Strauss HW, Pitt B: Idiopathic hypertrophic subaortic stenosis: detection by thallium-201 myocardial perfusion imaging. N Engl J Med 293:1113-1116, 1975.

15. Wackers F, Schnitzer J, Geha G, Zaret B, Laks H: Effect of acute increase of right ventricular (RV) afterload on RV thallium-201 uptake. Circulation 60: suppl II, II-61, abstract 231, 1979.

16. Schnitzer J, Wackers F, Laks H, Zaret B: Effects of pressure and volume overload of the right ventricle on myocardial blood flow and thallium-201 uptake. Clin Res 27:568A, 1979.

17. Cohen HA, Baird MG, Rouleau JR, Fuhrmann CF, Bailey IK, Summer WR, Strauss HW, Pitt B: Thallium-201 myocardial imaging in patients with pulmonary hypertension. Circulation 54:790-795, 1976.

18. Kondo M, Kubo A, Yamazaki H, Ohsuzu F, Hondo S, Tsugu T, Masaki H, Kinoshita F, Hashimoto S: Thallium-201 myocardial imaging for evaluation of right-ventricular overloading. J Nucl Med 19:1197-1203, 1978.

19. Khaja F, Alam M, Goldstein S, Anbe DT, Marks DS: Diagnostic value of visualization of the right ventricle using thallium-201 myocardial imaging. Circulation 59:182-188, 1979.

20. Trobaugh GB, Wackers FJTh, Busemann Sokole E, DeRouen TA, Ritchie JL, Hamilton GW: Thallium-201 myocardial imaging: an interinstitutional study of observer variability. J Nucl Med 19.359-363, 1978.

21. DeRouen TA, Murray JA, Owen W: Variability in the analysis of coronary arteriograms. Circulation 55:324-328, 1977

5. TECHNETIUM-99m-PYROPHOSPHATE MYOCARDIAL IMAGING

ROBERT W. PARKEY, FREDERICK J. BONTE, SAMUEL E. LEWIS
and JAMES T. WILLERSON

Technetium-99m is the most widely used radioisotope in nuclear medicine presently. It has nearly ideal decay characteristics, including a half-life of 6 hr, monoenergetic and highly abundant gamma rays (140 keV, 90%) and absence of beta or alpha particle emission [1]. It is also easy to produce and readily available in generator form. It has the ability to complex with many organic and inorganic compounds [1]. Technetium-99m is the daughter product of ^{99}Mo. Molybdenum-99 has a half-life of 67 hr and undergoes both gamma and beta decay, the beta-decay leading to its daughter product ^{99m}Tc. Technetium-99m can be separated easily from its parent product by simple solvent extraction with methylethylketone under basic conditions or by column chromatography on an alumina column. Simple elution with isotonic saline brings ionic pertechnetate (^{99m}TcO$_4$) through the column, leaving ^{99m}Mo behind, which, by its subsequent decay, generates more ^{99m}Tc that can be eluted later. Technetium-99m stannous pyrophosphate was chosen as a potential imaging agent to identify acute myocardial infarcts with the rationale being that pyrophosphate might complex with calcium which is deposited in irreversibly damaged myocardial cells following acute myocardial infarction [2, 3].

Patients suspected of having acute myocardial infarcts may undergo ^{99m}Tc-pyrophosphate myocardial scintigraphy for purposes of detecting and localizing the infarct [2-10]. The myocardial scintigrams can be obtained in the intensive care unit at the patient's bedside using a portable gamma camera or the patient may be moved to the nuclear cardiology facility if the distances involved are short and the patient is considered stable. If patients are moved, it is necessary to provide appropriate electrocardiographic monitoring and to have available emergency drugs, a defibrillator and the necessary medical and nursing personnel.. Critically ill patients who cannot be transported are best imaged at their bedside and even stable cardiac patients are subjected to less risk if the imaging can be done in the intensive care unit. A portable camera-computer system thus becomes a powerful tool in evaluating acutely ill cardiac patients. An associated computer allows one to process the ^{99m}Tc-pyrophosphate myocardial scintigrams which is helpful in 10-15% of patients in determining whether an acute myocardial infarct is present. The computer system may also allow one to calculate ventricular volumes and ejection fractions so that one may identify the presence or absence of an acute myocardial infarct and then establish the functional impact of old and new infarcts on ventricular performance using this scintigraphic approach. Electrocardiographic gating the ^{99m}Tc-pyrophosphate myocardial scintigrams also helps to separate bone uptake from abnormal myocardial uptake with small myocardial lesions that are situated close to bony structures. Computer processing helps to sharpen infarct margins and allows one to subtract some of the bone background; this may also help where small infarcts and/or those situated close to bone structures are present.

The procedure that we use for obtaining ^{99m}Tc-pyrophosphate myocardial scintigrams is described in Table 5-1. It is particularly important to check representative batches of the radiopharmaceutical that is injected to insure that excessive free ^{99m}Tc-pertechnetate is not present. This is done at our institution by the method shown in Table 5-2. If free ^{99m}Tc-pertechnetate is

Table 5-1. Proper procedure for obtaining a ^{99m}Tc-pyrophosphate myocardial scintigram

1. Ensure proper labeling of pyrophosphate with ^{99m}Tc by checking either all or representative batches of material for free ^{99m}Tc.
2. Careful intravenous injection into a vein (not into plastic intravenous tubing) with good flush.
3. Obtain ^{99m}Tc-pyrophosphate myocardial images in at least four projections, including the anterior, left anterior oblique (40° and 70°), and left lateral ones; images are routinely obtained at 2 hr following IV injection, but if there is any question concerning whether a particular image represents a blood pool scintigram, repeat images should be obtained at 3 to 4 hr after intravenous injection. Blood pool scintigrams due to delayed renal clearance (severe renal disease, etc.) or severely deranged ventricular function should clear within that time. However, those due to in vivo labeling of red blood cells because of excessive free ^{99m}Tc-pertechnetate in the injectate will not clear within that time periode, and one will have to wait until the next day to repeat the test again.
4. In positioning the patient and interpreting the ^{99m}Tc-pyrophosphate myocardial scintigrams, one needs to be certain that the position of the heart in the chest is known and that the imaging projections have allowed one to adequately visualize the various regions of the heart. In particular, one needs to be certain that the inferior wall of the heart has been well visualized.

Table 5-2. A method to determine the amount of free ^{99m}Tc-pertechnetate in ^{99m}Tc-pyrophosphate

1. Silica gel chromatographic paper is cut into 5 by 20 mm strips and dried in desiccator.
2. Small drop of ^{99m}Tc-pyrophosphate is placed one-half inch on opposite end of paper held with forceps; allow drop to dry in N$_2$ atmosphere.
3. Set dried paper strip in a bottle with approximately one-quarter inch of methylethylketone; drop remains above the level of MEK.
4. Thirty seconds later, remove and allow to dry. Then either (a) image the strip or (b) cut paper into pieces and count in a well counter.
5. It is best to discard ^{99m}Tc-pyrophosphate batch if there is significant migration of ^{99m}Tc-pertechnetate away from the drop.

present in the injectate in excess, it will be taken up in red cells and result in a persistent radionuclide blood pool scintigram for the half life of the radio-siotope (6 hr)[11]. This makes interpretation of the ^{99m}Tc-pyrophosphate myo-cardial scintigrams impossible as regards the documentation of the presence or absence of an acute myocardial infarct.

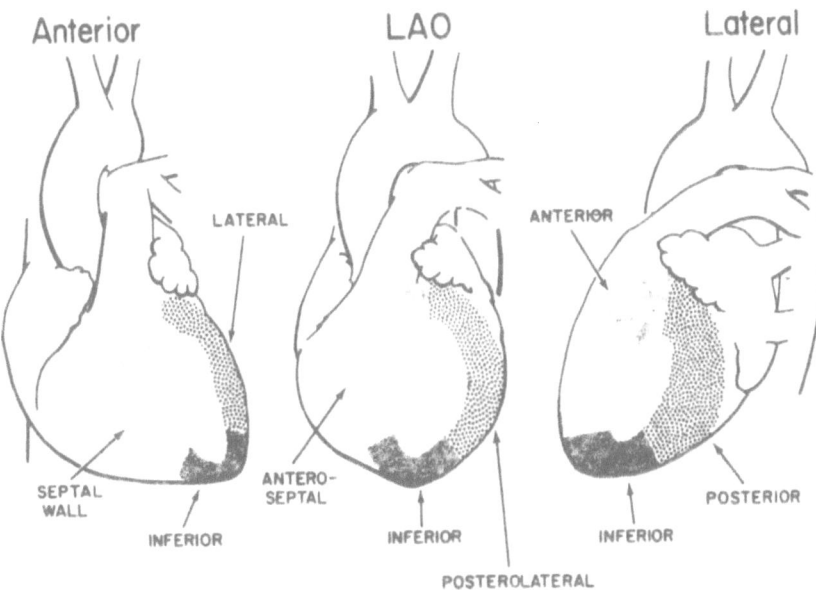

Figure 5-1. The line drawings showing the projections of the left ventricular muscle in the three standard imaging views: anterior, left anterior oblique (LAO) and left lateral. The medial portion of the ring of activity is predominantly septal wall on the anterior view and becomes the anterior wall as the patient is rotated into a left lateral projection. The myocardium perpendicular to the line of sight of the camera is seen best because of an end-on effect, with increased depth providing increased radioactivity. Reproduced from Parkey et al.: J Nucl Med 17: 17:771, 1976, by permission.

Technetium-99m-pyrophosphate myocardial scintigrams are obtained in the anterior, 30° to 40° and 70° left anterior oblique and left lateral positions (Figure 5-1). Occasionally, we also obtain a right anterior oblique image in order to evaluate the diaphragmatic aspect of the heart in yet an additional imaging view. These views are obtained with the patient in the supine position. The lateral view is obtained with the patient positioned on the edge of the bed. Thus, the lateral view is obtained with the left side up since there is a shorter distance between the camera face and the left ventricle. Figure 5-2 demonstrates how these views are used to locate an anterior wall myo-cardial infarct.

At our institution, at least 300,000 counts are collected in each imaging view. A larger total count collection improves resolution but this has to be

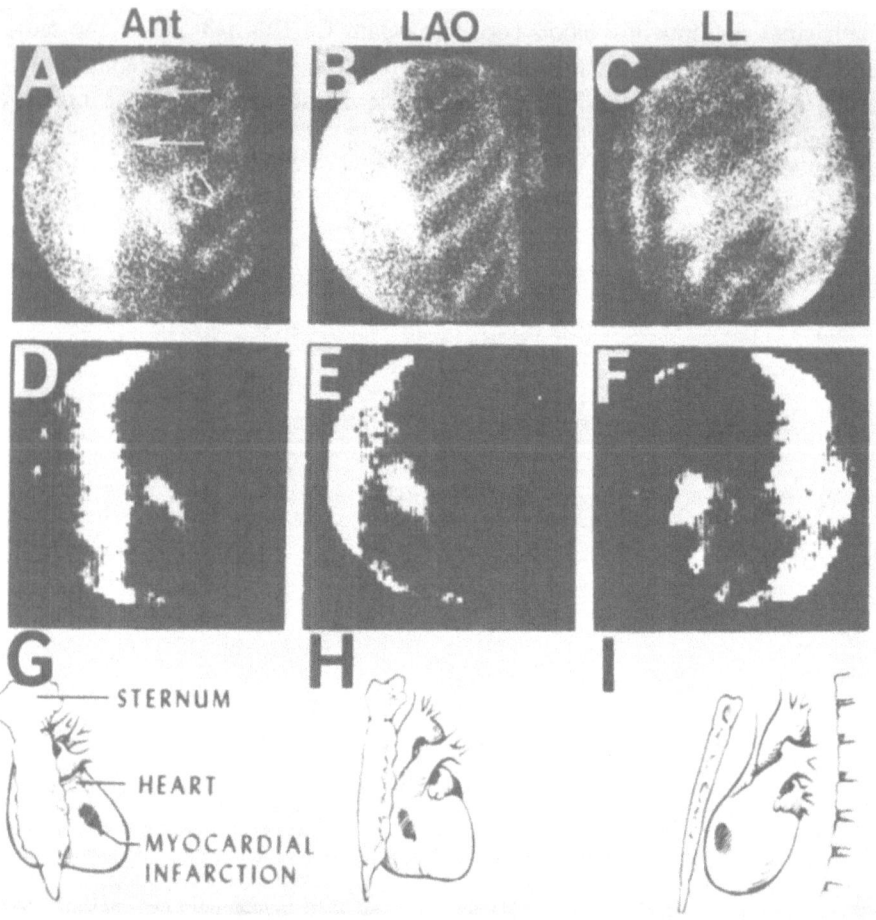

Figure 5-2. An anterior transmural myocardial infarct as detected by ^{99m}Tc-pyrophosphate myo-cardial scintigraphy is shown. The top three panels demonstrate the anterior (panel A), left anterior oblique (panel B), and left lateral (panel C) imaging views. The middle panels (panels D-F) represent the same imaging views but demonstrate the helpfulness of computer processing of the lesions. The bottom three panels (G-I) demonstrate the artist's schematic representation of the site of damage of the heart as it is rotated in the various imaging projections.

balanced against decreased resolution caused by increased patient motion secondary to the increased imaging time. Total counts ranging from 300,000 to 500,000 counts can be used depending upon the type of gamma camera and the patient's ability to cooperate. Centering each view is relatively easy when the sternum is well visualized. Anterior and left anterior oblique views are centered over the myocardium with the sternum imaged to the right side. Lateral views are ordinarily centered between the sternum and the spine. Lateral views are the most common ones that are mispositioned, and this usually is due to positioning either too low (and visualizing a kidney), or too

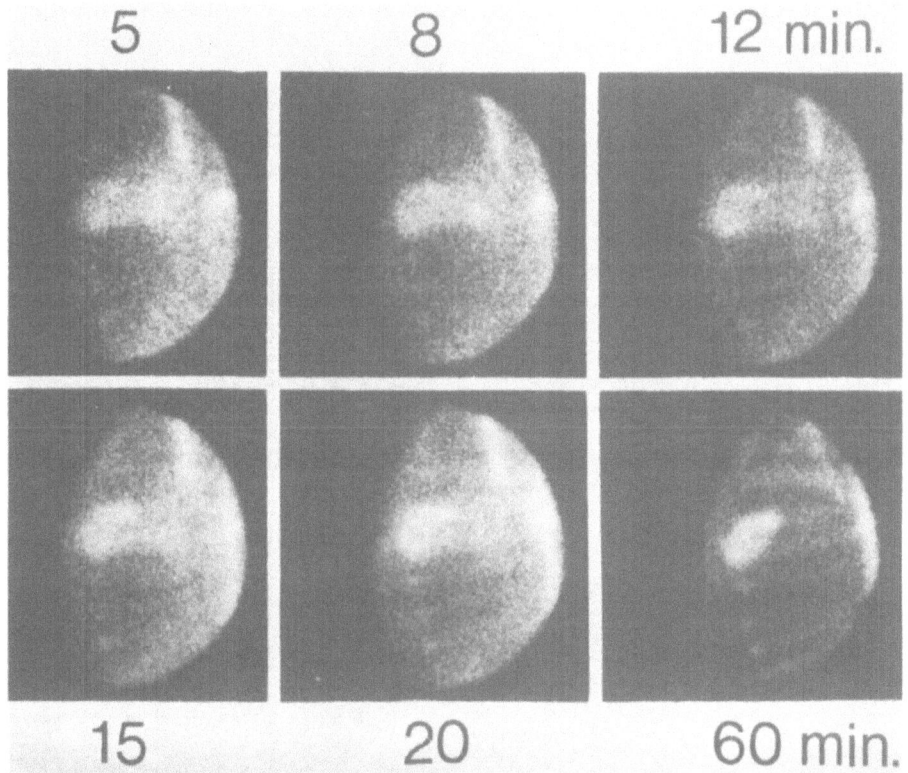

Figure 5-3. Approximately 1 hr is required following the intravenous injection of ^{99m}Tc-pyrophosphate for the cardiovascular blood pool to clear allowing one to determine whether acute myocardial infarction is present. In some patients, as long as 2–3 hr may be required and this is particularly true for those with severe renal insufficiency and those with importantly deranged left ventricular function.

high which may result in missing a myocardial infarct (particularly inferior ones) which otherwise could be visualized. Markers placed on the sternum and lateral chest wall are sometimes helpful. The imaging time post injection of ^{99m}Tc-pyrophosphate is ordinarily 2 to 3 hr after injection. In some patients, delayed clearance of the cardiovascular blood pool occurs because of severe renal insufficiency and/or deranged left ventricular function so that repeat images at 3 to 4 hr after the ^{99m}Tc-pyrophosphate injection may be necessary. Consequently, imaging at 2 to 3 hr after intravenous injection of the radiopharmaceutical is the preferred time. Figure 5-3 demonstrates the effect of radionuclide blood pool in obscuring the presence of a myocardial infarct until approximately 1 hr after the intraveneous injection of the radiopharmaceutical. However, if a persistent radionuclide blood pool occurs and is due to the presence of excessive technetium pertechnetate in the injectate, then one will

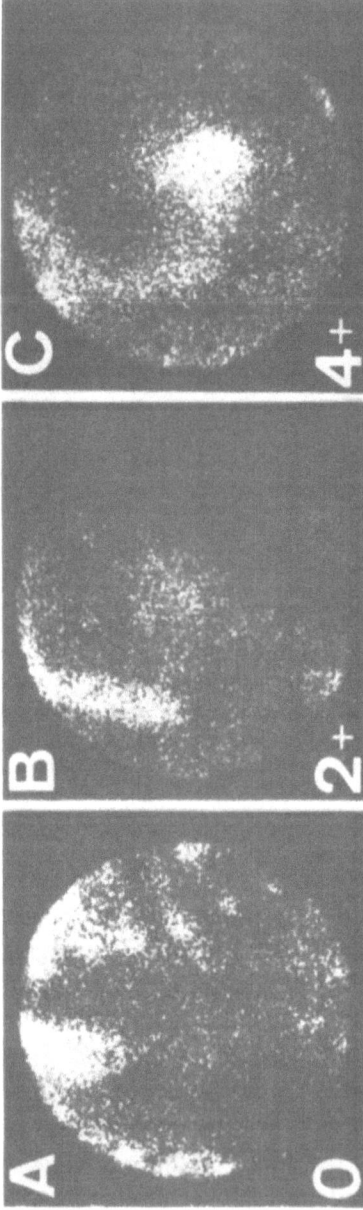

Figure 5-4. The grading scheme that we utilize for the interpretation of ^{99m}Tc-pyrophosphate myocardial scintigrams is shown. We consider ^{99m}Tc-pyrophosphate myocardial scintigrams that are "2–4+" in uptake as abnormal and reflecting the presence of acute myocardial necrosis. Reproduced from Willerson JT et al.: Circulation 51:1046, 1975, by permission.

not be able to obtain reliable images for infarct definition until the next day.

Technetium-99m-pyrophosphate myocardial scintigrams at our institution are presently graded o−4+, depending upon the activity over the myocardium. (Figure 5-4)[7–9]. Grading refers to visibility of the suspected lesion and not the size or configuration of the area. Zero represents no activity, "1+" indicates minimal activity felt to be due to blood pool or chest wall activity but not abnormal myocardium uptake, "2+" definite myocardial uptake that is less intense than immediately adjacent bone, "3+" activity equal to bone activity, and "4+" activity greater than adjacent bone activity. This system is arbitrary but, when used clinically, has shown an excellent correlation with electrocardiographic and enzyme criteria that are used to determine the presence of infarction. It should be emphasized, however, that the amount of ^{99m}Tc-pyrophosphate that localizes in an area of myocardial necrosis is dependent upon blood flow to the damaged area as well as the mass of tissue

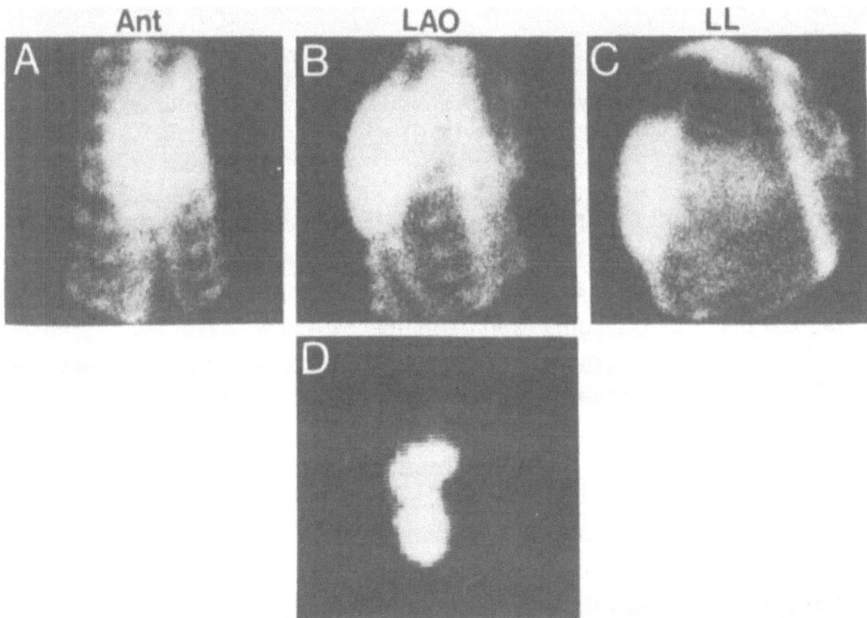

Figure 5-5. Skeletal muscle and myocardial necrosis that occurs in a closed chest animal receiving multiple doses of electrical cardioversion is shown. Panels A through C demonstrate the importance of skeletal muscle damage and increased ^{99m}Tc-pyrophosphate uptake that occurs following cardioversion. This animal received approximately 2000 W-sec as 200 W-sec given ten times over a 30 min period. Panels C through D demonstrate increased myocardial ^{99m}Tc-pyrophosphate uptake which is indicative of the presence of acute myocardial necrosis. Panels A through C demonstrate the anterior, left anterior oblique and left lateral imaging views in the closed chest animal. Panel D demonstrates the ^{99m}Tc-pyrophosphate myocardial images of the isolated heart in this animal.

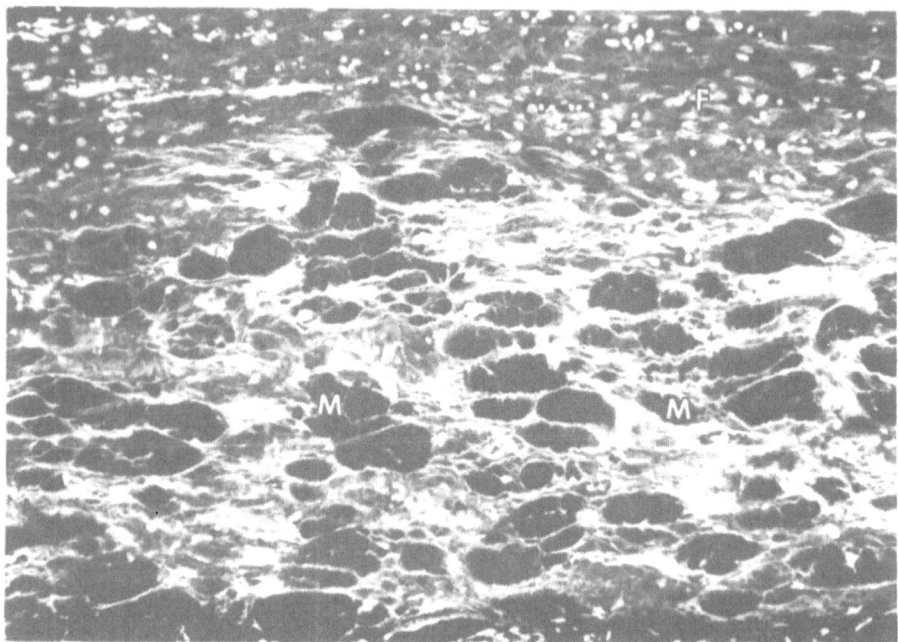

Figure 5-6. The severe myocytolysis (M) and fibrosis (F) present in a dyskinetic segment resected from a patient with unstable angina pectoris are shown.

injured. The majority of patients with acute transmural myocardial infarcts have "3+" or "4+" ^{99m}Tc-pyrophosphate myocardial scintigrams if serial myocardial scintigrams are obtained [8]. However, in patients with acute subendocardial infarcts, only approximately 40-50% have such intensely abnormal ^{99m}Tc-pyrophosphate myocardial scintigrams; the remainder have "2+" and less well localized ^{99m}Tc-pyrophosphate uptake [7, 12].

It should also be emphasized that increased ^{99m}Tc-pyrophosphate uptake occurs in the chest wall if there has been skeletal muscle damage and/or in bone if skeletal damage occurs. Skeletal muscle labels with the phosphates in a manner similar to myocardial muscle. By using at least three different imaging views, skeletal muscle localization of ^{99m}Tc-pyrophosphate can usually be shown to be separate from the myocardium. Chest wall muscle damage from surgery or burns caused by multiple cardioversions (Figure 5-5) can lead to "false positive" scintigrams [13]. Abnormal activity in bones from trauma or tumor is ordinarily relatively easy to separate from true myocardial necrosis.

REFERENCES

1. Kulkarni P: Radiopharmaceuticals in nuclear cardiology. In: Clinical nuclear cardiology, p 65. Parkey RW, Bonte FJ, Buja LM and Willerson JT, eds. New York: Appleton-Century-Crofts, 1979.
2. Willerson JT, Parkey RW, Buja LM, et al.: Detection of acute myocardial infarcts using myocardial scintigraphic techniques. In: Clinical nuclear cardiology, p 141, Parkey RW, Bonte FJ, Buja LM and Willerson JT, eds. New York: Appleton-Century-Crofts, 1979.
3. Bonte FJ, Parkey RW, Graham KD, et al.: A new method for radionuclide imaging of acute myocardial infarction in humans. Radiology 110:473, 1974.
4. Bruno FP, Cobb FR, Rivas F, et al.: Evaluation of ^{99m}technetium stannous pyrophosphate as an an imaging agent in acute myocardial infarction. Circulation 54:71, 1976.
5. Buja LM, Parkey RW, Stokely EM, et al.: Pathophysiology of technetium-99m stannous pyrophosphate and thallium-201 scintigraphy of acute anterior myocardial infarcts in dogs. J Clin Invest 57:1508, 1976.
6. Buja LM, Tofe AJ, Kulkarni PV, et al.: Site and mechanisms of localization of technetium-99m phosphorus radiopharmaceuticals in acute myocardial infarcts and other tissues. J Clin Invest 60:724, 1977.
7. Willerson JT, Parkey RW, Bonte FJ, et al.: Acute subendocardial myocardial infarction in patients; its detection by Tc-99m stannous pyrophosphate myocardial scintigrams. Circulation 51:436, 1975.
8. Willerson JT, Parkey RW, Bonte FJ, et al.: Technetium stannous pyrophosphate myocardial scintigrams in patients with chest pain of varying etiology. Circulation 51: 1046, 1975.
9. Parkey RW, Bonte FJ, Meyer SL, et al.: A new method for radionuclide imaging of acute myocardial infarction in humans. Circulation 50:540, 1974.
10. Willerson JT, Parkey RW, Buja LM, et al.: Are technetium-99m stannous pyrophosphate myocardial scintigrams clinically useful? Clin Nucl Med 2: 137, 1977 (editorial).
11. Stokely EM, Parkey RW, Bonte FJ, et al.: Gated blood pool imaging following technetium-99m phosphate scintigraphy. Radiology 120:433, 1976.
12. Rude RE, Rubin HS, Stone MJ, et al.: Radioimmunoassay of serum creatine kinase B isoenzyme: correlation with technetium-99m stannous pyrophosphate myocardial scintigraphy in the diagnosis of acute myocardial infarction. Am J Med, 68:405, 1980.
13. Pugh BR, Buja LM, Parkey RW, et al.: Cardioversion and its potential role in the production of "false positive" technetium-99m stannous pyrophosphate myocardial scintigrams. Circulation 54:399, 1976.

ACUTE MYOCARDIAL INFARCTION

6. THALLIUM-201 MYOCARDIAL IMAGING IN ACUTE MYOCARDIAL INFARCTION

FRANS J. TH. WACKERS, K.I. LIE, ELLINOR BUSEMANN SOKOLE, HEIN J.J. WELLENS, GERARD SAMSON and JAN B. VAN DER SCHOOT

Thallium-201 scintigraphy has proven to be an early and highly sensitive technique to detect myocardial perfusion abnormalities in patients with acute myocardial infarction [1, 2]. During the early phase of acute myocardial infarction, patients may be hemodynamically and electrically unstable. Therefore, scintigraphy is performed preferably at the bed side in the Coronary Care Unit using a mobile gamma camera. Additionally, in order to shorten imaging time in these often critically ill patients, we recommend injecting no less than 2 mCi of ^{201}Tl. Using this dosage, the imaging time per view will be approximately five minutes. Routinely, three views are taken: the first view is a supine 45° left-anterior-oblique view, followed by a supine anterior view and finally a left-lateral view, the latter with the patient turned on the right side [3].

READING OF THALLIUM-201 SCINTISCANS

All results presented in this and following chapters are based on the interpretation of analogue unprocessed images. In our laboratory we usually read the ^{201}Tl scintiscans as positive, questionable or normal. The judgement concerning diminished or absent regional ^{201}Tl activity is made qualitatively by comparison of ^{201}Tl accumulation in different areas of the left ventricular myocardium.

The scintiscans read as *positive*, show a consistent area of definite diminished ^{201}Tl activity (*perfusion defect*), equal or less than lung activity, on all three views. *Questionable* scans represent either a consistent area with diminished activity but slightly higher than background activity on all three views or a defect on only one view. *Normal* scans show homogeneous uptake of the radiopharmaceutical in the left ventricle on all three views.

Since even among experienced readers considerable interobserver variability may exist [4], all scans are read by at least two observers and the results presented are the consensus of the observers.

SCINTIGRAPHIC IMAGES IN ACUTE MYOCARDIAL INFARCTION

Myocardial infarction is visualized on ^{201}Tl scintiscans as an area with markedly reduced uptake of the radionuclide. The three views routinely obtained usually are sufficient to detect and localize the anatomic extent of

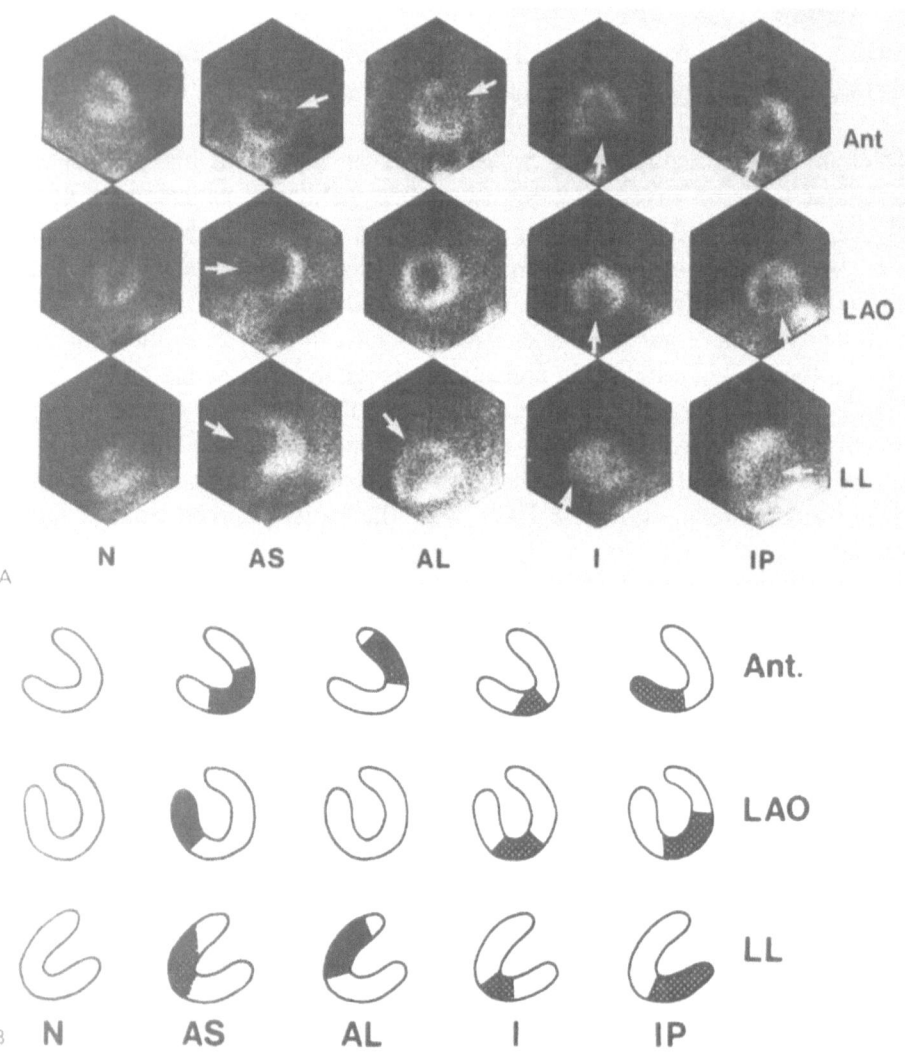

Figure 6-1. (A) Typical examples of acute myocardial infarctions demonstrated with ^{201}Tl myocardial imaging in anterior (Ant), 45° left-anterior-oblique (LAO) and left-lateral (LL) projections. The first column shows a normal (N) ^{201}Tl scan. The second to fourth columns show defects (arrows) caused by acute myocardial infarction involving the anteroseptal (AS), anterolateral (AL), inferior (I) and inferoposterior (IP) walls. (B) Schematic representations of the images. Reproduced with permission from Ref. [2].

the perfusion defects. Typical scintigraphic images can be recognized for infarctions at various anatomic locations [2, 5]. Examples of typical ^{201}Tl scintiscans in patients with acute myocardial infarction are shown in Figure 6-1.

Anterolateral infarction

An anterolateral infarction usually will display perfusion defects on both the anterior and left-lateral views. On the 45° left-anterior-oblique view often no perfusion defect will be seen. This is because in the latter view the anterior wall is parallel to the plane of view and imaged *en face*, which in normal subjects results in a central area of diminished activity outlining the ventricular cavity. When the activity of the overlying anterior wall is lost as the consequence of anterior wall infarction, it often can be appreciated that the "ventricular cavity" is darker, while the doughnut of myocardium is nicely visualized.

Occasionally, a definite defect may be present only on the left-lateral view (Figure 6-2). This may occur in patients with pure anterior myocardial infarction without extension into the lateral free wall. This is explained since the anterior wall is projected mainly on the left-lateral view, whereas the (antero)lateral wall is visualized as the cranical portion of the horseshoe on the anterior view. In contrast to the solitary defects described in chapter 4, p. 89, solitary defects of the anterior wall in the left-lateral view invariably are abnormal.

Anteroseptal infarction

An anteroseptal infarction usually will display perfusion defects on all three views. The defects on the anterior and left-lateral views will be similar to those seen in anterolateral myocardial infarction. The involvement of the septum can be best appreciated on the 45° left-anterior-oblique view, in which the septum is perpendicular to the plane of view and free of overlying structures. Frequently, the anterior view also will display a perfusion defect in the caudal segment of the "horseshoe". However, such a perfusion defect also may reflect diminished uptake in the inferior wall. Again the 45° left-anterior-oblique view will make it possible to determine whether there is septal or inferior wall involvement, or both (Figure 6-3).

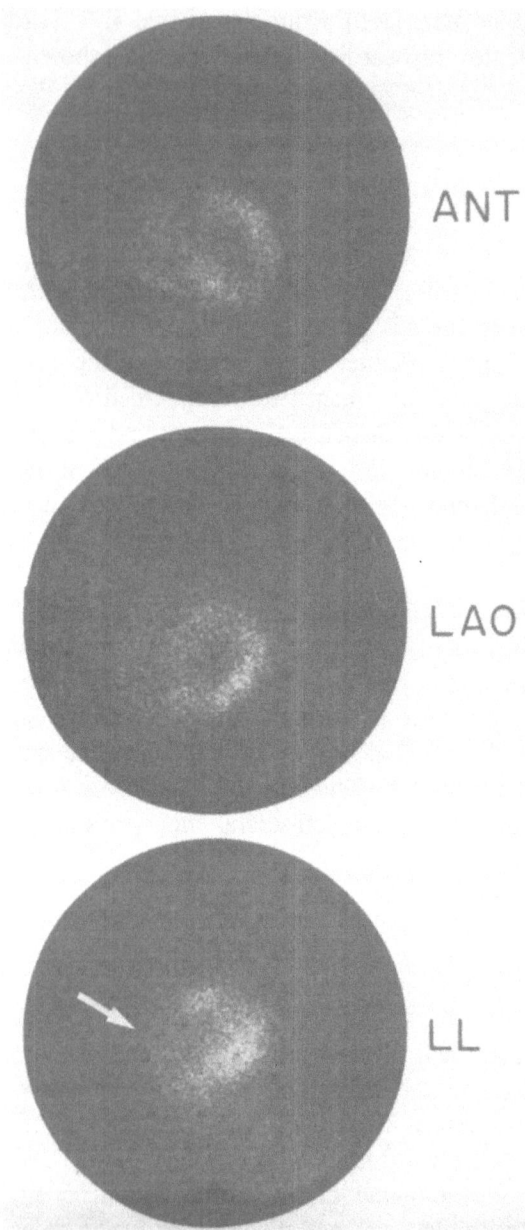

Figure 6-2. Thallium-201 scintiscans in a patient with anterior wall infarction. Although slightly decreased activity is present on the anterior (Ant) and the 45° left-anterior-oblique (LAO) projections at the apex and septum, a definite and diagnostic defect is present only on the left-lateral (LL) view.

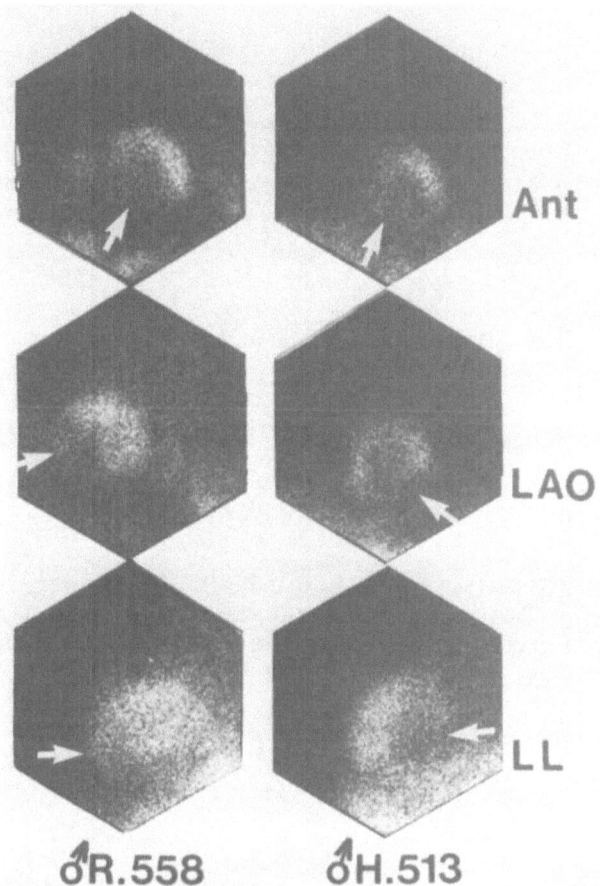

Figure 6-3. Thallium-201 scintiscans of a patient with apicalseptal myocardial infarction (Left) and a patient with inferoposterior myocardial infarction (right). The anterior projection in both patients displays similar images. The left-anterior-oblique views demonstrate the location of the ^{201}Tl perfusion defects to be predominantly septal in one patient (left) and posterior in the other patient (right). Reproduced with permission from Ref. [5].

Inferoposterior infarction

A pure inferior wall infarction will display perfusion defects on all three views. These defects extend from the apex along the inferior wall. Sometimes these defects may be difficult to distinguish from *normal apical defects*. This may be particularly difficult on the 45° left-anterior-oblique view. However, on the anterior and left-lateral views it can be appreciated that the defect is not aligned with the left ventricular long axis as a normal apical defect, but extends along the inferior part of the "horseshoe".

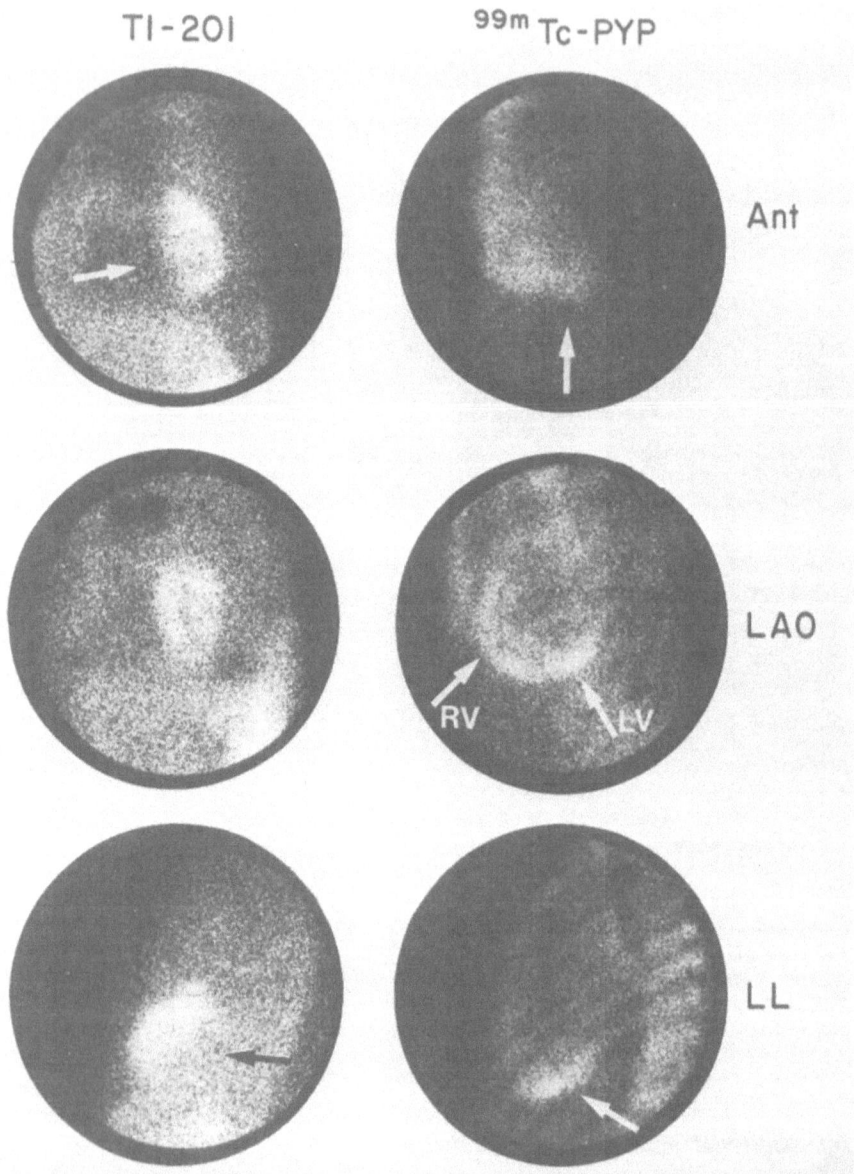

TI-201 ^{99m}Tc-PYP

Ant

LAO

RV   LV

LL

Figure 6-4. Myocardial scintigraphy with ^{201}Tl and ^{99m}Tc-pyrophosphate in a patient with acute inferior wall infarction and right ventricular involvement. At the time of study the patient was hypotensive with disproportionally elevated right ventricular pressure as compared to pulmonary wedge pressure. The ^{201}Tl scintiscans show a moderate size inferoposterior wall perfusion defect. In a patient in cardiogenic shock, it is remarkable that the left ventricle is not dilated and normal in size. The ^{99m}Tc-pyrophosphate study shows definite accumulation in the cardiac region. Although there is accumulation of ^{99m}Tc-pyrophosphate in the inferior wall of the left ventricle, more of the activity is located in the inferolateral wall of the right ventricle. Abbreviations: LV = left ventricle; RV = right ventricle; S = site of interventricular septum.

For the recognition of posterior myocardial infarction a technically correct left-lateral image is of critical importance[3]. The exact extent of infero-posterior wall infarctions can best be appreciated on this left-lateral view. An inferoposterior myocardial infarction displays a typical ^{201}Tl image; on the 45° left-anterior oblique view there is a defect in the left lower quadrant of the doughnut; on the left-lateral view only the anterior wall is visualized display-ing a banana-shaped image and the anterior view will display a perfusion defect in the caudal portion of the horseshoe.

Right ventricular infarction

Since the right ventricle is not visualized by ^{201}Tl under resting conditions, the diagnosis of right ventricular infarction cannot be made directly from the scintiscans. However, right ventricular infarction occurs almost exclusively in patients with inferior wall infarction[6], and in many of these patients the septum is involved which can easily be appreciated on ^{201}Tl scans[7]. Certain-ly right ventricular infarction should be suspected in a patient in cardiogenic shock showing a normal, and not dilated, left ventricle with a rather small inferior wall perfusion defect on the ^{201}Tl scans (Figure 6-4). Combined imaging with ^{99m}Tc-Sn-pyrophosphate[7] or gated blood pool imaging[8] will be extremely helpful for the correct diagnosis (also see chapter 9).

SCINTIGRAPHIC LOCATION OF MYOCARDIAL INFARCTION

Accurate location of acute myocardial infarction has clinical relevance, since the location of infarction has prognostic significance. It is well known that patients with an anterior wall infarction have a poorer prognosis than patients with an inferior wall infarction[9]. Moreover, involvement of the septum in anterior wall infarction often indicates massive infarction and is associated with a three times higher mortality than in infarction at other loca-tions[10].

Since with ^{201}Tl scintigraphy the normally perfused myocardium is well visualized precise anatomic location of the infarction is often possible. The correlation of electrocardiographic location and ^{201}Tl scintigraphic location in 200 patients with acute myocardial infarction is shown in Table 6-1. A good correlation exists for anteroseptal, anterior and inferior location. However 3/4 of the patients with inferior wall infarction on the electrocardiogram, dis-played extension into the posterior wall on the ^{201}Tl scintiscans. On the other hand, 1/6 of the patients with electrocardiographic anteroseptal infarcts (QS complex in the precordial lead V_1) displayed visualization of the septum on

Table 6-1. Correlation between ECG and scintigraphic localization of infarction in 200 patients

		Scintigraphy			
		As	A	I	IP
ECG	AS	59	1		
	A	11	35	2	
	I		1	14	35
	IP			3	39

Abbreviations: AS = anteroseptal; A = anterior; I = inferior; IP = inferoposterior

the ^{201}Tl scintiscans, indicating that at least the posterior portion of the septum probably was still perfused. Other investigators [11-17] reported similar correlation between electrocardiographic and scintigraphic location of infarction. However, it is well known that the electrocardiogram is not a very reliable method to locate myocardial infarction. The correlation with location at post mortem is at best only fair [18]. The correlation of ^{201}Tl scintigraphic location of infarction with actual location at post mortem is shown in Table 6-2. These data are derived from 23 patients who died from complications of transmural infarction a few days of scintigraphy with ^{201}Tl [19]. In 22/ 23 (91%) patients there was an excellent agreement for location between ^{201}Tl images and post mortem findings. Minor disagreement concerned the extent of the infarction. In five patients, who died within two days after injection of ^{201}Tl, transverse slices of the heart were studied by scintigraphy for comparison with *in vivo* images. Figure 6-5 shows an example of one of these patients. The other four cases also showed excellent agreement. However, in one patient there was complete disagreement. The ^{201}Tl scintiscans in this patient showed an extensive inferoposterior perfusion defect (Figure 6-7)

Table 6-2. Localization of infarction in 23 patients [19]

		Scintigraphy				ECG			
		AS	A	I	IP	AS	A	I	IP
Postmortem	AS	11			1	7	2		
	A		2			1	1		
	I				1				1
	IP				8		2	6	
ECG *	AS	7	1						
	A	1	1		1				
	I				1				
	IP				8				

* In three patients ECG localization was not possible. Abbreviations: A = anterior; AS = anteroseptal; I = inferior; IP = inferoposterior

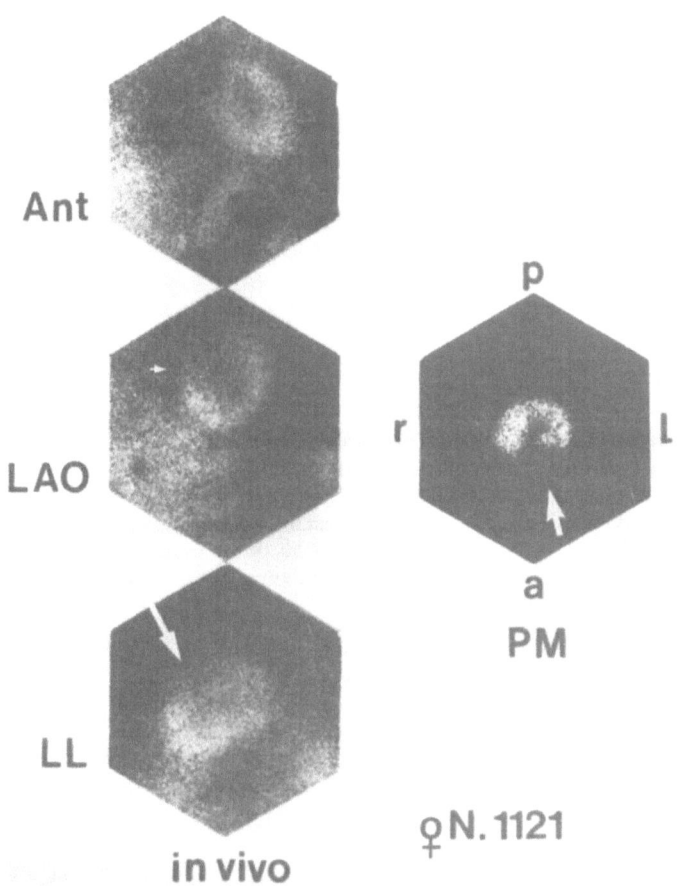

Figure 6-5. Thallium-201 scintiscans obtained *in vivo* and at post mortem of a transverse slice (patient # 15). *In vivo* diminished activity is noted at the anterior wall and probably the high septum (arrows). The image at post mortem shows close agreement in distribution of ^{201}Tl: an evident region of absent activity is present at the anterior wall. Abbreviations: Ant = anterior; LAO = 45° left-anterior-oblique; LL = left-lateral; a = anterior; p = posterior; r = right; l = left; PM = post mortem. Reproduced with permission from Ref. [19].

which, at autopsy, was found to represent the initial acute infarction. A fresh extension of infarction involving one-third of the septum occurred after scintigraphy (Figure 6-8).

In contrast to the excellent correlation with ^{201}Tl scintigraphy, the correlation with electrocardiographic location of infarction was not as good in these patients. In three of 23 patients electrocardiographic location was not possible. In two patients, the electrocardiogram showed nondiagnostic ST segment changes and in the third complete left bundle branch block was present. In only 14 of 20 patients (70%) was there complete agreement between electrocardiographic location of infarction and post mortem findings.

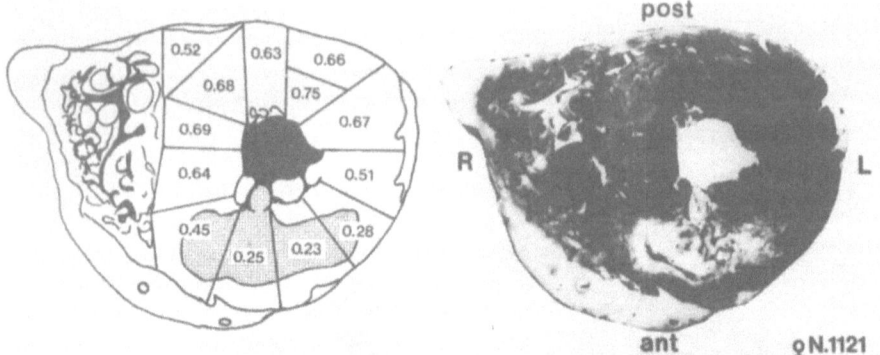

Figure 6-6. Thallium-201 distribution (left) in the same slice as in Figure 6-5 and the adjacent transverse slice stained with Nitrobluetetrazolium (right). The normal myocardium is stained darkly: the anterior infarction remained unstained. The shaded area in the diagram indicates an approximation of the extent of the infarction. Thallium-201 distribution is expressed as fraction of administered activity per gram tissue $\times 10^5$. The relative higher ^{201}Tl concentration (0.45) in the septal area is due to the presence of a relatively large amount of normal myocardium next to infarcted myocardium. Significant difference ($P < 0.05$) exists between mean values of ^{201}Tl distribution in normal and infarcted myocardium. Abbreviation: ant = anterior; post = posterior; r = right; L = left. Reproduced with permission from Ref. [19].

Thallium-201 myocardial distribution at post mortem

Thallium-201 myocardial tissue distribution was studied in 10 patients who died within five days after injection of ^{201}Tl. The specific radioactivity of ^{201}Tl was measured in a transverse slice of the heart containing the infarct. The myocardium was cut into small pieces of approximately 1 g, and specific radioactivity was determined in a well counter and expressed as a fraction of administered ^{201}Tl. Figure 6-6 illustrates the distribution of ^{201}Tl in the same transverse slice as in Figure 6-5. A significant difference ($P < 0.05$) existed between mean values of normal and infarcted myocardium. Table 6-3 gives the ^{201}Tl distribution in the myocardium of 10 patients. The data are expressed as fractions of administered radioactivity per gram tissue $\times 10^5$ (average values) at time of death. In all patients (except patient 10 who had a large circumferential infarction) there was significant difference ($P < 0.05$) between ^{201}Tl activity in normal and in infarcted myocardium. The ratios of mean values for normal and infarcted myocardium ranged from 1.5 to 6.6:1.

Figure 6-9 shows a Nitrobluetetrazoleum (NBT) stained slice [20] of the heart of patient 19 and the scintigraphic image of the adjacent slice. Macroscopically a definite transitional zone could be identified both in the septum and the lateral wall as a zone of partly stained myocardium. Microscopically this region revealed patchy necrosis intermingled with normal myocardial fibers. Measurements of ^{201}Tl distribution revealed a definite transitional zone (val-

Table 6-3. Distribution * of ^{201}Tl in myocardium at post mortem [19] ($n = 10$)

	#5†	#19	14#	#23	#10	#16	#22	#15	#18	#20
Death after inj. Tl-201	1½ hr	1¼ hr	3 hr	3½ hr	8½ hr	14 hr	2 days	2 days	4 days	5 days
Normal myocardium	8.05	12.07	15.6	(1.0)	7.7	6.1	3.1	0.64	0.43	0.66
Infarction	5.5	1.82	9.9	(0.63)	6.8	3.2	1.8	0.30	0.25	0.43
Normal: infarction ratio	1.5	6.6	1.6	1.6	1.1*	1.9	1.7	2.1	1.7	1.5

* Data in fraction of administered activity per gram tissue $\times 10^5$ (average values) at the time of death
† Patient numbers
** Large circumferential infarction
( ) Only relative measurements

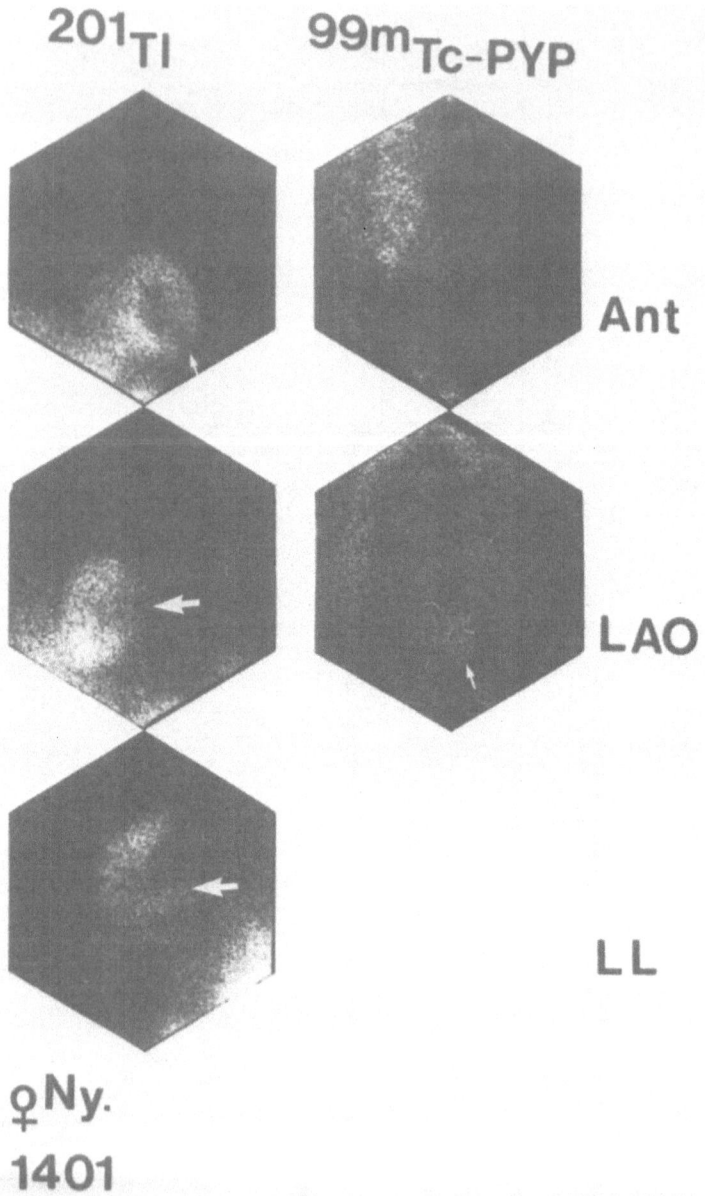

Figure 6-7. Thallium-201 scintiscans obtained *in vivo* in patient #20 with acute inferior wall infarction. A definite perfusion defect can be noted at the inferoposterior and lateral wall. Several days after scintigraphy the patient's condition deteriorated, probably due to infarct extension. The patient subsequently died.

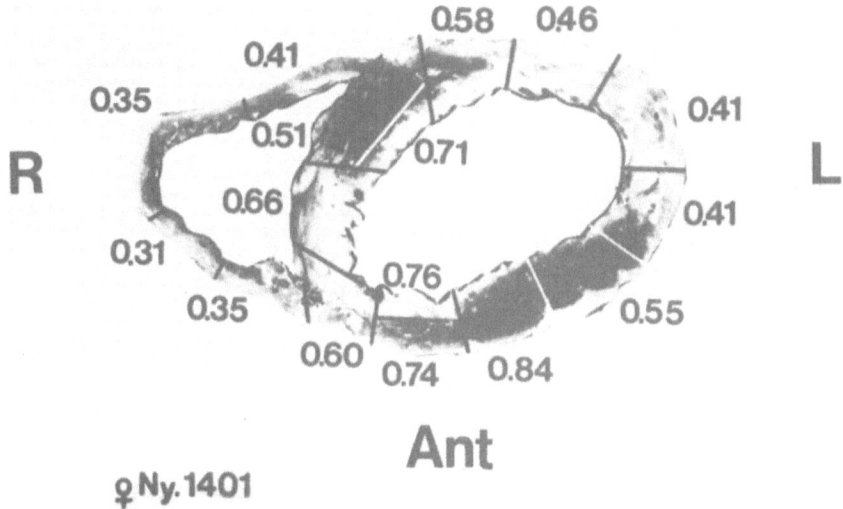

Figure 6-8. Thallium-201 distribution in a transverse slice of the heart of the patient shown in Figure 6–7. The slice is stained with Nitrobluetetrazolium. In addition to the inferolateral infarction (unstained), which is in agreement with the scintigraphic perfusion defect *in vivo*, an anteroseptal infarct is present. Significant difference $(P<0.05)$ exists between mean values of ^{201}Tl distribution in the two sites of infarction. While the concentration of ^{201}Tl in the inferolateral infarction is significantly $(P<0.05)$ lower the normal (darkly stained) myocardium, such a difference is not present between the anteroseptal infarction and the normal myocardium. This finding is consistent with the clinical impression that extension of infarction occurred after scintigraphy. Data are expressed as fraction of administered activity per gram tissue $\times 10^5$. Abbreviations: Ant = anterior; R = right; L = left. Reproduced with permission from Ref. [19].

ues 3.26-7.75) between normal and macroscopically infarcted myocardium. The differences in mean values for ^{201}Tl activity in three zones were statistically significant $(P<0.05)$. One could explain this finding by assuming that severely ischemic myocardium at the time of scintigraphy progressed into infarction. In view of the short time interval ($1\frac{3}{4}$ hr) between scintigraphy and death in this patient, the possibility exists that no sharp demarcation in ^{201}Tl uptake at the border of an infarction occurs. In experimental infarction in dogs, Buja et al. [21] observed a similar ^{201}Tl accumulation in the outer periphery of acute myocardial infarct. Since ^{201}Tl concentrates in the myocardium primarily according to regional perfusion [22, 23], it was surprising that ^{201}Tl activity was measurable also in the *center* of necrotic tissue. At autopsy, the ratios of activity per gram tissue in normal myocardium versus infarcted myocardium varied (Table 6-3). Due to the time interval between scintigraphy and death, it is conceivable that the relatively low ratios may not reflect the actual ratios at the time of scintigraphy. Thallium-201 may have entered the necrotic tissue by passive diffusion or by subsequently developed collateral flow [41, 42]. In this study, autopsy was never performed earlier than 10 hr

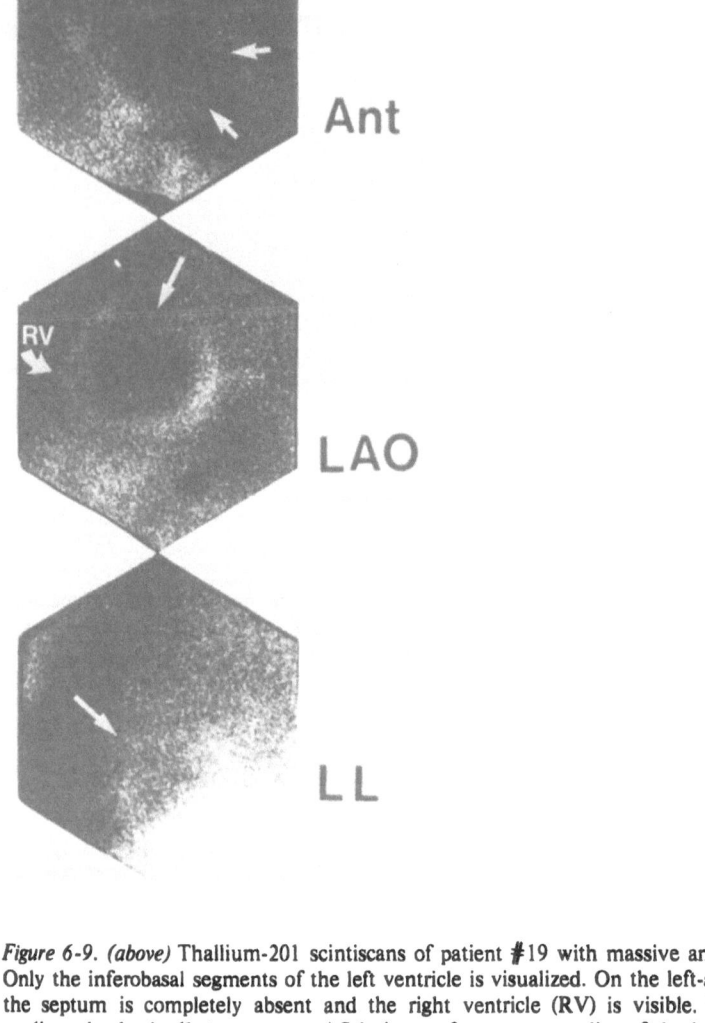

Figure 6-9. (above) Thallium-201 scintiscans of patient #19 with massive anteroseptal infarction. Only the inferobasal segments of the left ventricle is visualized. On the left-anterior-oblique view the septum is completely absent and the right ventricle (RV) is visible. The patient died in cardiogenic shock. *(facing page: top)* Scintiscan of a transverse slice of the heart *at postmortem* of patient #19. A large anteroseptal area with almost absent ²⁰¹Tl activity can be noted. *(facing page: bottom)* Nitrobluetetrazolium stained transverse slice of the heart of patient #19. Close agreement exists between ²⁰¹Tl distribution on the scintigraphic studies and the pattern of staining of the myocardium. Measurements of ²⁰¹Tl distribution (expressed as fraction of administered activity per gram tissue $\times 10^5$) revealed three zones (values 1.08–2.73; 3.26–6.75; and 10.90–12.96). Significant differences ($P < 0.05$) exist between the mean value of each of the three zones. The intermediate zone revealed microscopically patchy necrosis intermingled with normal myocardial fibers. Reproduced with permission from Ref. [19].

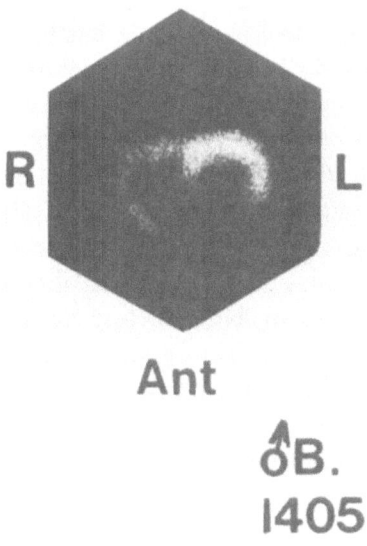

R L

Ant

♂B.
1405

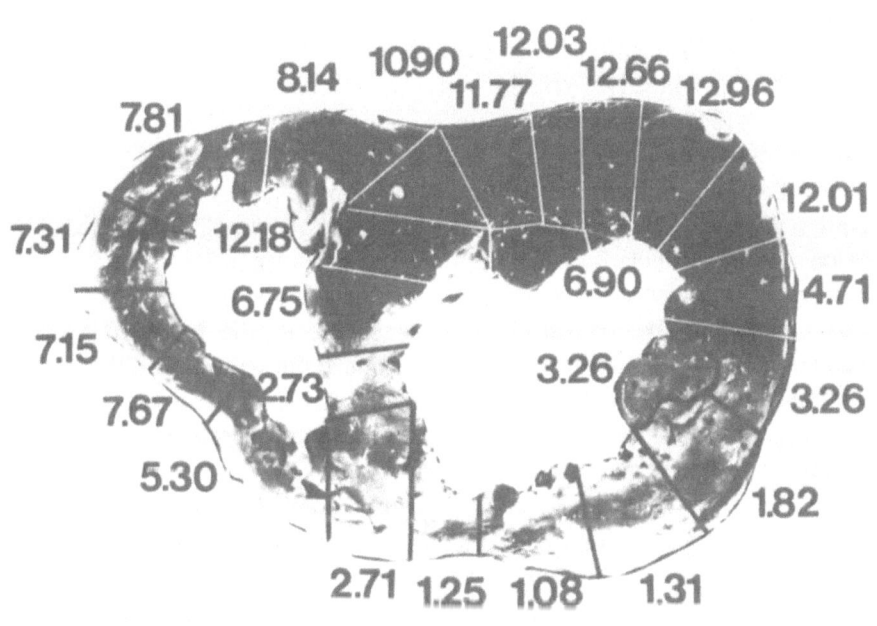

♂B.1405

after death. Figure 6-8 shows a Nitrobluetetrazoleum-stained slice of the heart of patient 20. When scintigraphy was performed five days before death, an inferoposterior defect was observed. On the third day after acute myocardial infarction, the patient's condition deteriorated, probably due to an extension of the infarction, as indicated by a new rise of enzyme levels. The electrocardiogram was not conclusive. At post mortem (6 days after acute infarction) the NBT stained slice demonstrated a posterolateral infarction with subendocardial extension into the anteroseptal region. A significant difference ($P < 0.05$) existed not only between the mean values of ^{201}Tl concentration in the posterolateral infarction and normal myocardium, but also between the posterolateral infarction and the anteroseptal infarction. No significant differences in mean values of ^{201}Tl concentration are found between the anteroseptal infarction and the normal myocardium. In view of the ^{201}Tl distribution it is conceivable that the septal infarction represents the secondary extension *after* scintigraphy was performed.

SIZE OF MYOCARDIAL INFARCTION

Since the earliest application of radionuclide techniques in patients with acute myocardial infarction, the potential value of these techniques to assess quantitatively and noninvasively the extent of myocardial damage has been of prime concern. The immediate prognosis of a patient with acute myocardial infarction is directly related to the total amount of damaged myocardium [24].

Experimental data suggest that the greatest opportunity to salvage ischemic myocardium occurs within the first 6 hr after infarction [25]. Thallium-201 scintigraphy provides a simple noninvasive way to visualize myocardial perfusion and is particularly sensitive during the early hours of infarction.

Since ^{201}Tl myocardial scintigraphy visualizes the normal myocardium, ^{201}Tl defects can be expressed as a percentage of the total left ventricle. Moreover, since ^{201}Tl scintiscans demonstrate both acute and old infarction, the total amount of lost myocardial mass can be determined. Thus ^{201}Tl imaging seems particularly suited for the assessment of infarct size. However, the following points have to be taken into consideration:

(1) Clearly, to determine the size of an infarction from two-dimensional projections without sophisticated three-dimensional reconstruction techniques, seems incorrect and doomed to failure. Moreover, the heart cannot be imaged from all angles due to technical difficulties such as patient positioning and photon absorption.

(2) The static ^{201}Tl images represent the integrated radioactivity distribution of a moving organ over a period of time. Electrocardiogram-gated ^{201}Tl

studies [26] have demonstrated that "blurring" of image caused by heart motion is especially present on the left-anterior-oblique images.

(3) In the acute phase of myocardial infarction ischemic myocardium is visualized in addition to the necrotic myocardium. However, if it may be possible to differentiate between the two by delayed imaging, then this lack of specificity may turn into an advantage allowing identification of ischemic and potentially viable myocardium [38, 39].

(4) As will be discussed later, changes of the size of scintigraphic perfusion defects may occur spontaneously during the first 24 hr after acute myocardial infarction [2]. After 24 hr, these changes occur less frequently and are of lesser magnitude. Thus, myocardial imaging early after infarction may tend to overestimate the extent of infarction.

(5) The determination of the outlines of scintigraphic abnormal areas is necessarily a subjective interpretation. Usually, there is no sharp demarcation between abnormal and normal myocardium. Additionally, areas of absent ^{201}Tl activity and areas with only slightly diminished ^{201}Tl activity, most probably reflect various degrees of impaired myocardial perfusion. A computerized method using circumferential profiles as proposed by Burow et al. [27] may be a better way to determine the extent of perfusion abnormalities.

(6) The "gold standard" for the actual size of infarction is the total extent of infarction and/or scar tissue, measured at post mortem. However, the assessment of infact size on post mortem specimens is also frought with uncertainties and potential sources of error. Macroscopic recognition of infarction from post mortem specimen requires a time interval of approximately 24 hr between onset of acute myocardial infarction and death. However, the use of Nitrobluetetrazoleum staining for dehydrogenase allows recognition as early as 8 hr post infarction [20]. Nonetheless, the deliniation of the extent of infarcted regions, with or without Nitrobluetetrazoleum staining or microscopic verification, from the post mortem specimen may still be only an approximation since the outerzones of an infarct may be irregular or poorly defined.

In spite of the above mentioned considerations, we found a reasonable correlation between size of infarction, as estimated from ^{201}Tl scintiscans and findings at post mortem [19].

Size of scintigraphic defect

We applied a simple planimetric method to determine the size of the perfusion defects on the ^{201}Tl scans (Figure 6-10). Schematic drawings of the scintigraphic images on three views were made. The areas with definite diminished ^{201}Tl activity, as compared to adjacent regions were outlined. It

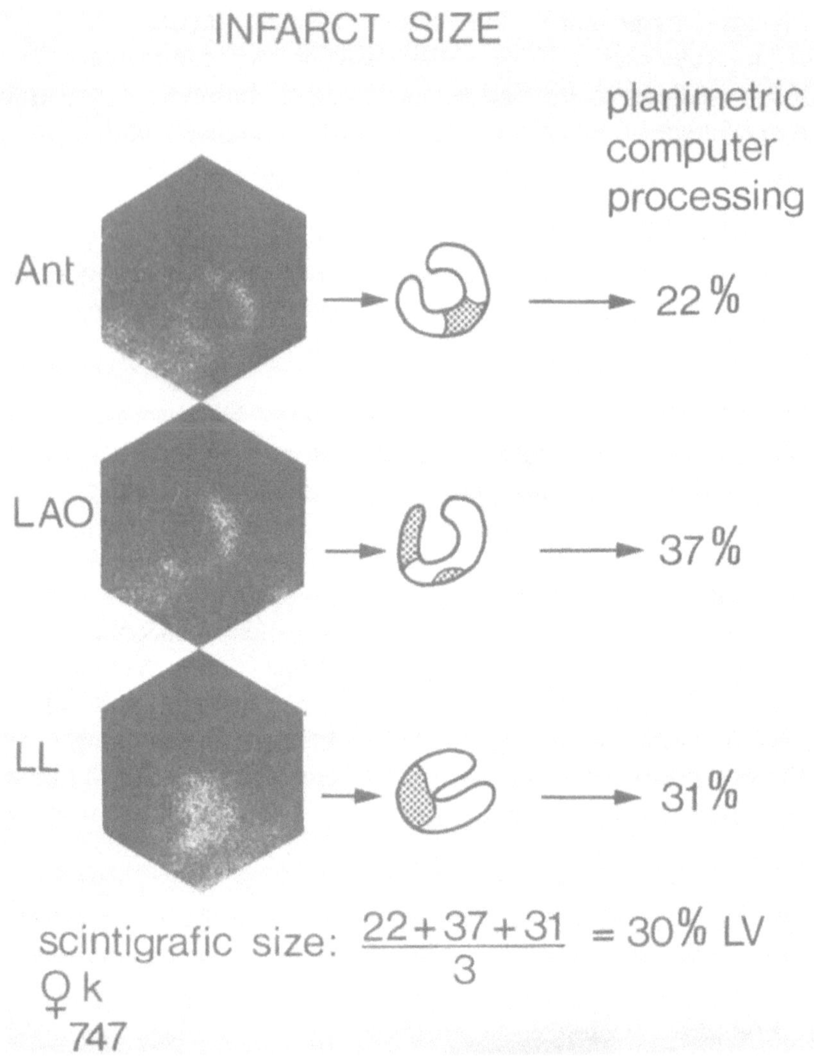

Figure 6-10. Thallium-201 scintiscans in a patient with anteroseptal infarction. Planimetric method to estimate the scintigraphic size of perfusion defects. For each view a schematic drawing of the total left ventricle and the perfusion defect is made and planimetered. The size of the defect is assessed for each view as a percentage of total left ventricle on that projection. The total size of the scintigraphically abnormal area is expressed as the arithmetic means of the percentages on three views. In the example shown, the scintigraphic size of infarction was estimated to involve 30% of the left ventricle.

was possible to do this, since in all patients the configuration of the entire left ventricle could be recognized on the unprocessed analogue images. The size of the malperfused area was determined by planimetry using a Quantimet 720D TV scanner and a Cyber 73 CDC computer. The total size of the scintigraphically abnormal area was expressed as the arithmetic mean of the percentage of scintigraphically abnormal area of the left ventricle in three views.

Size of infarction at post mortem

At autopsy, the extent of infarction was established after cutting the heart transversely into 1 cm thick slices. These slices were stained with Nitroblue-tetrazoleum dehydrogenase staining for macroscopic demonstration of the infarcted myocardium in the slices. When considered necessary, macroscopic inspection was supplemented by microscopic study. The extent of the infarction in the transverse slices was determined by three investigators without

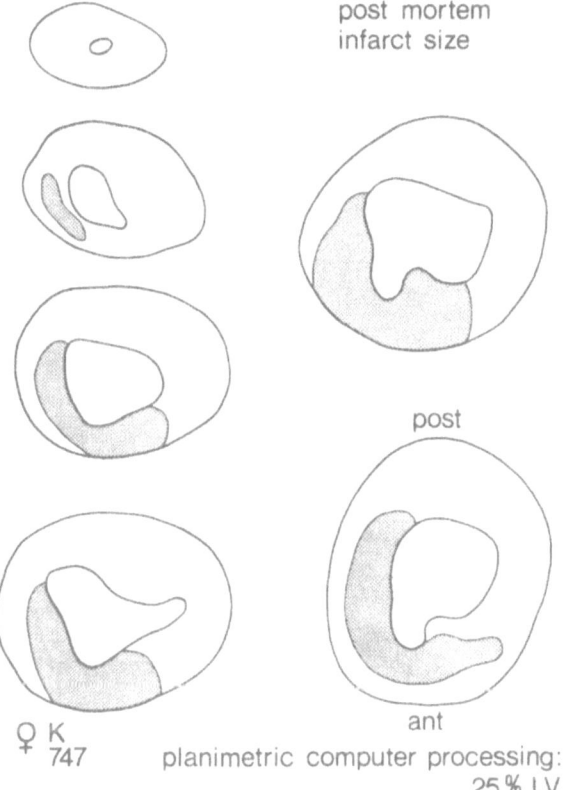

post mortem
infarct size

post

ant

♀ K
♂ 747

planimetric computer processing:
25 % LV

Figure 6-11. Schematic drawings of transverse slices of the heart of the patient in Figure 6-10. The slices were stained with Nitrobluetetrazolium for better delineation of the infarct. The infarction (shaded area) and the total left ventricle are planimetered. The postmortem size of infarction is expressed as percentage of total left ventricle. In the example shown, the size of infarction *at postmortem* was 25%, compared to 30% on the basis of ^{201}Tl scintigraphic data.

knowledge of the scintigraphic results. Schematic drawings were made of the infarction, including scar tissue of old infarction, when present. These drawings were again processed by planimetry using a Quantimet 720D TV scanner and a Cyber 73 CDC computer. The infarcted area was expressed as a percentage of the total left ventricular mass (Figure 6-11). In two patients post mortem assessment of the size of infarction was not possible. The latter two patients showed macroscopically extensive infarction, but patchy necrosis was equally intermingled with normal myocardial fibers. Therefore, definite delineation of the extent of infarction was not readily possible.

Correlation of thallium-201 scintiscans with post mortem findings

The correlation between the size of scintigraphic perfusion defects and size of infarction at post mortem in 19 patients is shown in Table 6-4 and Figure 6-12. The linear correlation coefficient for the whole group ($n = 19$) was 0.72. For the different infarct locations, the correlation coefficients were 0.91 for six

Table 6-4. Size of infarction estimated from ^{201}Tl scintiscans (CSC%) and determined at postmortem [19] – (PM%)

Pt	CSC%	PM%	Time of SC after AMI
1	36	29	10 days
2	33	29	2½ days
3	28	18	5½ hr
4	33	?	6 hr
5	45	26	5 hr
6	33	33	1½ hr
7	29	28	6 hr
8	40	35	5 hr
9	49	?	10 hr
10	46	60	17 hr
11	28	27	13 hr
12	30	25	9 hr
13	29	18	2 days
14	29	21	7½ hr
15	13	15	2 days
16	51	49	5 hr
17	44	61	3½ hr
18	59	55	1½ day
19	56	30	8¼ hr
20	41	28 *	28 hr
21	28	22	3 days

* Only inferoposterolateral infarction measured. Abbreviations: CSC% = computer calculated size of scintigraphic abnormal area as percentage of left ventricle; PM% = computer calculated size of infarction on basis of postmortem slices of the heart; SC = scintigraphy; AMI = acute myocardial infarction; ? = delineation of infarction not possible

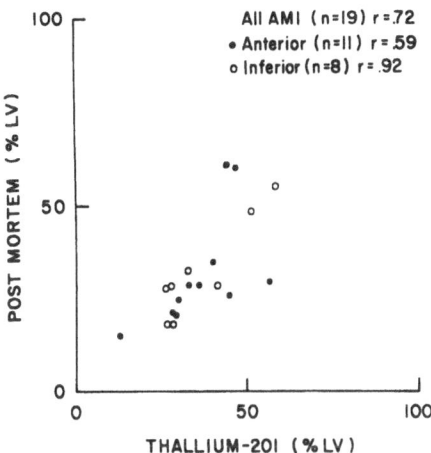

Figure 6-12. Relationship between size of infarction determined on the basis of postmortem findings and the size of scintigraphic abnormalities, assessed as demonstrated in Figures 6–10 and 6–11. n = 19; $y = (0.88 \pm 0.21)\, x - (0.36 \pm 7.89)$.

patients with anterior wall infarct, 0.97 for six patients with inferior infarct and 0.86 for seven patients with antero-posterior-infarct.

Since 16 of 19 patients in this study died within 5 days after onset of acute myocardial infarction and the scintigraphic study, it seems likely that the extent of infarction at the time of autopsy did not differ significantly from that present at the time of scintigraphy.

In this study the correlation was not influenced by the time of scintigraphy after infarction or the time interval between scintigraphy and death. This seems in contradiction of our earlier observations that especially during the first hours after acute myocardial infarction ^{201}Tl scintiscans may overestimate the actual size of infarction by visualizing surrounding ischemia[2]. These observations of decreasing size of defects were most impressive in small infarctions. The 19 patients in whom we correlated infarct size at post mortem with *in vivo* [201]Tl scintiscans, all had moderate to large transmural infarctions and all patients died from complications of their infarctions. Therefore, the results of this correlative study might not necessarily apply to the general population of patients with acute myocardial infarction.

However, recently Niess et al. [28] reported a significant quantitative relationship between the size of ^{201}Tl defects and angiographic percent abnormally contracting segments of the left ventricle in patients who sustained myocardial infarction. In this study myocardial infarction had occurred 6 days – 69 months (mean 7 ± 2 months) previously. Using a computerized planimetry system, the size of the ^{201}Tl defects was expressed as a percentage of total potential ^{201}Tl uptake. Scintigraphic defects were present in only four of 10 patients (40%) with less than 6% abnormal wall motion, but defects were

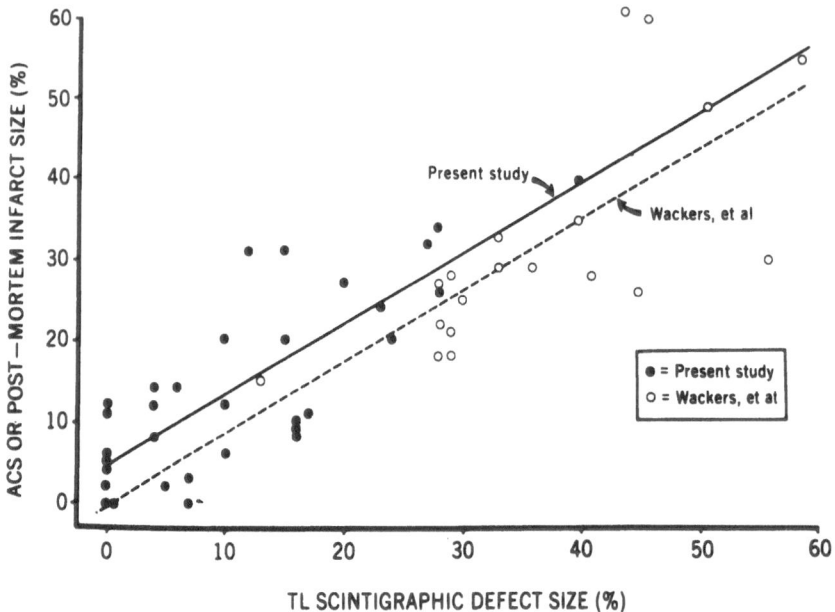

Figure 6-13. Comparison of size of ²⁰¹Tl defect with angiographic (present study: Neiss et al.) [28] and postmortem (Wackers et al.) [19] infarct size. A statistical comparison of the regression line from Wackers' data $(y = (0.88 \pm 0.21) \; x - (0.36 \pm 7.89))$ and the line from Niess' data $(y = (0.86 \pm 0.12) \; x + (4.41 \pm 1.81))$ shows no significant difference between slopes and intercepts. The linear correlation coefficient between percent abnormally contracting segment (%ACS) and ²⁰¹Tl scintigraphic size of defect was 0.80. Reproduced with permission from Ref. [28].

present in 20 of 22 patients (91%) with more than 6% abnormally contracting segments ($P<0.01$). The size of ²⁰¹Tl deflects correlated only marginally with angiographic left ventricular ejection fraction ($r = -0.60$), but correlated closely (Figure 6-13) with angiographic percent abnormally contracting segments ($r = 0.80$). The size of the ²⁰¹Tl defects was similar among patients with one, two or three vessel coronary artery disease ($>70\%$ stenosis), but ²⁰¹Tl defect size was larger in patients with electrocardiographic transmural infarction ($P<0.01$) or pulmonary wedge pressure >12 mmHg ($P<0.001$). Henning et al. [11] reported a reasonable semiquantitative relationship between mean CK curve area and ²⁰¹Tl scintigraphic defects.

The clinical implication of these data is that the extent of ²⁰¹Tl perfusion defects in patients with acute myocardial infarction probably reflects accurately the extent of necrotic and/or jeopardized myocardium.

Recently Burrow et al. [27] described a relatively simple computer-aided circumferential profile technique to quantitate ²⁰¹Tl perfusion defects (Figure 6-14). Bulkley et al. [29] used this method for the assessment of the size of infarction. They did not find a good correlation between the computer score for size of defects and the actual size of infarction at post mortem. However, the clinical course in these patients suggested that in addition to necrosis

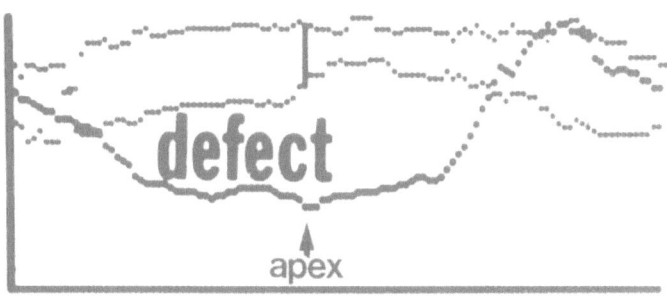

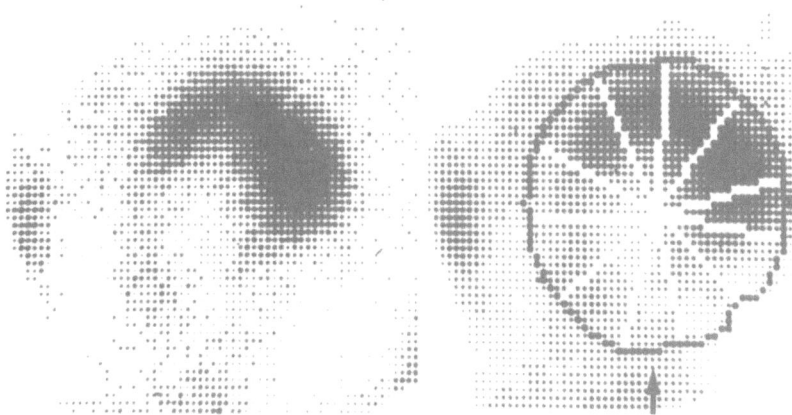

Figure 6-14. Circumferential profile method of quantitating ^{201}Tl scintigraphic defects. On the lower right is an example of a ^{201}Tl image with superimposed computer-constructed outlines and radii. Above is a ^{201}Tl activity curve as a function of radii. The ordinate is activity normalized to the highest radial value. The two lines joined by the white bar represent the standard activity band (derived from 13 volunteers, representing the mean ± 2 SD for each radius).

The lower curve shows the activity from the ^{201}Tl scan in this figure. The defect score is obtained by integrating the area of discordance between the ^{201}Tl scan curve and the standard activity band (percent abnormal radii × average amount below normal for these radii. Reproduced with permission from Ref. [29].

important areas with severe ischemia were visualized Silverman et al. [30] correlated in 42 hemodynamically stable patients with acute myocardial infarctions the subsequent clinical course to the computer score of ^{201}Tl defects using circumferential profiles. Two clinical subgroups could be identified on the basis of the size of defects. Thallium-201 defects involving at least 40% of the left ventricular circumference was noted in 13 patients. In these patients, the mortality in-hospital was 46%, at 6 months 63% and at last follow-up (mean 9 months) 92%. In contrast, in the remaining 29 patients with smaller defects the corresponding values for mortality were 3%, 7% and 7% respectively, ($P < 0.001$ for all). In this study a large ^{201}Tl defect had a higher predictive value for poor prognosis than prior myocardial infarction, anterior location of infarction or peak $CK > 1000$ IU/L. These results suggest that ^{201}Tl scintigraphy may provide an accurate and relatively simple non-invasive method for separating high risk and low risk subgroups of hemodynamically stable patients with acute myocardial infarction in the early hours after the onset of chest pain. Botvinick et al. [31] reported similar preliminary results in 65 patients with acute myocardial infarction.

It is conceivable that the application of multiplanar emission tomography using a multiple pinhole collimator, as recently described by Vogel et al. [32], may improve the results of quantitation of ^{201}Tl by perfusion defects in patients with myocardial infarction. However, recently the usefulness of this method for assessment of the size of perfusion defects has been questioned [33]. The lack of resolution in depth may be an important limitation. Holman et al. [34] reported the feasibility of single photon transaxial emission computed tomography using ^{201}Tl. Yet single photon emission tomography also is, to some extent, limited by varying resolution in depth and radiation attenuation by interposed tissues, which introduces image distortion and may make quantitative assessment more complicated. Another promising approach to overcome these technical problems is the use of positron emitting radionuclides. Excellent results have already been reported [35]. Moreover, since positrons can be incorporated in true substrates of myocardial metabolism positron emission transaxial tomography has the exciting potential to delineate in a quantitative way ischemic but viable myocardium form infarcted tissue [36].

SENSITIVITY TO DETECT ACUTE MYOCARDIAL INFARCTION

Thallium-201 scintigraphy is an extremely sensitive and reliable method to detect acute myocardial infarction, when imaging is performed with understanding of the temporal sequence and accuracy of the technique.

We assessed the value and limitations of ^{201}Tl scintigraphy for the diagnosis of acute myocardial infarction in two different patient populations:
a) patients with electrocardiographically and biochemically proven acute myocardial infarction [2];
b) patients referred to the Coronary Care Unit to rule out myocardial infarction [45].

PATIENTS WITH PROVEN ACUTE MYOCARDIAL INFARCTION

The sensitivity of ^{201}Tl scintigraphy to detect acute myocardial infarction was determined in 200 consecutive patients with proven myocardial infarction [2].

In all patients acute myocardial infarction was documented by diagnostic electrocardiographic changes and typical rise and fall of serum enzymes. The electrocardiographic location of infarction was anteroseptal in 60 patients, anterior in 46 patients, inferior in 50 patients and posterior in 42 patients, and uncertain in two patients. The myocardial infarction was transmural in 153 patients and nontransmural in 47 patients. There were 139 patients with biochemically large infarction (maximal rise of SGOT > 3.5 times upper limit of normal) and 61 patients with biochemically small infarctions. Twenty-nine patients had recurrent infarction.

For the purpose of blinded reading, the ^{201}Tl scans of the 200 patients with infarction were mixed with 100 ^{201}Tl scans obtained during the same time period. The scans were read by three observers without knowledge of the clinical data. The results reported here represent a consensus.

Overall, positive ^{201}Tl scans were obtained in 165 of 200 patients (82%). Of the patients with biochemically large infarction 131 (94%) had positive scans; of the patients with biochemically small infarction this occurred in 35 (57%). Of the patients with transmural infarction 135 (88%) had positive scans; of the patients with nontransmural infarction this occurred in 30 (63%). These results are summarized in Table 6-5.

Table 6-5. Results of ^{201}Tl scintigraphy in 200 patients with acute myocardial infarction (MI). Relationship to size of infarction

	Positive scintiscans
All MI (*n* = 200)	165 (82%)
Large MI * (*n* = 139)	131 (94%)
Small MI † (*n* = 61)	35 (57%)
Transmural MI (*n* = 153)	135 (88%)
Nontransmural MI (*n* = 47)	30 (63%)

* Serum SGOT > 3.5 times upper limit of normal
† Serum SGOT < 3.5 times upper limit of normal

Thallium-201 scintiscans and time of infarction

There was a clear relationship between results of scintigraphy and the time of scintigraphy after onset of symptoms (Figure 6-15 and Table 6-6). All 44 patients studied within 6 hr of onset of chest pain had positive ^{201}Tl scans. Of those studied between 6 and 24 hr after chest pain (*n* = 52) 88% had perfusion defects, while of those studied later than 24 hr after onset of symptoms (*n* = 104) only 72% had definite image defects. Accordingly, the number of studies read as questionable or normal increased with time after infarction.

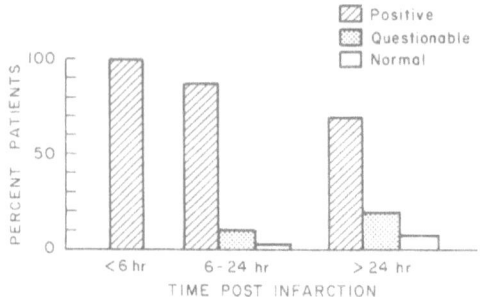

THALLIUM-201 IN ACUTE MYOCARDIAL
INFARCTION

Figure 6-15. Results of ^{201}Tl scintigraphy in 200 patients with acute myocardial infarction in relation to time interval after onset of chest pain.

Table 6-6. Results of ^{201}Tl scintigraphy in 200 patients with acute myocardial infarction [2]

Time of scintigraphy * (hr)	No. of patients	Scintiscans		
		Defect	Questionable	Negative
<6	44	44	—	—
6-24	52	46	5	1
>24	104	75	21	8

* After onset of symptoms

Thallium-201 scintiscans and size of infarction

As shown in Figures 6-16 and 6-17, and Tables 6-7 and 6-8, the results were also directly related to the biochemical size of myocardial infarction and to whether the infarction was transmural or nontransmural (Tables 6-9 and 6-10).

All patients with biochemically large infarctions, studied within the first 24 hr after onset of chest pain (71 of 139 patients) had positive scans. When

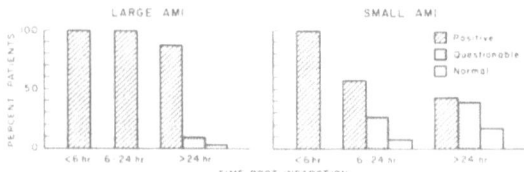

Figure 6-16. Result of ^{201}Tl scintigraphy in patients with biochemically large and biochemically small acute myocardial infarction in relation to time interval after onset of chest pain.

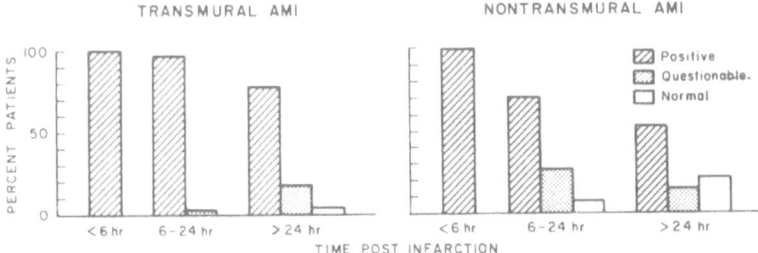

Figure 6-17. Result of ^{201}Tl scintigraphy in patients with transmural and nontransmural acute myocardial infarction in relation to time interval after onset of chest pain.

Table 6-7. Results of ^{201}Tl scintigraphy in 139 patients with SGOT >3.5 times upper limit of normal [2]

Time of scintigraphy * (hr)	No. of patients	Scintiscans		
		Defect	Questionable	Negative
<6	33	33	—	—
6-24	38	38	—	—
>24	68	60	7	1

* After onset of symptoms

Table 6-8. Results of ^{201}Tl scintigraphy in 61 patients with SGOT <3.5 times upper limit of normal [2]

Time of scintigraphy * (hr)	No. of patients	Scintiscans		
		Defect	Questionable	Negative
<6	11	11	—	—
6-24	14	8	5	1
>24	36	15	14	7

* After onset of symptoms

Table 6-9. Results of ^{201}Tl scintigraphy in 153 patients with acute transmural infarction [2]

Time of scintigraphy * (hr)	No. of patients	Scintiscans		
		Defect	Questionable	Negative
<6	39	39	—	—
6-24	35	34	1	—
>24	79	62	14	3

* After onset of symptoms

Table 6-10. Results of ^{201}Tl scintigraphy in 47 patients with acute nontransmural infarction [2]

Time of scintigraphy * (hr)	No. of patients	Scintiscans		
		Defect	Questionable	Negative
<6	5	5	—	—
6-24	17	12	4	1
>24	25	13	7	5

* After onset of symptoms

scintigraphy was performed after 24 hr in these patients with large infarctions, seven patients had questionable scans and in one patient false negative scans were obtained on the third day after infarction. Of the patients with transmural infarction all 41 patients studied within 6 hr had positive scans. Between 6 and 24 hr after infarction 97% had positive scans. After 24 hr positive scans were obtained in 78%, questionable scans in 18% and negative scans in 4% of these patients.

In the patients with biochemically small infarctions and nontransmural infarctions all patients studied within 6 hr had abnormal images. Between 6 and 24 hr after infarction positive scans were obtained in 57% of the patients with small infarcts and in 70% of the patients with nontransmural infarcts. The earliest false negative image was obtained in a patient with a small nontransmural infarction at 12 hr after onset of chest pain.

Later than 24 hr positive scans were obtained in 42% of the patients with biochemically small infarcts and in 52% of the patients with nontransmural infarcts. The results of scintigraphy were not influenced by the presence or absence of previous infarction (Table 6-11).

Table 6-11. Results of ^{201}Tl scintigraphy in 29 patients with recurrent acute myocardial infarction [2]

Time of scintigraphy * (hr)	No. of patients	Scintiscans		
		Defect	Questionable	Negative
<6	3	3	—	—
6-24	9	7	2	—
>24	17	11	5	1

* After onset of symptoms

Serial thallium-201 scintigraphy

The obvious relationship between results of ^{201}Tl scintigraphy and the time of scintigraphy after onset of symptoms was further evaluated by repeated ^{201}Tl imaging in 28 patients. For each repeated study the patient received a new dose of ^{201}Tl. Table 6-12 shows the results of repeated scintigraphy. Comparison of ^{201}Tl images obtained early (within 6 hr) after onset of infarction with those obtained later (24 hr or 4–10 days) in the same patient, revealed that the size of scintigraphic defects often changed with time. Although four patients studied early showed an increase in the size of the defects, there was a clear tendency for defects to decrease in size as the time between onset of symptoms and imaging increased. Changes in size of scintigraphic defects occurred significantly more frequently within 24 hr of infarction than later ($P<0.05$). Although not statistically different in this relative small number of patients, changes tended to occur more often in patients with viochemically small infarcts.

Table 6-12. Results of repeated scintigraphy in 28 patients with acute myocardial infarction[2]

Compared scintiscans	No. of patients	Patients with scintigraphic defect		
		Increase	Decrease	Similar
Group A *	13	4	7	2
Hroup B †	9	—	9	—
Group C ‡	15	—	7	8

* At 6 hr vs 24 hr after onset of symptoms
† At 6 hr vs 4-10 days after onset of symptoms
‡ At 24 hr vs 4-10 days after onset of symptoms

Examples of such changes are shown in Figures 6-18, 6-19 and 6-20. In Figure 6-18 the ^{201}Tl scans at $4\frac{1}{2}$ hr after chest pain were clearly abnormal, demonstrating an inferoposterior wall defect. By 24 hr the image on the 45° left-anterior-oblique view is essentially normal while on the left-lateral view decreased activity still can be appreciated. By 8 days the images were similar to those at 24 hr after acute infarction.

Figure 6-19 demonstrates repeated imaging in another patient with a small nontransmural infarction. An evident anteroseptal defect was present at $2\frac{1}{2}$ hr after chest pain. By 24 hr the defect was still present, although less impressive and by 8 days the ^{201}Tl scintiscans were essentially normal. Thus, in these patients positive, questionable or false negative ^{201}Tl scintiscans could have been obtained, depending on the timing of scintigraphy after the onset of chest pain. Figure 6-20 is of interest since it shows (re)visualization of the septum, when studied after 7 days, whereas during the acute phase there was a septal defect. This study also demonstrates that ^{201}Tl images reveal *relative* uptake of the radioisotope: a previous inferior wall infarction was masked initially because ^{201}Tl uptake was relatively more impaired in the septal region than in the scar tissue.

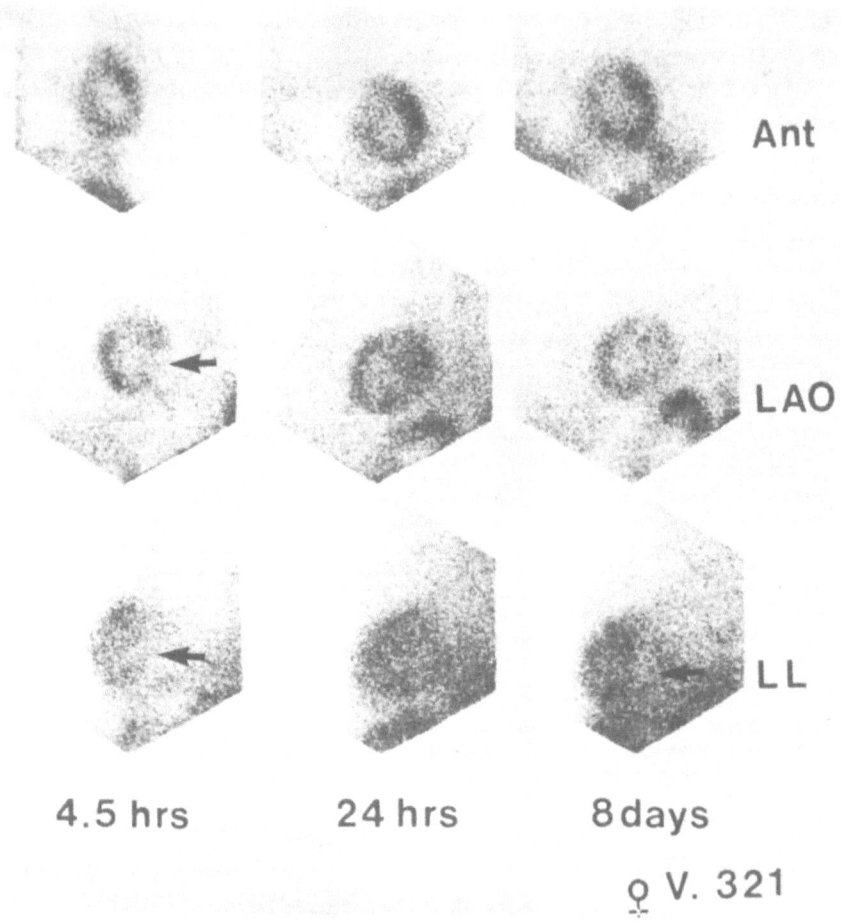

Figure 6-18. Repeated ^{201}Tl scintigraphy in a patient with acute inferoposterior wall infarction (peak SGOT level 4× upper limit of normal). At 4½ hr after onset of chest pain a clearly visible defect is present (arrows). Scintigraphic abnormalities diminished at repeated studies, especially on the left-anterior-oblique view. Reproduced with permission from Ref. [2].

These temporal changes following acute myocardial infarction have been confirmed in an experimental canine model by Umbach et al. [37]. These investigators performed ^{201}Tl imaging at 4 hr and 24 hr after closed-chest anterior wall infarction. A decrease in size of ^{201}Tl defects was noted in 10 of 13 dogs. These studies demonstrated two important factors that influence the results of ^{201}Tl scintigraphy in patients with acute myocardial infarction. Firstly, it is important to perform imaging as early as possible after the onset of symptoms, since the sensitivity to detect perfusion defect decreases as time from infarction increases. Secondly, the size of infarction is of importance. Small or nontransmural infarctions may account for false negative results.

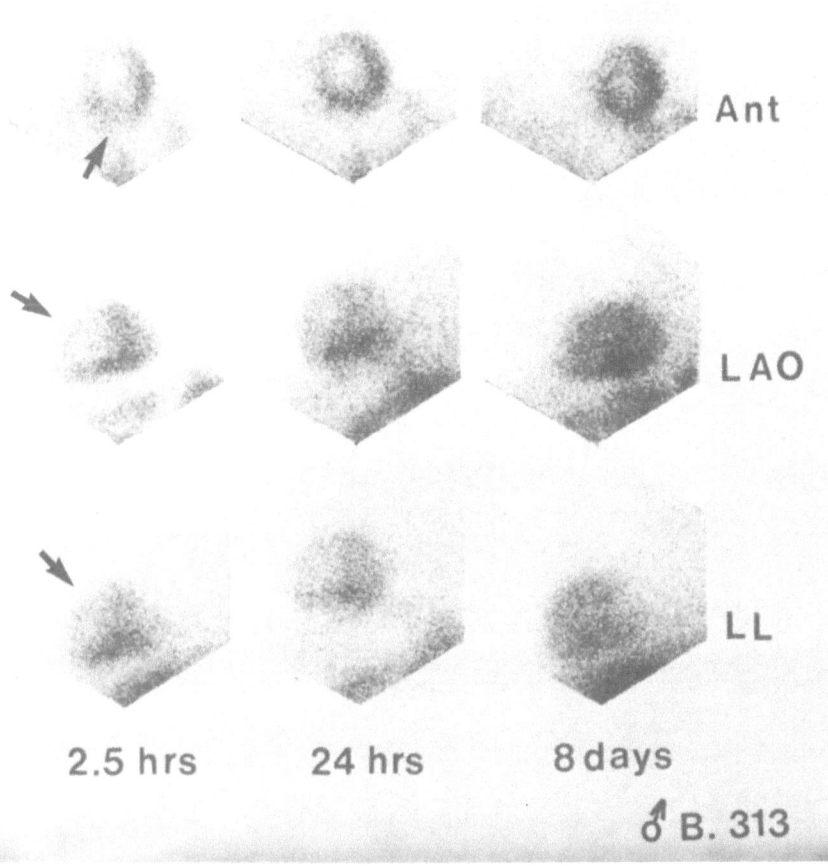

Figure 6-19. Repeated ²⁰¹Tl scintigraphy in a patient with anteroseptal infarction (peak SGOT level 4 × upper limit of normal). An evident anteroseptal perfusion defect (arrows) is present at 2½ hr after onset of chest pain – especially on the left-anterior-oblique view. At 24 hr the area of diminished activity is still present. At eight days after onset of symptoms the scintiscans have returned almost to normal. Reproduced with permission from Ref. [2].

However, when imaging is performed early, positive images will be obtained in almost all patients.

After this initial study we have reproduced the above described results in over 1000 patients with acute myocardial infarction. False negative results during the first 6 hr after acute infarction are extremely rare. In our patient material collected after the above described study, we obtained early false negative results in patients with left ventricular hypertrophy and in a few patients with small nontransmural infarctions. A similar sensitivity to detect

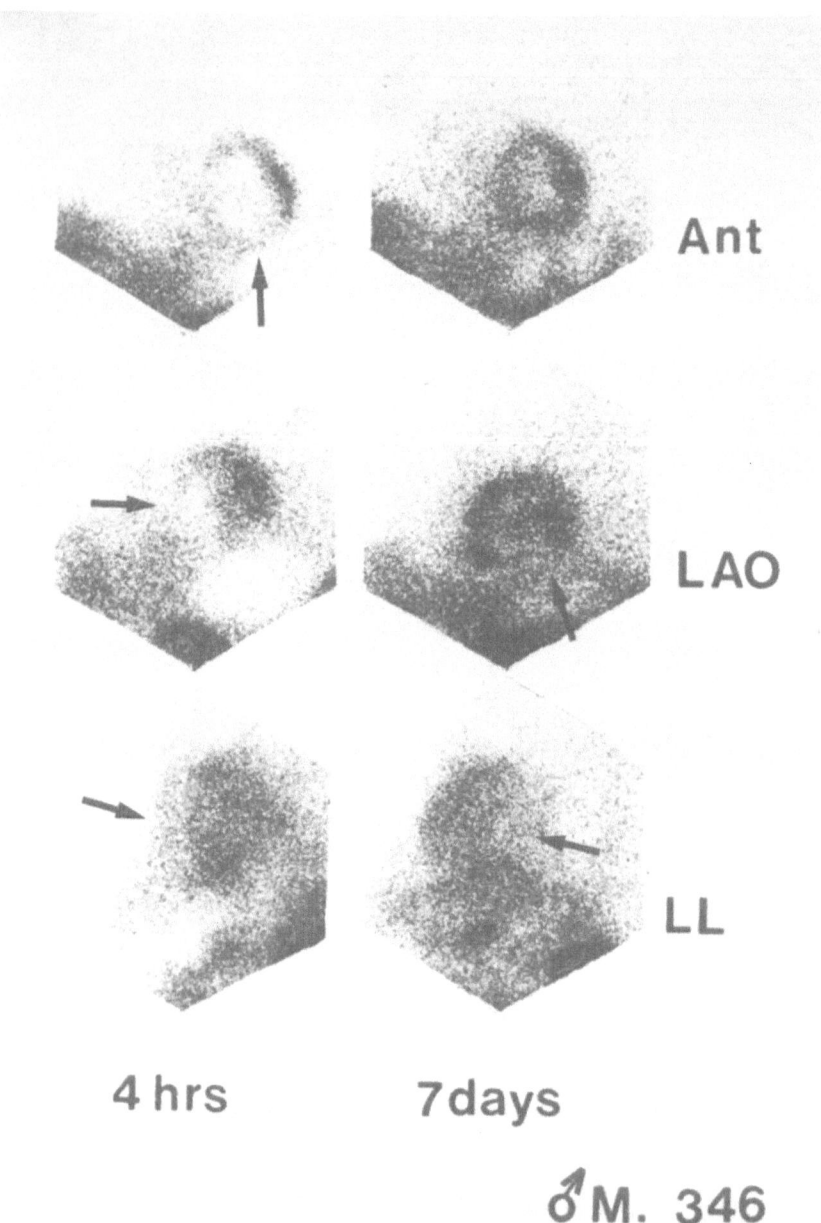

Figure 6-20. Repeated ²⁰¹Tl scintigraphy in a patient with acute nontransmural anteroseptal infarction (peak SGOT 3 × upper limit of normal). At 4 hr after chest pain an evident anteroseptal perfusion defect (arrows) is present. After 7 days the septal area is revisualized; the clear defect in the inferoposterior region at day 7 represents a previous infarction. Reproduced with permission from Ref. [2].

acute myocardial infarction was obtained by Henning et al. [11]. Berger et al. [14] reported the results of ^{201}Tl imaging in 80 patients during the subacute (>24 hr, average 6 days) phase of infarction, using a multicrystal computerized gamma camera. In this study it was noted that the sensitivity to detect acute myocardial infarction was different for anterior and inferior infarcts. All patients with anterior wall transmural infarction had positive scans, while only 85% of the patients with inferior or lateral transmural infarcts had positive ^{201}Tl scans. We never noted any difference in the sensitivity to detect myocardial infarction in relation to the site of infarction. A likely explanation for this difference is that Berger et al. [14] obtained only two views (anterior and left-anterior-oblique) in their patient series. It is especially the left-lateral view, which is of diagnostic importance to recognize inferoposterior wall abnormalities [3]. Berger et al. [14] reported an overall sensitivity of 88% in patients with nontransmural infarcts when studied during the subacute phase.

Recently Smitherman et al. [38] reported on serial myocardial imaging after a single dose of ^{201}Tl in 10 patients studied within 6 hr of acute myocardial infarction. In eight of 10 patients the perfusion defects on the redistribution images (mean 5.7 hr after injection) appeared to have decreased in size. These eight patients had uncomplicated infarction, the two remaining patients had extension of the infarction clinically. These two patients showed increased size of perfusion defects on redistribution images. Zir et al. [39] reported preliminary results of redistribution studies in a small group of patients with acute myocardial infarction. In nine of 16 patients delayed images demonstrated decrease of the size of the initial perfusion defects. The latter patients had a higher left ventricular ejection fraction by multiple gated cardiac blood pool imaging than the remaining seven patients who had no change in the delayed images (58.2% and 46.5%, respectively $P<0.01$).

There may be several explanations for the changes in size of perfusion defect as observed by repeated imaging. The pathophysiologic mechanisms of temporal changes of ^{201}Tl perfusion defects may very well be different for imaging after repeated injections and delayed or redistribution imaging after a single dose [40]. Nonetheless, these data suggest that in a considerable number of patients, during the actue phase of myocardial infarction, a definite zone of ischemic myocardium exists surrounding the actual area of necrosis. Since on one single ^{201}Tl study no differentiation can be made between ischemia and necrosis even in patients with small infarcts, the scintiscans may initially display definite defects (Figure 6-21).

In the canine model significant increase in blood flow to the infarct zone has been demonstrated during the first 24 hr after infarction [41, 42]. Thus, an increase of collateral flow during the imaging sequence could result in increased flow-related ^{201}Tl uptake in previously ischemic regions. In patients

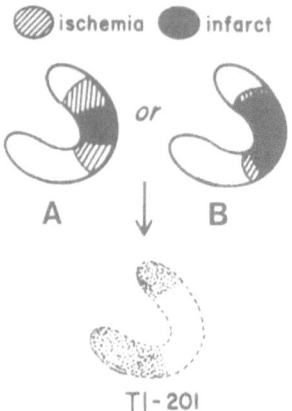

Figure 6-21. Thallium-201 perfusion defects may represent either ischemia, necrosis or the combination of the two. The schematic drawing illustrates that on one single study shortly after injection of ^{201}Tl it is not possible to distinguish between a relatively small infarct with considerable surrounding ischemia (A) and a larger infarct with a small zone of ischemia (B). Although the initial images may be similar, delayed imaging after 4 hr may demonstrate a decrease in size of defect in A, but not in B.

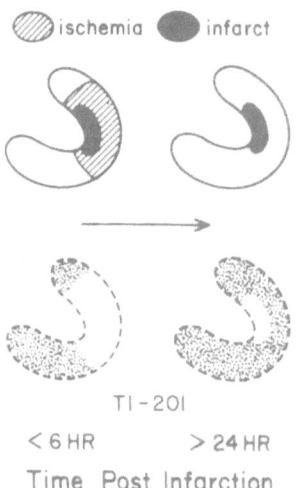

Figure 6-22. Schematic representation of possible mechanism for decrease in size of ^{201}Tl defects in patients with small acute myocardial infarction. Left, the situation early after onset of chest pain, right, after 24 hr. Initially, a relatively large region of "myocardium at risk" exists, composed of partly irreversible ischemic myocardium, resulting in a definite defect on the ^{201}Tl scintiscans. After 24 hr, myocardial blood flow has stabilized leaving a relatively small infarction, which may be too small to be detected with certainty by the gamma camera.

with small and/or nontransmural infarctions the actual area of necrosis and decreased ^{201}Tl uptake may then be too small to be detected by the currently available gamma cameras, resulting in questionable or false negative results (Figure 6-22). Mueller et al. [43] found in dogs with experimental infarctions that the minimal mass of hypoperfused myocardium detectable on ^{201}Tl scintiscans was 4.9 g, with decreased perfusion of at least 45% of normal.

Changes in cardiac dimensions also may explain the changes noted on sequential ^{201}Tl images. Recently, Gewirtz et al. [44], demonstrated that changes in myocardial images can be the result of alterations in left ventricular geometry and wall motion, independent of any change in tracer distribution. Myocardial perfusion images were obtained in dogs after intraatrial injection of ^{99m}Tc-labeled microspheres. Control images were compared to those obtained after partial aortic occlusion (to increase left ventricular volume); after ligation of the coronary vasculature supplying the apex (to produce regional dyskinesis) and after nitropruside induced hypotension and preload reduction (to decrease left ventricular volume). Partial conclusion of the aorta produced increases in size of the left ventricle and apparent (antero) apical defects on the scintiscans. Similarly, anteroapical defects were obtained after coronary ligation. With nitroprusside the defects tended to decrease in size. These myocardial image changes occurred despite the constancy of myocardial tracer distribution per unit mass of tissue, documented by post mortem scintillation well counting. It was felt that the appearance of myocardial defects could be explained by the decline of counts per unit area by stretching and thinning of the ventricular wall. These data offer another potential explanation for the changes observed in sequential ^{201}Tl imaging following acute myocardial infarction. In the clinical situation, improvement in segmental wall motion and in myocardial perfusion are often inseparable. However, changes in left ventricular dimension may not always be readily recognized on two-dimensional images.

Thus, two important factors determine the results of ^{201}Tl scintigraphy in acute myocardial infarction: first, the time of scintigraphy after onset of chest pain, and second, the size of the myocardial infarct. Thallium-201 scintigraphy is extremely sensitive in detecting perfusion abnormalities during the first 6-10 hr after onset of symptoms. After this time interval the sensitivity may decrease, especially in patients with small or nontransmural infarcts.

SENSITIVITY AND SPECIFICITY OF THALLIUM-201 SCINTIGRAPHY IN PATIENTS ADMITTED TO RULE OUT ACUTE MYOCARDIAL INFARCTION

In the previous section of this chapter we evaluated the sensitivity of ^{201}Tl scintigraphy in patients with proven acute myocardial infarction. However, to determine more realistically the practical value of ^{201}Tl scintigraphy for the detection of acute myocardial infarction we studied a selected subgroup of patients in whom, at the time of admission, the diagnosis was uncertain since they had an atypical history and nondiagnostic electrocardiograms [45]. These patients were admitted to rule out acute myocardial infarction.

In these patients the sensitivity, specificity and diagnostic accuracy was evaluated. The *sensitivity* of ^{201}Tl scintiscans was defined as:

$$\frac{\text{True Positives (TP)}}{\text{TP + False Negatives (FN)}} \times 100$$

The *specificity* was defined as:

$$\frac{\text{True Negatives (TN)}}{\text{TN + False Positives (FP)}} \times 100$$

The *predictive accuracy* of positive ^{201}Tl scintiscans was defined as:

$$\frac{\text{TP}}{\text{TP + FP}} \times 100$$

A total of 203 patients was studied. All patients had ^{201}Tl scintigraphy as soon as possible after admission to the coronary care unit. The time interval between the last episode of chest pain and scintigraphy did not exceed 10 hr. The results of this study will be discussed more in detail in chapter 12. In the present context we will only discuss the results in the patients who sustained acute myocardial infarction. Of the 203 patients 34 (17%) had acute myocardial infarction at time of scintigraphy, as apparent from enzyme elevation in blood samples obtained at the time of admission. Thallium-201 scintiscans were positive in 30 (88%) of these patients and read as questionable in the remaining four patients.

Positive scans were also obtained in 10 of 47 patients with unstable angina and in nine of 24 patients with previous myocardial infarction. Seventy-three patients were considered to have atypical complaints. None of the latter patients had positive ^{201}Tl scintiscans, although questionable scintiscans were obtained in 12 patients.

From these results, in a highly selected group of patients in whom neither the electrocardiogram nor history were contributory for the diagnosis, the practical value of ^{201}Tl as an additional aid for the detection of acute myocardial infarction can be assessed. Positive ^{201}Tl scintiscans had a sensitivity to detect acute myocardial infarction of 88% and a specificity of 88%. Positive scans had a 61% predictive accuracy to detect acute myocardial infarction. The potential value of ^{201}Tl scintigraphy as a means to select patients for the coronary care unit will be discussed in chapter 12.

Detection of previous myocardial infarction

A major disadvantage of ^{201}Tl scintigraphy is its lack of specificity. No differentiation can be made between acute and old myocardial infarction.

Only limited data exist with regard to the incidence of positive ^{201}Tl scintiscans in patients with prior myocardial infarction.

Our data in patients with acute myocardial infarction suggest that some patients with small or nontransmural infarction may have normal scans when the infarct is old. Also in patients with larger infarcts the defects, although still definitely present, tend to become less prominent with time (Figure 6-23). It is also not unusual in our experience that prior infarction can be recognized only as a thinner and/or irregular myocardial segment (Figures 4-15, 6-24 and 6-25). In the literature, the incidence of positive ^{201}Tl scans in patients with prior infarction is only mentioned in the context of studies with other specific aims. Hamilton et al. [46] reported positive rest scans in 10 of 11

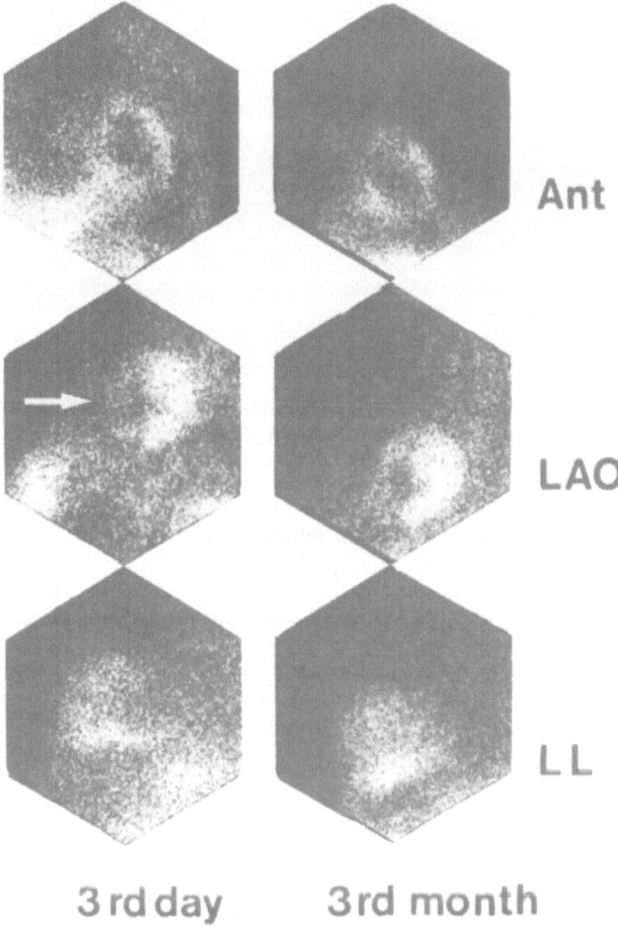

Ant

LAO

LL

3rd day   3rd month

Figure 6-23. Thallium-201 scintiscans on the 3rd day and 3rd month after infarction. An anteroseptal perfusion defect is present on both studies, although less prominent (especially septum) after 3 months. Reproduced with permission from Ref. [5].

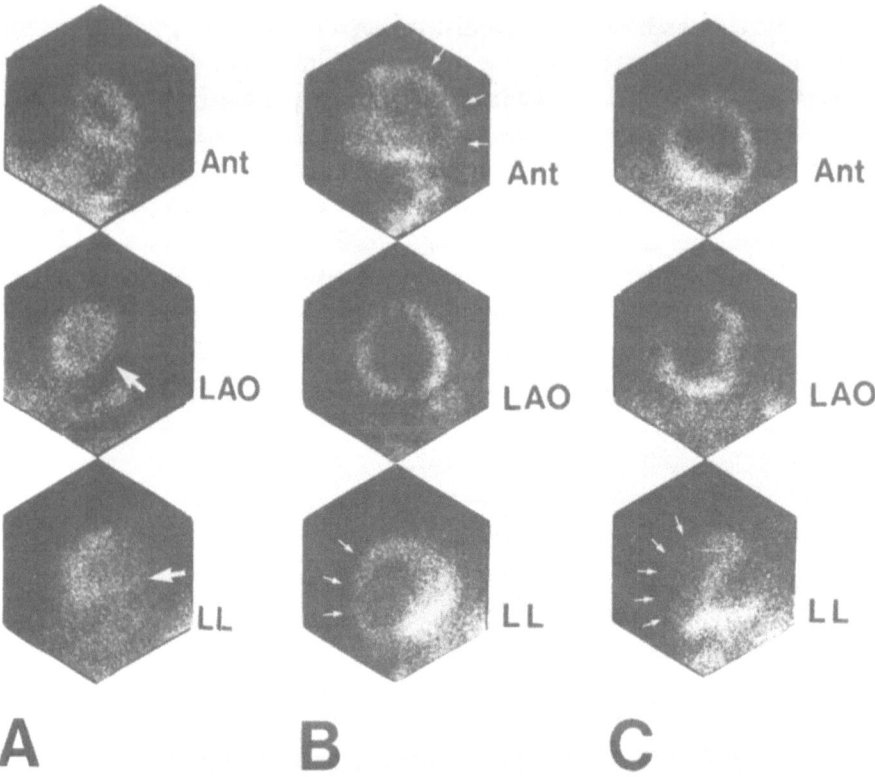

Figure 6-24. Thallium-201 Studies in patients with previous myocardial infarction. (A) Documented previous inferoposterior wall infarction. The site of the previous infarct is hardly recognizable. Without knowledge of the patient's history, the subtle area of diminished activity (arrows) is not diagnostic. (B) Documented previous anterior wall infarction. The left ventricle is markedly enlarged and dilated. No true defect is present. Without the patient's history it is difficult to determine whether there was a previous infarction or not, since the image is compatible with nonischemic congestive cardiomyopathy. In view of the patient's history, it is likely that the thin anterolateral wall represents the old infarction. (C) Documented previous anteroseptal infarction and aneurysm. The left ventricle is markedly enlarged and dilated. The left-lateral view displays definitely abnormal images: large anterior wall defect. Note, the increased contribution to the image by normal myocardium adjacent to the aneurysm. The anterior and left-anterior-oblique views demonstrate no defect but extremely "dark cavity", since aneurysm is viewed *en face*.

patients with prior myocardial infarction, who had rest and exercise ^{201}Tl scintigraphy. Verani et al. [47] observed complete filling in of exercise-induced perfusion defects by redistribution in only five of 27 patients. Thus, in 22 patients the remote infarction was still demonstrable. Blood et al. [48] found perfusion defects in 15 rest studies and 26 redistribution studies, both performed in 28 patients with prior infarcts. We obtained positive rest scans in nine of 24 patients with old infarction [45].

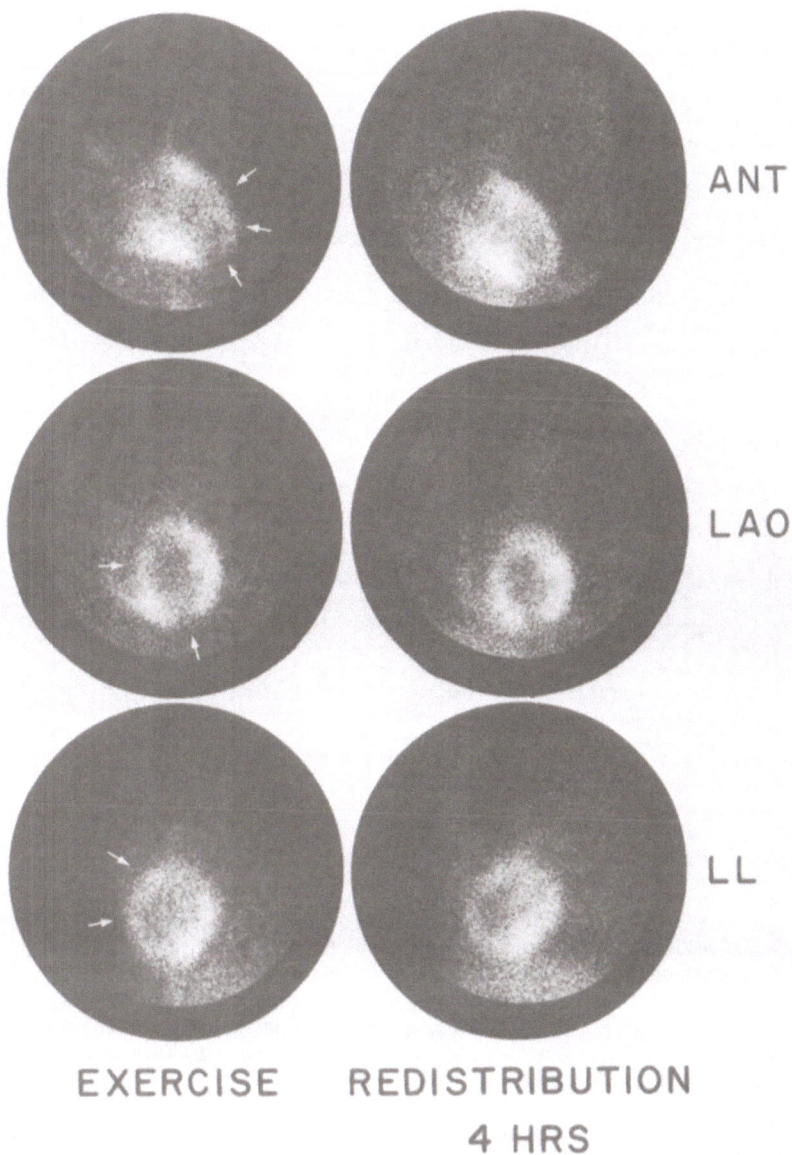

ANT

LAO

LL

EXERCISE   REDISTRIBUTION
4 HRS

Figure 6-25. Thallium-201 scintigraphy following exercise and 4 hr redistribution in a patient with documented prior anteroseptal infarction. The study immediately post-exercise demonstrates decreased activity and thinned walls in the anteroseptal region. No true defects are present. The delayed images demonstrate no major change, except for some increased uptake in the antero-apical (anterior view) and septal (left-anterior-oblique view) regions.

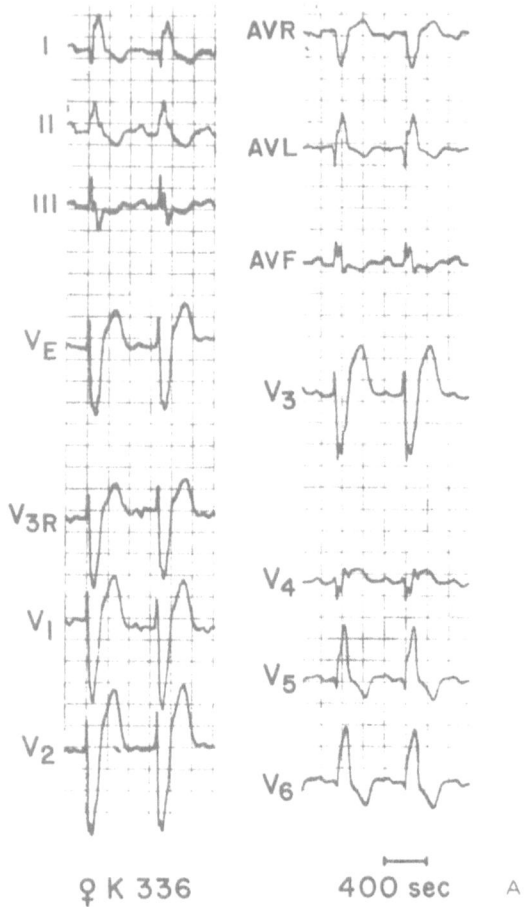

I   AVR

II   AVL

III AVF

V_E

V_3

V_{3R}

V_4

V_1

V_5

V_2

V_6

♀ K 336   400 sec   A

Figure 6-26. Thallium-201 scintiscans in a patient with left bundle branch block (LBBB) and acute myocardial infarction. (*above*: A) Electrocardiogram showing complete LBBB. The diagnosis and site of infarction cannot be made with certainty from this electrocardiogram. Remarkable are the narrow Q waves in leads I, aVL, V_{5-6}; the relatively large R in V_{1-3}; the notching of the QRS in leads III, aVF, V_4 and ST segment elevation in V4. (*facing page*: B) Thallium-201 scintiscans clearly demonstrate an anteroseptal and apical defect.

Thus, the incidence of positive scans in selected patient groups with previous myocardial infarcts, as reported in the literature, varies from 37% to 91%. Although we never studied this particular problem systematically in a larger and unselected series of patients, we tend to believe that the incidence (54%) as reported in the study by Blood et al. [48] is probably the most realistic. In approximately half of the patients with old infarction ^{201}Tl scintiscans may become normal. Typically, this may occur in a resting ^{201}Tl study in a patient with an old nontransmural inferior wall infarction. In the latter

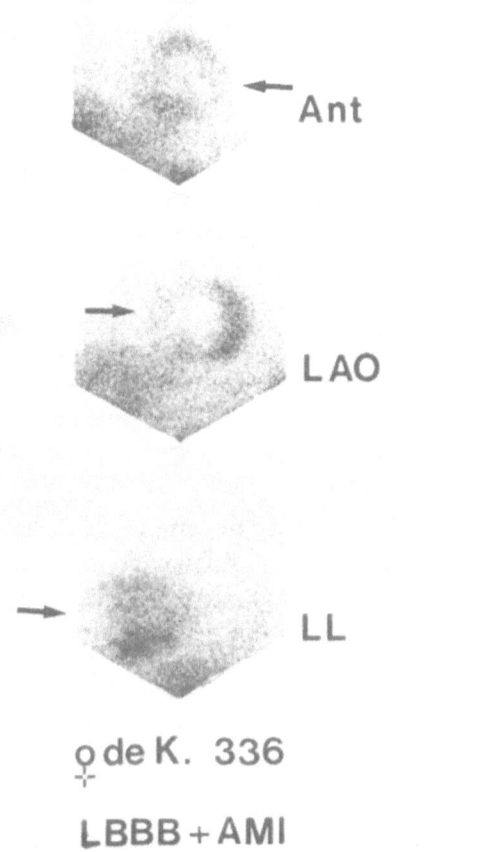

Ant

LAO

LL

♀ de K. 336

LBBB + AMI

B

patients the relatively high subdiaphragmatic activity adjacent to the inferior wall may obscure perfusion defects. As suggested by Blood et al. [48] redistribution myocardial perfusion scintiscans following exercise are significantly more sensitive than rest scintiscans to detect prior myocardial infarction.

On the other hand, since a fair number of patients may have normal ^{201}Tl scintiscans in the presence of prior infarction, ^{201}Tl scintigraphy is not *a priori* meaningless when these patients sustain a new attack of acute chest pain suggestive for acute infarction.

CLINICAL APPLICATION OF THALLIUM-201 SCINTIGRAPHY
TO DETECT ACUTE MYOCARDIAL INFARCTION

In many patients admitted to the coronary care unit the history and initial electrocardiogram will provide sufficient information to be able to make the diagnosis of acute myocardial infarction at the time of hospital arrival. In these patients there may be no need for ^{201}Tl scintigraphy. However, in patients with complete left bundle branch block (Figure 6-26), Wolf-Parkinson-White Syndrome or pacemaker rhythm, the electrocardiographic diagnosis of acute myocardial infarction may be very difficult or impossible. In this limited number of patients, ^{201}Tl scintigraphy will be very helpful [49].

The best and most practical application of ^{201}Tl scintigraphy is without doubt in patients with an atypical history and nondiagnostic electrocardiogram, in whom acute myocardial infarction has to be ruled out. In the latter group of patients it is of crucial importance that imaging is performed within 10–18 hr after the last episode of chest pain.

Furthermore, ^{201}Tl scintigraphy allows accurate anatomic localization of the infarction. It also provides a potentially important means to judge the relative size of the malperfused or infarcted myocardium. As demonstrated recently by Becker and his associates [30], measuring the size of ^{201}Tl deflects on the scintiscans of patients with acute myocardial infarcts permits early stratification of patients in high and low risk subgroups.

REFERENCES

1. Wackers FJTh, van der Schoot JB, Busemann Sokole E, Samson G, Niftrik GJC, Lie KI, Durrer D, Wellens HJJ: Noninvasive visualization of acute myocardial infarction in man with thallium-201. Br Heart J 37:741-744, 1975.
2. Wackers FJTh, Busemann Sokole E, Samson G, van der Schoot JB, Lie KI, Liem KL, Wellens HJJ: Value and limitations of thallium-201 scintigraphy in the acute phase of myocardial infarction. N Engl J Med 295:1-5, 1976.
3. Johnstone DE, Wackers FJTh, Berger HJ, Hoffer PB, Kelley MJ, Gottschalk A, Zaret BL: Effect of patient positioning on left lateral thallium-201 myocardial images. J Nucl Med 20:183-188, 1979.
4. Trobaugh GB, Wackers FJTh, Busemann Sokole E, DeRouen TA, Ritchie JL, Hamilton GW: Thallium-201 myocardial imaging: an interinstitutional study of observer variability. J Nucl Med 19:359-363, 1978.
5. Wackers FJTh, Busemann Sokole E, Samson G, van der Schoot JB: Atlas of ^{201}Tl myocardial scintigraphy. Clin Nucl Med 2:64-74, 1977.
6. Isner JM, Roberts WC: Right ventricular infarction complicating left ventricular infarction secondary to coronary heart disease: frequency, location, associated findings and significance from analysis of 236 necropsy patients with acute or healed myocardial infarction. Am J Cardiol 42:885-894, 1978.
7. Wackers FJTh, Lie KI, Busemann Sokole E, van der Schoot JB, Durrer D: Prevalence of right ventricular involvement in inferior wall infarction assessed with myocardial imaging with thallium-201 and technetium-99m pyrophosphate. Am J Cardiol 42:358-362, 1978.
8. Rigo P, Murray M. Taylor DR, Weisfeldt ML, Kelly DT, Strauss HW, Pitt B: Right ventricular dysfunction detected by gated scintiphotography in patients with acute inferior myocardial infarction. Circulation 52:268-274, 1975.

9. Kannel WB, Sorlie P, McNamara PM: Prognosis after initial infarction. The Framingham study. Am J Cardiol 44:53-59, 1979.

10. Lie KI, Wellens HJ, Schuilenburg RM, Becker AE, Durrer D: Factors influencing prognosis of bundle branch block complicating acute antero-septal infarction. The value of His bundle recordings. Circulation 50:935-941, 1974.

11. Henning H, Schelbert HR, Righetti A, Ashburn WL, O'Rourke RA: Dual myocardial imaging with technetium-99m pyrophosphate and thallium-201 for detecting, localizing and sizing acute myocardial infarction. Am J Cardiol 40:147-155, 1977.

12. Strauss HW, Pitt B: Common procedures for the noninvasive determination of regional myocardial perfusion, evaluation of regional wall motion and detection of acute infarction. Am J Cardiol 38:731-746, 1976.

13. Ritchie JL, Zaret BL, Strauss HW, Pitt B, Berman DS, Schelbert HR, Ashburn WL, Berger HJ, Hamilton GW: Myocardial imaging with thallium-201: a multicenter study in patients with angina pectoris or acute myocardial infarction. Am J Cardiol 42:345-350, 1978.

14. Berger HJ, Gottschalk A, Zaret BL: Dual radionuclide study of acute myocardial infarction: comparison of thallium-201 and technetium-99m stannous pyrophosphate imaging in man. Ann Intern Med 88:145-154, 1978.

15. Zaret BL: Myocardial imaging with radioactive potassium and its analogs. Prog Cardiovasc Dis 20:81-94, 1977.

16. Parkey RW, Bonte FJ, Stokely EM, Lewis SE, Graham KD, Buja, LM, Willerson JT: Acute myocardial infarction imaged with ^{99m}Tc-stannous pyrophosphate and ^{201}Tl: a clinical evaluation. J Nucl Med 17:771-779, 1976.

17. Pabst HW, Hör G, Lichte H, Sebening H, Kriegel H: Experience with ^{201}thallium in detection of myocardial infarction. Eur J Nucl Med 1:19-25, 1976.

18. Sullivan W, Vlodaver Z, Tuna N, Long L, Edwards JE: Correlation of electrocardiographic and pathologic findings in healed myocardial infarction. Am J Cardiol 42:724-732, 1978.

19. Wackers FJTh, Becker AE, Samson G, Busemann Sokole E, van der Schoot JB, Vet AJTM, Lie KI, Durrer D, Wellens H: Location and size of acute transmural myocardial infarction estimated from thallium-201 scintiscans: a clinicopathological study. Circulation 56:72-78, 1977.

20. Ramkissoon RA: Macroscopic identification of early myocardial infarction by dehydrogenase alterations. J Clin Path 19:479-481, 1966.

21. Buja LM, Parkey RW, Stokely EM, Bonte FJ, Willerson JT: Pathophysiology of technetium-99m stannous pyrophosphate and thallium-201 scintigraphy of acute anterior myocardial infarcts in dogs. J Clin Invest 57:1508-1522, 1976.

22. Strauss HW, Harrison K, Langan JK, Lebowitz E, Pitt B: Thallium-201 for myocardial imaging: relation of thallium-201 to regional myocardial perfusion. Circulation 51:641-645, 1975.

23. DiCola VC, Downing SE, Donabedian RK, Zaret BL: Pathophysiological correlates of thallium-201 myocardial uptake in experimental infarction. Cardiovasc Res 11:141-146, 1977.

24. Page DL, Caulfield JB, Kastor JA, DeSantis RW, Sanders CA: Myocardial changes associated with cardiogenic shock. N Engl J Med 285:134, 1971.

25. Maroko PR, Braunwald E: Effects of metabolic and pharmacologic intervention on myocardial infarct size following coronary occlusion. Circulation 53:(Suppl 1) 162-168, 1976.

26. Hamilton GW, Narahara KA, Trobaugh GB, Ritchie JL, Williams DL: Thallium-201 myocardial imaging: characterization of the ECG-synchronized images. J Nucl Med 19:1103-1110, 1978.

27. Burow RD, Pond M, Scharer AW, Becker L: "Circumferential profiles": a new method for computer analysis of thallium-201 myocardial perfusion images. J Nucl Med 20:771-777, 1979.

28. Niess GS, Logic JR, Russell RO, Rackley CE, Rogers WJ: Usefulness and limitations of thallium-201 myocardial scintigraphy in delineating location and size of prior myocardial infarction. Circulation 50:1010-1019, 1979.

29. Bulkley BH, Silverman K, Weisfeldt ML, Burow R, Pond M, Becker LC: Pathologic basis of thallium-201 scintigraphic defects in patients with fatal myocardial injury. Circulation 60:785-792, 1979.

30. Silverman KJ, Becker LC, Bulkley BH, Burow RD, Mellits ED, Kallman CH, Weisfeldt ML.: Value of early thallium-201 scintigraphy for predicting mortality in patients with acute myocardial infarction. Circulation 61:996-1003, 1980.

31. Botvinick E, Perez-Gonzalez J, Ports T, Rahimtoola S, Parmley W, Holly A: Prognostic implications of quantitative scintigraphic studies in acute myocardial infarction. Circulation 60:suppl II, II-69, abstract 264, 1979.

32. Vogel RA, Kirch D, LeFree M, Steele P: A new method of multiplanar emission tomography using a seven pinhole collimator and an Anger scintillation camera. J Nucl Med 19:648-654, 1978.

33. Williams DL, Ritchie JL, Harp GC, Hamilton GW: In vivo simulation of thallium-201 myocardial scintigraphy by seven pinhole emission tomography. Circulation 60:suppl. II, II-60, abstract 228, 1979.

34. Holman BL, Hill TC, Wynne J, Lovett RD, Zimmerman RE, Smith EM: Single-photon transaxial emission computed tomography of the heart in normal subjects and in patients with infarction. J. Nucl Med 20:736-740, 1979.

35. Sobel BE, Weis ES, Welch MJ, Siegel BA, Ter-Pogossian MM: Detection of remote myocardial infarction in patients with positron emission transaxial tomography and intravenous ^{11}C-palmitate. Circulation 55:853-857, 1977.

36. Weiss ES, Siegel BA, Sobel BE, Welch MJ, Ter-Pogossian MM: Evaluation of myocardial metabolism and perfusion with positron-emitting radionuclides. Prog Cardiovasc Dis 20:191-206, 1977.

37. Umbach RE, Lange RC, Lee JC, Zaret BL: Temporal changes in sequential quantitative thallium-201 imaging following myocardial infarction in dogs: comparison of four and twenty-four hour infarct images. Yale J Biol Med 51:597-603, 1978.

38. Smitherman TC, Osborn RC, Narahara KA: Serial myocardial scintigraphy after a single dose of thallium-201 in men after acute myocardial infarction. Am J Cardiol 42:177-182, 1978.

39. Zir LM, Strauss HW, Gewirtz H, Shea WH, Forwand SA, Voukydis PC, Pohost GM: Tl-201 redistribution in patients with acute myocardial infarction. J Nucl Med 20:649, 1979.

40. Beller GA, Watson DD, Pohost GM: Kinetics of thallium distribution and redistribution: clinical applications in sequential myocardial imaging. In: Cardiovascular nuclear medicine 2nd edition, pp 225-242, Strauss HW, Pitt B, eds. St. Louis: Mosby 1979.

41. Rivas F, Cobb FR, Bache RJ, Greenfield JC: Relationship between blood flow to ischemic regions and extent of myocardial infarction. Serial measurement of blood flow to ischemic regions in dogs. Circulation Res 30:439-447, 1976.

42. Schwartz JS, Ponto RA, Forstrom LA, Bache RJ: Mechanism of decrease in scintigraphic defect size after coronary occlusion. Circulation 60:suppl II, II-173, abstract 675, 1979.

43. Mueller TM, Marcus ML, Ehrhardt JC, Chaudhuri T, Abboud FM: Limitations of thallium-201 myocardial perfusion scintigrams. Circulation 54:640-646, 1976.

44. Gewirtz H, Grotte GJ, Strauss HW, O'Keefe DD, Akins CW, Daggett WM, Pohost GM: The influence of left ventricular volume and wall motion on myocardial images. Circulation 59:1172-1177, 1979.

45. Wackers FJTh, Lie KI, Liem KL, Busemann Sokole E, Samson G, van der Schoot J, Durrer D: Potential value of thallium-201 scintigraphy as a means of selecting patients for the coronary care unit. Br Heart J 41:111-117, 1979.

46. Hamilton GW, Trobaugh GB, Ritchie JL, Williams DL, Weaver WD, Gould KL: Myocardial imaging with intravenously injected thallium-201 in patients with suspected coronary artery disease. Am J Cardiol 39:347-354, 1977.

47. Verani MS, Jhingran S, Attar M, Rizk A, Quinones MA, Miller RR: Poststress redistribution of thallium-201 in patients with coronary artery disease, with and without prior myocardial infarction. Am J Cardiol 43:1114-1122, 1979.

48. Blood DK, McCarthy DM, Sciacca RR, Cannon PJ: Comparison of single-dose and double-dose thallium-201 myocardial perfusion scintigraphy for the detection of coronary artery disease and prior myocardial infarction. Circulation 58:777-788, 1978.

49. Wackers FJTh, Busemann Sokole E, Samson G, van der Schoot JB, Lie KI, Durrer D, Wellens HJJ: Thallium-201 for visualization of acute myocardial infarction in the presence of left bundle branch block. Herz 2:163-166, 1977.

7. TECHNETIUM-99m-PYROPHOSPHATE MYOCARDIAL IMAGING IN ACUTE MYOCARDIAL INFARCTION

JAMES T. WILLERSON, ROBERT W. PARKEY, FREDERICK J. BONTE, SAMUEL E. LEWIS, ERNEST STOKELY and L. MAXIMILIAN BUJA

The recognition of acute myocardial infarcts is not always easily accomplished. Infarct recognition is especially difficult using electrocardiography in individuals who had previous myocardial infarcts, those with left bundle branch block, those who have been cardioverted, and those with acute non-transmural (subendocardial) myocardial infarcts. Even the most sophisticated enzymatic techniques presently available have certain limitations in identifying the presence of absence of acute myocardial infarcts in patients including: (1) there is a temporal dependency in the ability of various enzyme markers to detect acute myocardial infarcts, and (2) certain clinical settings preclude using traditional enzyme techniques (including creatine kinase – MB isoenzyme) for infarct recognition and to be emphasized in this regard is the perioperative and postoperative setting after coronary artery revascularization. Therefore, it is important to have additional relatively noninvasive means that allow infarct detection, localization and provide some estimate of the size of the lesion.

We have extensively evaluated "hot spot" myocardial imaging using ^{99m}Tc-stannous-pyrophosphate for these purposes. This imaging technique has been extensively evaluated in experimental animals and in patients with acute myocardial infarcts at our institution[1–19].

Shen and Jennings[20] and D'Agostino[21] suggested the potential for using ^{99m}Tc-pyrophosphate myocardial scintigraphy to recognize acute myocardial necrosis when they demonstrated that calcium is deposited in crystalline and subcrystalline form in irreversibly damaged myocardial cells. These observations led Bonte and associates to question whether ^{99m}Tc-pyrophosphate might be capable of identifying irreversibly damaged myocardial cells on the basis of pyrophosphate complexing with the calcium deposited in these cells[1]. Subsequently, we have carried out an extensive evaluation in patients and in large numbers of experimental animals to examine the ability of this imaging agent to identify irreversibly damaged myocardium and to further elucidate pathophysiologic factors involved in the uptake and concentration of ^{99m}Tc-pyrophosphate in injured myocardium[1–19]. Studies performed in experimental animals and in patients using this imaging technique have emphasized that the most important determinants of ^{99m}Tc-pyrophosphate myocardial uptake in the heart are: (1) the presence of acute myocardial necrosis, (2) persistent residual coronary blood flow into the area(s) of irreversible cellular damage, and (3) the time elapsed after the onset of myocardial damage prior to obtaining the ^{99m}Tc-pyrophosphate myocardial scintigrams [1–19]. These observations have been generally confirmed by others [22–24]. Using contemporary imaging cameras and two-dimensional scintigraphic information, at least 3 g of myocardial necrosis must be present to consistently identify acute myocardial infarcts in experimental animals and patients with permanent coronary artery occlusion using this imaging technique [13–15, 17, 25]. Technetium-99m-pyrophosphate myocardial uptake is greatest in myocardial regions in which coronary blood flow is reduced to levels of 10–40% of normal with fixed coronary artery occlusion and experimental myocardial infarction. Technetium-99m-pyrophosphate scintigrams become abnormal within 10-12 hr after infarction but they generally become increasingly abnormal in the first 24-72 hr after infarction (Figures 7-1 and 7-2). The development of an abnormal ^{99m}Tc-pyrophosphate myocardial scintigram and the increasing uptake of the radiopharmaceutical correlate temporally and topographically with increasing calcium deposition in the regions of myocardial necrosis [6, 7, 15]. Ordinarily, the scintigrams fade and/or become negative at approximately 13-14 days in experimental animals with acute myocardial infarcts and by 6 days in patients (Figure 7-2). It should be emphasized, however, that some patients retain "persistently positive" ^{99m}Tc-pyrophosphate myocardial scintigrams for months (Figure 7-3) [26]. An occasional patient first develops an abnormal ^{99m}Tc-pyrophosphate myocardial scintigram 5-6 days after infarction [27]. Consequently, there is a need for serial myocardial imaging to differentiate persistently "abnormal" ^{99m}Tc-pyrophosphate myocardial scintigrams and to detect the occasional patient who first develops

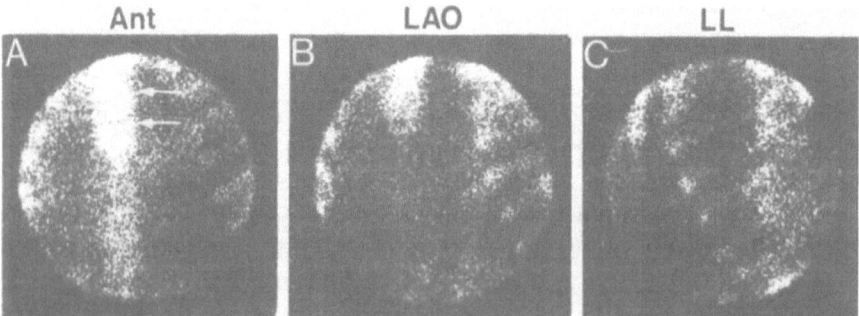

Figure 7-1. A normal ^{99m}Tc-pyrophosphate myocardial scintigram is shown. Note the uptake of the radionuclide agent in skeletal structures but there is no important uptake in the region of the heart. The closed arrows mark ^{99m}Tc-pyrophosphate uptake in the sternum. The imaging projections shown are panel A. the anterior view; panel B, the left anterior oblique view; and panel C, the left lateral view.

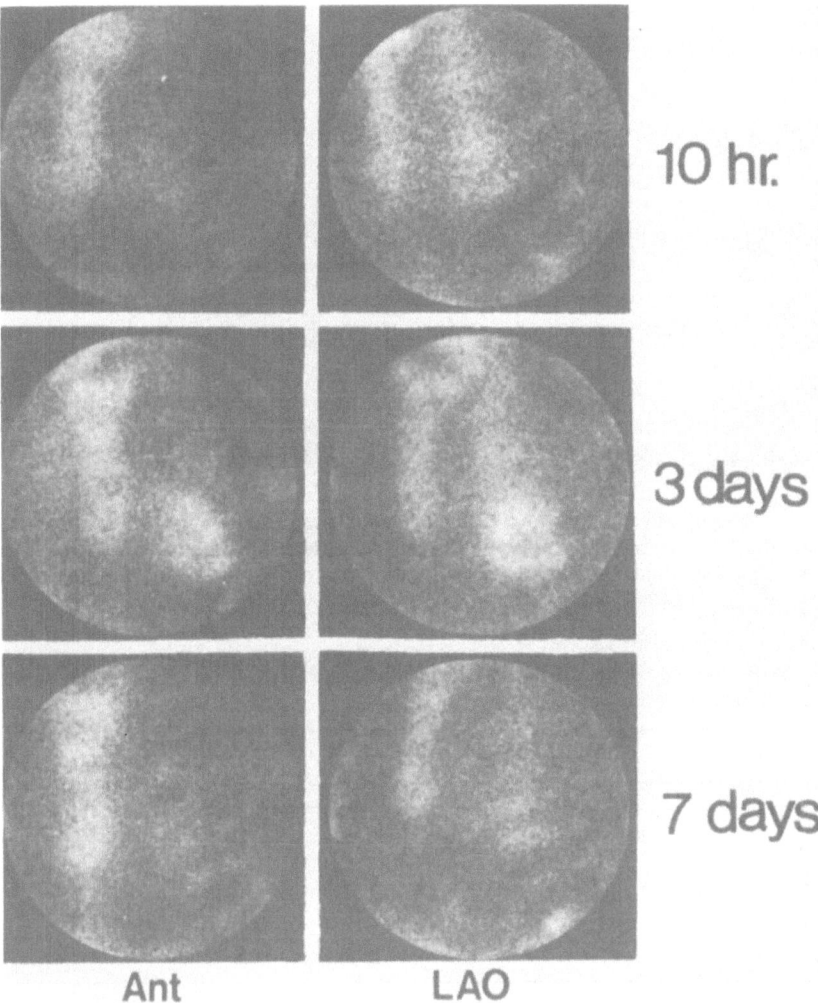

Figure 7-2. The changes in ^{99m}Tc-pyrophosphate uptake that occur following acute myocardial infarction with the passage of time are shown. The views are from left to right: the anterior view and the left anterior oblique one. Note that by three days, there is considerably more ^{99m}Tc-pyrophosphate activity in the anterolateral and apical myocardial infarct as compared to ^{99m}Tc-pyrophosphate uptake 10 hr after the onset of symptoms suggestive of infarction. By 6 to 7 days, the scintigrams have generally faded and/or become negative.

an abnormal ^{99m}Tc-pyrophosphate myocardial scintigram 5-6 days after acute myocardial infarction [28].

When the appropriate imaging technique and time periods for study are utilized, one finds excellent sensitivity for this imaging test in the detection of acute myocardial infarcts (Table 7-1)[18]. Figure 7-4 demonstrates the scintigraphic appearance of the various types of acute transmural myocardial

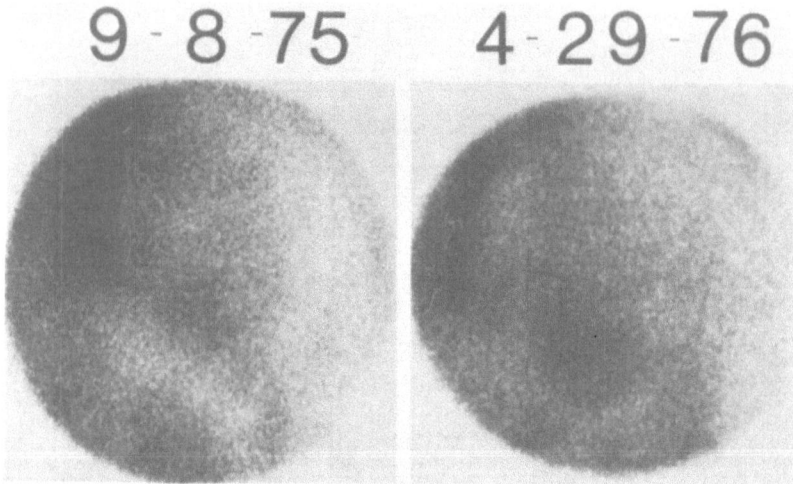

Figure 7-3. A "persistently abnormal" ^{99m}Tc-pyrophosphate myocardial scintigram is shown. In this patient, the ^{99m}Tc-pyrophosphate uptake persisted for at least 6 months following infarction and the scintigraphic abnormality was associated with ongoing persistent and severe angina pectoris.

Table 7-1. Predictive indices for the recognition of myocardial necrosis by ^{99m}Tc-pyrophosphate myocardial scintigraphy for 59 clinical events in 52 patients *

Predictive indices	Microscopic or gross necrosis	Gross myocardial infarct
Prevalence	78%	53%
Sensitivity	89%	94%
Specificity	100%	57%
Predictive value		
Positive scan	100%	71%
Negative scan	72%	98%

* This table is reproduced from Ref. [18]

infarcts using the ^{99m}Tc-pyrophosphate myocardial imaging techniques. Figure 7-5 demonstrates the grading scheme that we use for the interpretation of ^{99m}Tc-pyrophosphate myocardial scintigrams. Scintigrams graded " 2+ to 4+ " are considered abnormal at our institution. Most transmural infarcts develop focal and intensely abnormal ^{99m}Tc-pyrophosphate myocardial scintigrams if serial myocardial imaging is utilized. However, many nontransmural (subendocardial) myocardial infarcts demonstrate a fainter and more poorly localized pattern of ^{99m}Tc-pyrophosphate uptake (Figure 7-6) [4,18,28,29].

We recommend that when using this technique, a ^{99m}Tc-pyrophosphate myocardial scintigram be obtained within 24–48 hr after symptoms suggestive of acute myocardial infarction. However, if clinical suspicion of myocardial

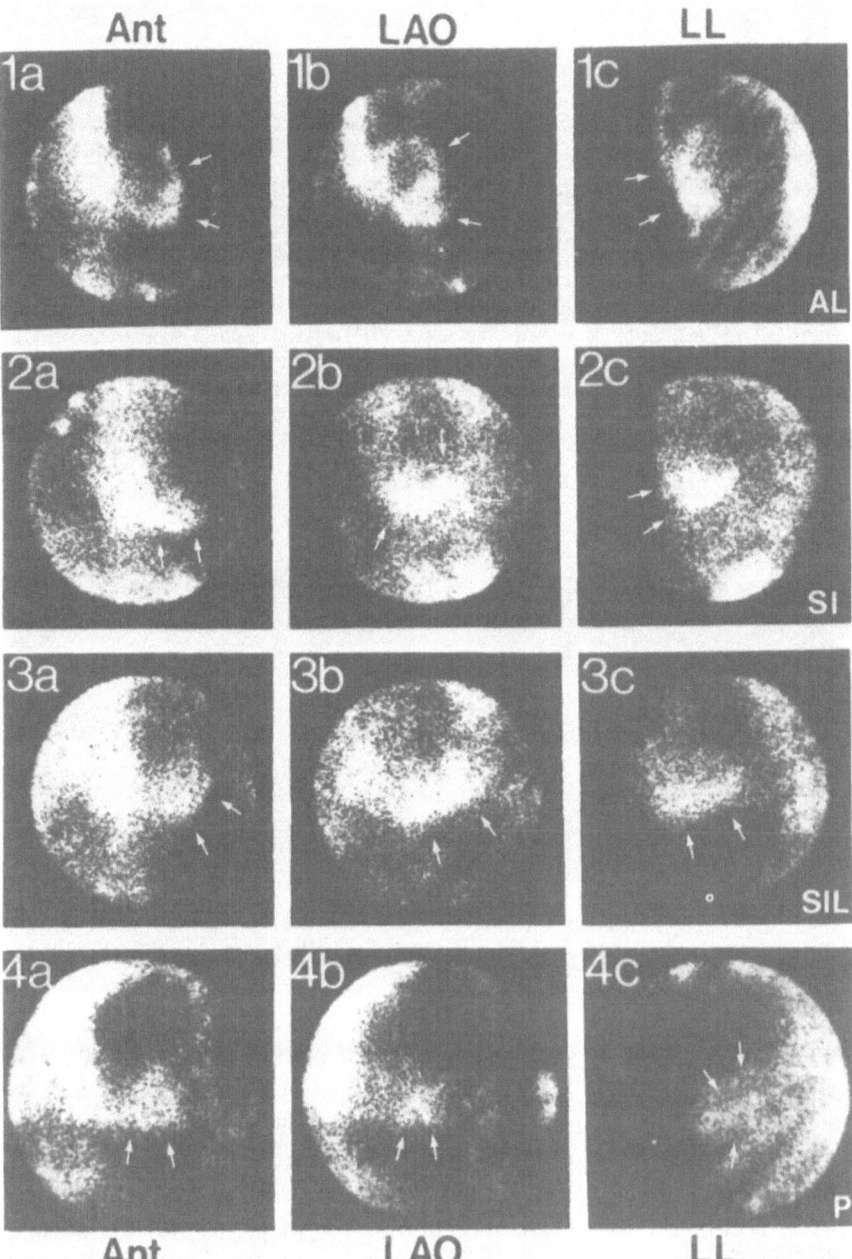

Figure 7-4. The various types of transmural acute myocardial infarction as identified by ^{99m}Tc-pyrophosphate myocardial scintigraphy are shown. Panels A through C demonstrate the anterior, left anterior oblique and left lateral views, respectively. Panels 1A through 1C demonstrate a large "doughnut" anterolateral (AL) myocardial infarct. Panels 2A through 2C demonstrate septal and inferior (SI) infarction; Panels 3A through 3C demonstrate septal, inferior and lateral (SIL) ^{99m}Tc-pyrophosphate uptake; and Panels 4A through 4C demonstrate a true posterior (P) myocardial infarct. Reproduced from Ref. [3] by permission.

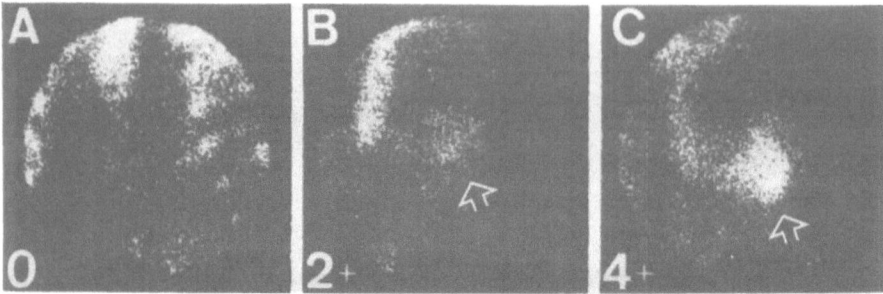

Figure 7-5. The grading scheme utilized for the interpretation of ^{99m}Tc-pyrophosphate myocardial scintigrams at our institution is shown. We regard ^{99m}Tc-pyrophosphate scintigrams that are "2+ to 4+" in intensity as being abnormal and reflecting the presence of acute myocardial necrosis. Many nontransmural (subendocardial) myocardial infarcts have a "2+" pattern while many transmural infarcts have "3+ to 4+" ^{99m}Tc-pyrophosphate uptake. Reproduced from Ref. [3] by permission.

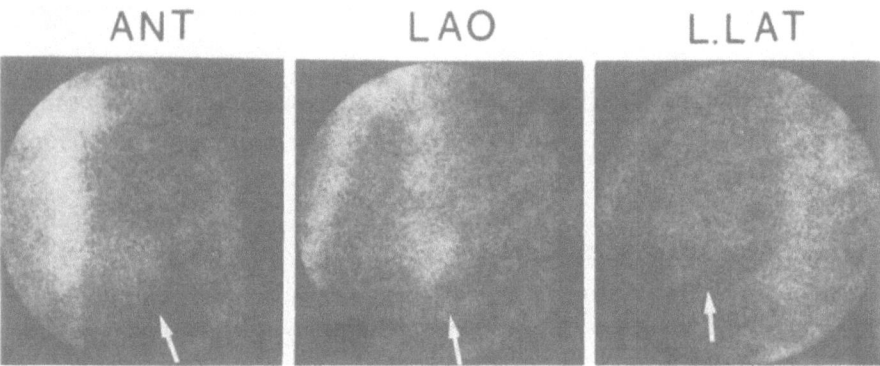

Figure 7-6. Technetium-99m-pyrophosphate scintigraphic appearance of an acute subendocardial myocardial infarct is shown. Note that the ^{99m}Tc-pyrophosphate uptake is fainter and somewhat less well localized than occurs for transmural infarcts.

infarction is strong and the initial scintigram negative or equivocal, then the test should be repeated at least once, approximately 96 hr after the onset of symptoms sugggestive of infarction [3, 4, 27, 28]. This serial imaging approach will allow detection of an occasional patient in whom the initial scintigram was negative but who develops abnormal test in a more delayed fashion than classically occurs [27]. Most patients requiring longer periods for the development of an abnormal ^{99m}Tc-pyrophosphate myocardial scintigram after acute infarction, have severe extensive coronary artery disease. Other technical factors important in the proper use of this imaging technique are outlined in chapter 5. We also wish to emphasize that any cause of acute myocardial necrosis that results in 3 g or more of irreversible cellular damage, when imaged in the proper time frame, will result in an abnormal ^{99m}Tc-pyrophos-

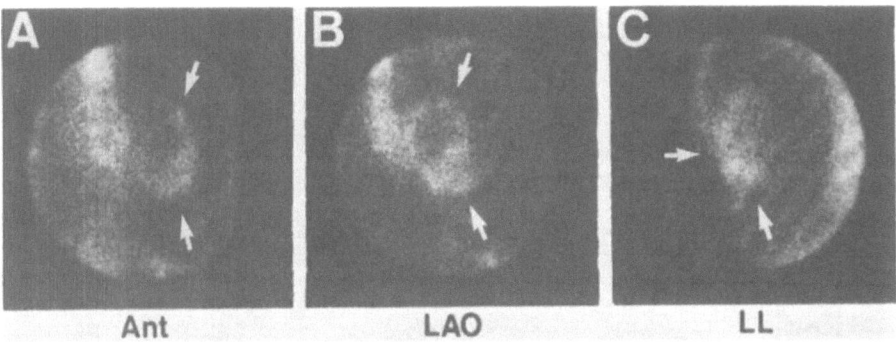

Figure 7-7. A large anterolateral "doughnut" ⁹⁹ᵐTc-pyrophosphate myocardial infarct is shown. These infarcts are approximately twice as large as «nondoughnut" anterior or anterolateral infarcts.

phate myocardial scintigram since dead and dying cells are the primary cell types that take up abnormal amounts of ⁹⁹ᵐTc-pyrophosphate following experimental and clinical myocardial infarcts [6, 7, 11, 12, 15, 18, 26].

There are two distinctive ⁹⁹ᵐTc-pyrophosphate scintigraphic patterns that deserve additional comment. One is the "doughnut" ⁹⁹ᵐTc-pyrophosphate myocardial scintigram [6, 7, 15, 19] and the "persistently abnormal" ⁹⁹ᵐTc-pyrophosphate myocardial scintigrams [26, 30]. "Doughnut" ⁹⁹ᵐTc-pyrophosphate myocardial scintigrams develop when very proximal coronary occlusion (usually left anterior descending coronary artery occlusion or severe narrowing) results in an acute anterolateral myocardial infarct (Figure 7-7). These infarcts are approximately twice as large as "nondoughnut" anterolateral myocardial infarcts; there is also a significant incidence of acquired left ventricular failure as a complication [19]. The central portion of the "doughnut" lesion is a region into which almost no coronary flow enters, no calcium is delivered and few polymorphonuclear leukocytes migrate within the first few hours after infarction. However, many hours to several days after the event, most patients and experimental animals demonstrate at least partial filling in of the central defect as collateral flow reaches central areas of damage [19]. The "persistently abnormal" ⁹⁹ᵐTc-pyrophosphate myocardial scintigrams appear to represent chronic and ongoing severe myocardial cellular injury from chronic myocardial ischemia [26] and the "persistently abnormal" myocardial scintigram correlates with clinical behaviour usually typified by severe and limiting angina pectoris and/or marked congestive heart failure [26, 31]. Thus, it may be that the "persistently abnormal" ⁹⁹ᵐTc-pyrophosphate myocardial scintigram will be an important prognostic marker of progressive chronic myocardial ischemia but larger numbers of patients from different institutions need to be studied to establish this point with more certainty.

168

^{99M}TC-PYP INFARCT SIZING IN DOGS

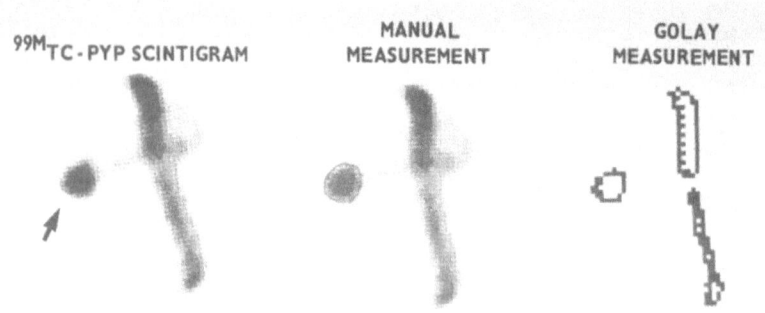

^{99M}TC-PYP SCINTIGRAM   MANUAL MEASUREMENT   GOLAY MEASUREMENT

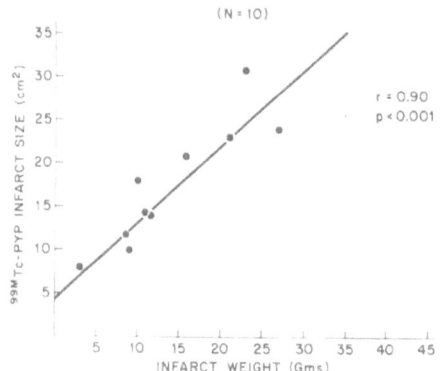

CORRELATION BETWEEN ^{99M}Tc-PYP SCINTIGRAPHIC INFARCT SIZE
AND HISTOLOGICAL INFARCT SIZE (cm^2)
(N = 10)

r = 0.90
p < 0.001

^{99m}Tc-PYP INFARCT SIZE (cm^2)

INFARCT WEIGHT (Gms)

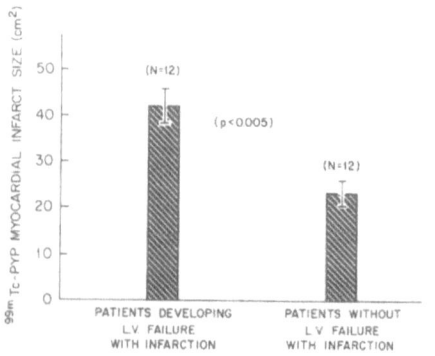

^{99m}Tc-PYP MYOCARDIAL INFARCT SIZE IN PATIENTS WITH
ACUTE ANTERIOR OR ANTEROLATERAL INFARCTS
(N = 24)

^{99m}Tc-PYP MYOCARDIAL INFARCT SIZE (cm^2)

(N=12)   (p<0005)   (N=12)

PATIENTS DEVELOPING
LV FAILURE
WITH INFARCTION

PATIENTS WITHOUT
LV FAILURE
WITH INFARCTION

It is possible to size acute transmural anterior or anterolateral myocardial infarcts with this imaging technique presently (Figure 7-8)[13, 14, 17]. However, it is not presently possible to size accurately acute inferior and nontransmural (subendocardial) myocardial infarcts with this imaging technique using two-dimensional measurements of infarct size. The explanation for this is that the true extent of inferior and nontransmural myocardial infarcts cannot be seen in two-dimensions and it will require three-dimensional imaging approaches to accurately size these lesions. Studies performed by Keyes et al. have suggested that tomographic imaging with gamma emitters may allow one to accurately size infarcts in these locations [32]. As commercially available tomographic systems become available, it will be interesting to determine how accurately inferior and subendocardial infarcts may be sized with ^{99m}Tc-pyrophosphate myocardial imaging techniques.

In summary, studies performed at our institution and elsewhere have indicated that ^{99m}Tc-pyrophosphate myocardial scintigraphy is a sensitive means to detect acute myocardial necrosis when the extent of irreversible cellular damage is at least 3 g of tissue. One has to pay proper attention to the appropriate imaging methodology and image within the proper time periods to obtain maximal sensitivity and specificity from this imaging technique. Further, one needs to keep in mind that trauma, infection, cardioversion, invasive tumor, etc. that result in acute myocardial necrosis may also produce abnormal ^{99m}Tc-pyrophosphate myocardial scintigrams [7, 11, 12, 15, 26]. Table 7-2 lists the clinical settings in which we believe ^{99m}Tc-pyrophosphate myocardial scintigraphy may be important in the detection of acute myocardial necrosis.

Figure 7-8. Upper panel: The method used for sizing ^{99m}Tc-pyrophosphate myocardial infarcts is shown. Computer processing of the scintigrams is utilized and then either manual outlining of the area of increased ^{99m}Tc-pyrophosphate uptake or computer measurements (such as the Golay measurement) are used to make ^{99m}Tc-pyrophosphate infarct size. *Middle panel:* The correlation between infarct size as measured by ^{99m}Tc-pyrophosphate myocardial scintigraphy and histological infarct weight in ten experimental animals with acute anterior or anterolateral transmural infarcts is shown. A close relationship between scintigraphic and histological infarct size for transmural anterior or anterolateral infarcts exist. *Bottom panel:* This figure demonstrates that patients with the largest ^{99m}Tc-pyrophosphate anterior or anterolateral transmural infarcts develop left ventricular failure as complications of their acute myocardial infarct. The bars represent mean values and the cross bars standard errors of the mean for the infarct sizes. Reproduced from Ref. [14] by permission.

Table 7-2. Clinical uses of ^{99m}Tc-pyrophosphate myocardial scintigrams to identify myocardial infarcts

Detect myocardial infarcts of 3 g or larger *	Often virtually essential to identifying presence or absence of myocardial infarct	May be helpful in future in predicting prognosis
Potentially all myocardial infarcts in man when myocardial imaging is performed between days 1 and 6 after onset of symptoms	Patients arriving at hospital 16 hr or later after onset of pain Patients with conduction abnormalities on ECG (especially left bundle branch block) Patients with acute subendocardial myocardial infarcts Patients undergoing coronary artery revascularization Patients with ECG evidence of old infarcts To detect in-hospital infarct extension	Sizing acute myocardial infarcts (progress has been made in this area, but ultimately depends on the availability of three-dimensional infarct sizing capability – either with tomographic cameras or suitable computer assisted reconstruction techniques) Persistently positive ^{99m}Tc-pyrophosphate myocardial scintigrams (present data suggest that at least some patients with persistently positive tests for 3 months or longer have unfavorable clinical courses subsequently

* Requires using serial myocardial imaging between days 1 and 6 after symptoms suggestive of infarction and the availability of scintigraphic cameras of high resolution. One must be certain that excessive free ^{99m}Tc-pertechnetate is not present in the ^{99m}Tc-pyrophosphate injectate

REFERENCES

1. Bonte FJ, Parkey RW, Graham KD, et al.: A new method for radionuclide imaging of acute myocardial infarcts. Radiology 110:473, 1974.
2. Parkey RW, Bonte FJ, Meyer SL, et al.: A new method for radionuclide imaging of acute myocardial infarction in humans. Circulation 50:540, 1974.
3. Willerson JT, Parkey RW, Bonte FJ, et al.: Technetium stannous pyrophosphate myocardial scintigrams in patients with chest pain of varying etiology. Circulation 51:1046, 1975.
4. Willerson JT, Parkey RW, Bonte FJ, et al.: Acute subendocardial myocardial infarcts detected by technetium-99m stannous pyrophosphate myocardial scintigrams. Circulation 51:436, 1975.
5. Willerson JT, Parkey RW, Bonte FJ, et al.: Technetium-99m stannous pyrophosphate myocardial scintigraphy: A new method of proven value for the diagnosis and localization of acute myocardial infarcts and for the detection of infarct extension in patients. Tex Med 72:61, 1976.
6. Buja LM, Parkey RW, Dees JH, et al.: Morphologic correlated of technetium-99m stannous pyrophosphate imaging of acute myocardial infarcts in dogs. Circulation 52:596, 1975.
7. Buja LM, Parkey RW, Stokely EM, et al.: Pathophysiology of technetium-99m stannous pyrophosphate and thallium-201 scintigraphy of acute anterior myocardial infarcts in dogs. J Clin Invest 57:1508, 1976.

8. Platt MR, Parkey RW, Willerson JT, et al.: Technetium-99m stannous pyrophosphate myocardial scintigrams in the recognition of myocardial infarction in patients undergoing coronary artery revascularization. Ann Thorac Surg 21:311, 1976.

9. Platt MR, Mills LJ, Parkey RW, et al.: Perioperative myocardial infarction diagnosed by technetium-99m stannous pyrophosphate myocardial scintigrams. Circulation 54 (Suppl III):24, 1976.

10. Donsky MS, Curry GC, Parkey RW, et al.: Unstable angina pectoris: Clinical, angiographic, and myocardial scintigraphic observations. Br Heart J 38:257, 1976.

11. Pugh BR, Buja LM, Parkey RW, et al.: Cardioversion and its potential role in the production of " false positive " technetium-99m stannous pyrophosphate myocardial scintigrams. Circulation 54:399, 1976.

12. Harford W, Weinberg M, Buja LM, et al.: Positive technetium-99m stannous pyrophosphate myocardial scintigram in a patient with carcinoma of the lung. Radiology 122:747, 1977.

13. Stokely EM, Buja Lm, Lewis SE, et al.: Measurement of acute myocardial infarcts in dogs with technetium-99m stannous pyrophosphate scintigrams. J Nucl Med 17:1, 1976.

14. Willerson JT, Parkey RW, Stokely EM, et al.: Infarct sizing with technetium-99m stannous pyrophosphate scintigraphy in dogs and man; the relationship between scintigraphic and precordial mapping estimates of infarct size in patients. Cardiovasc Res 11:291, 1977.

15. Buja LM, Tofe AJ, Kulharni PV, et al.: Sites and mechanisms of localization of technetium-99m phosphorus radiopharmaceuticals in acute myocardial infarcts and other tissues. J Clin Invest 60:724, 1977.

16. Parkey RW, Bonte FJ, Stokely EM, et al.: Acute myocardial infarction imaged with technetium-99m stannous pyrophosphate and thallium 201: a clinical evaluation. J Nucl Med 17:771, 1976.

17. Lewis M, Buja LM, Saffer S, et al.: Experimental infarct sizing utilizing computer processing and a three-dimensional model. Science 197:167, 1977.

18. Poliner LR, Buja LM, Parkey RW, et al.: Clinicopathologic findings in 52 patients studied by technetium-99m stannous pyrophosphate myocardial scintigrams. Circulation 59:257, 1979.

19. Rude R, Parkey RW, Bonte FJ, et al.: Clinical implications of the "doughnut" pattern of uptake in technetium-99m stannous pyrophosphate myocardial scintigrams in patients with acute myocardial infarction. Circulation 59:721, 1979.

20. Shen AC, and Jennings RB: Myocardial calcium and magnesium in acute ischemic injury. Am J Pathol 67:417, 1972.

21. D'Agostino AN: An electron microscopic study of cardiac necrosis produced by 9 a-fluorocortisol and sodium phosphate. Am J Pathol 45:633, 1964.

22. Perez LA: Clinical experience: technetium 99m labeled phosphates in myocardial imaging. Clin Nucl Med 1:2, 1976.

23. Bruno FP, Cobb FR, Rivas F, et al.: Evaluation of ^{99m}technetium stannous pyrophosphate as an imaging agent in acute myocardial infarction. Circulation 54:71, 1976.

24. Zaret BL, DiCola VC, Donabedian RK, et al.: Dual radionuclide study of myocardial infarction. Relationship between myocardial uptake of potassium-43, technetium-99m stannous pyrophosphate, regional myocardial blood flow and creatine phosphokinase depletion. Circulation 53:422, 1976.

25. Poliner LR, Buja LM, Parkey RW, et al.: Comparative evaluation of several different noninvasive methods of infarct sizing during experimental myocardial infarction. J Nucl Med 18:517, 1977.

26. Buja LM, Poliner L, Parkey RW, et al.: Clinicopathologic findings in patients with persistently positive technetium-99m stannous pyrophosphate myocardial scintigrams and myocytolytic degeneration after acute myocardial infarction. Circulation 56:1016, 1977.

27. Falkoff M, Parkey RW, Bonte FJ, et al.: Technetium-99m Stannous pyrophosphate myocardial scintigraphy: the need for serial imaging to detect myocardial infarcts in patients. Clin Cardiol 1:163, 1978.

28. Rude RE, Rubin HS, Stone MJ, et al.: Radioimmunoassay of serum creatine kinase B isoenzyme: Correlation with technetium-99m stannous pyrophosphate myocardial scintigraphy in the diagnosis of acute myocardial infarction. Am J Med 68:405, 1980).

29. Pulido JI, Parkey RW, Lewis SE, et al.: Acute subendocardial myocardial infarction: Its detection by technetium-99m stannous pyrophosphate myocardial scintigraphy. Clin Nucl Med 5:191, 1980.
30. Willerson JT, Parkey RW, Buja LM, et al.: Technetium-99m stannous pyrophosphate "hot spot" imaging to detect acute myocardial infarcts. In: Nuclear cardiology, p 139, Willerson JT, ed. Philadelphia: F.A. Davis, 1979.
31. Lyons KP, Olson HG, et al: Persistence of an abnormal pattern of ^{99m}Tc pyrophosphate myocardial scintigraphy following acute myocardial infarction. Clin Nucl Med 1:253, 1976.
32. Keyes JW Jr, Orlandea N, Heetclerks WJ, et al.: The humongotron – a scintillation camera transaxial tomograph. J Nucl Med 18:381, 1977.

8. COMPARATIVE VALUE AND LIMITATIONS OF THALLIUM-201 AND TECHNETIUM-99m-PYROPHOSPHATE MYOCARDIAL IMAGING IN ACUTE MYOCARDIAL INFARCTION

FRANS J. TH. WACKERS, ROBERT W. PARKEY, FREDERICK J. BONTE and JAMES T. WILLERSON

Comparing the results of ^{201}Tl and ^{99m}Tc-pyrophosphate myocardial imaging in patients with acute myocardial infarction, it is evident that both imaging techniques provide different information and each has its own advantages and disadvantages. For the practical application in the coronary care unit, it is essential to realize that each method yields its best results at different time intervals after onset of myocardial infarction (Figure 8-1).

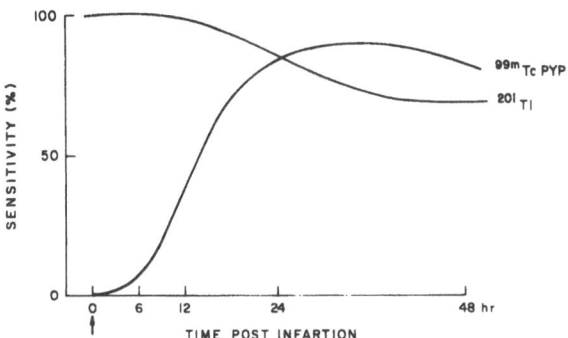

Figure 8-1. Schematic representation of the overall relative sensitivity of ^{201}Tl and ^{99m}Tc-pyrophosphate scintigraphy to detect acute myocardial infarction in relation to onset of infarction. Whereas during the first 6–10 hr after infarction the sensitivity of ^{201}Tl scintigraphy is close to 100%, this declines to 75% after the second day of infarction. Using ^{99m}Tc-pyrophosphate scintigraphy 90% of all infarcts will be detected between 24 and 48 hr of infarction.

Thallium-201 myocardial imaging is highly sensitive during the acute phase after infarction[1, 2], whereas ^{99m}Tc-pyrophosphate imaging yields the best results during the subacute phase (24–72 hr) after infarction[3].

In patients with large infarcts the scintiscans will be abnormal in all instances by ^{201}Tl imaging[1] and also in most patients by ^{99m}Tc-pyrophosphate imaging. In a rare patient very large infarction, the ^{99m}Tc-pyrophosphate studies may be negative in the initial study since the radiopharmaceutical did not reach the infarcted myocardium due to insufficient and/or delayed development of collateral flow into the area of irreversible damage. In the latter patients serial imaging with ^{99m}Tc-pyrophosphate is of utmost importance to demonstrate the infarction. This occurs rarely, however (<5% of patients studied).

The sensitivity of ^{201}Tl scintigraphy to detect small (<4 g) and/or nontransmural infarcts is less than for large infarcts. Myocardial infarcts smaller than 3 g in size will also not be consistently detected by ^{99m}Tc-pyrophosphate scintigraphy, but there is no difference in the sensitivity of ^{99m}Tc-pyrophosphate in the detection of transmural and nontransmural infarcts. It is in the subgroup of patients with small and nontransmural infarcts that correct timing of the study is particularly crucial to obtain optimal results. Since, in these patients, both imaging techniques are less sensitive, dual imaging with ^{201}Tl and ^{99m}Tc-pyrophosphate may be extremely helpful, if the clinical suspicion for infarction is high.

Another disadvantage of ^{201}Tl myocardial imaging is that no distinction can be made between old and new infarction. In the latter situation ^{99m}Tc-pyrophosphate imaging will be of diagnostic importance. However, a subgroup of patients (approximately 10-20%) may demonstrate persistently abnormal ^{99m}Tc-pyrophosphate scintiscans after previous myocardial infarction; this pattern appears to be a marker of ongoing ischemic damage in these patients [4].

The scintigraphic studies by each method are not just complementary, but provide different pathophysiologic information. A ^{201}Tl myocardial perfusion defect may represent either myocardial ischemia [5] or myocardial necrosis [1, 6], whereas myocardial accumulation of ^{99m}Tc-pyrophosphate indicates irreversible myocardial damage [7–9].

The size and pattern of scintigraphic abnormalities by both imaging techniques may provide important information with regard to prognosis in patients with acute myocardial infarction. Table 8-1 lists the clinically relevant characteristics for ^{201}Tl and ^{99m}Tc-pyrophosphate myocardial imaging.

In summary, both imaging techniques provide clinically important answers concerning the presence of acute infarction, its location and its extent. The selection of one or the other imaging technique is mainly dependent on the timing of scintigraphy after acute myocardial infarction and whether or not the patient sustained a previous infarction. Under certain circumstances scintigraphy with both imaging agents consecutively may be beneficial and enhance diagnostic accuracy, as will be discussed in chapter 9.

In comparison to the conventional diagnostic methods such as the electrocardiogram and serum enzyme determinations, myocardial imaging provides different and additional information in patients with acute myocardial infarcts. The imaging techniques should not be envisaged as competitive but rather each method should be employed with an understanding of its own

Table 8-1. Characteristics of ^{201}Tl and ^{99m}Tc-pyrophosphate myocardial imaging in acute myocardial infarction

	Thallium-201	^{99m}Tc-pyrophosphate
Scintigraphic pattern	"Cold spot"	"Hot spot"
Highest sensitivity relative to onset of infarction	<6 hr	24-72 hr
Imaging p. injection	5 min	1½-3 hr
Size infarct	Percentage total LV	Area cm^2
Location infarct	Detailed, accurate	accurate
False negatives	After 24 hr	<12-24 hr > 7 days
	Small infarction (<4.9 g) Nontransmural infarction LV hypertrophy	Small infarction (<3 g)
False positives	Unstable angina	Unstable angina
	Variant angina	Persistantly positive after previous myocardial infarct
	Previous infarct	Non-ischemic myocardial damage
	Asymmetrical septal hypertrophy	

particular strengths and limitations. Although at present an extensive experience already exists with myocardial imaging in patients with acute chest pain syndromes, the techniques are still relatively new. It can be expected that our insight into the clinical application has to be updated and better defined in the near future on the basis of new and broader clinical experience. On the other hand, present limitations of planar myocardial imaging, caused by anatomic overlap of normal and abnormal myocardium, can be expected to be overcome by further development of computer techniques and imaging systems capable of three dimensional analysis that may be used with single photon emission tomography [10–12].

In addition, it can be anticipated that new radionuclides will be developed allowing evaluation of more specific aspects of myocardial pathophysiology than is presently possible.

REFERENCES

1. Wackers FJT, Busemann Sokole E, Samson G, van der Schoot JB, Lie KI, Liem KL, Wellens HJJ: Value and limitations of thallium-201 scintigraphy in the acute phase of myocardial infarction. N Engl J Med 295:1-5, 1976.
2. Wackers FJT, van der Schoot J, Busemann Sokole E, Samson G, van Niftrik GJC, Durrer D, Wellens HJJ: Noninvasive visualization of acute myocardial infarction in man with thallium-201. Br Heart J 37:741-744, 1975.
3. Parkey RW, Bonte FJ, Meyer SL, Atkins JM, Curry GL, Stokely EM, Willerson JT: A new method for radionuclide imaging of acute myocardial infarction in humans. Circulation 50:540-546, 1974.

4. Buja LM, Poliner LR, Parkey RW, Pulido JI, Hutcheson D, Platt MR, Mills LJ, Bonte FJ, Willerson JT: Clinicopathologic study of persistently positive technetium-99m stannous pyrophosphate myocardial scintigrams and myocytolytic degeneration after myocardial infarction. Circulation 56: 1016-1023, 1977.

5. Wackers FJT, Lie KI, Liem KL, Busemann Sokole E, Samson G, van der Schoot JB, Durrer D: Thallium-201 scintigraphy in unstable angina pectoris. Circulation 57:738-742, 1978.

6. Wackers FJT, Becker AE, Samson G, Busemann Sokole E, van der Schoot JB, Vet AJTM, Lie KI, Durrer D, Wellens H: Location and size of acute transmural myocardial infarction estimated from thallium-201 scintiscans. Circulation 56:72-78, 1977.

7. Buja LM, Parkey RW, Stokely EM, Bonte FJ, Willerson JT: Pathophysiology of technetium-99m stannous pyrophosphate and thallium-201 scintigraphy of acute anterior myocardial infarcts in dogs. J Clin Invest 57:1508-1522, 1976.

8. Buja LM, Tofe AJ, Kulkarni PV, Mukherjee A, Parkey RW, Francis MD, Bonte FJ, Willerson JT: Sites and mechanisms of localization of technetium-99m phosphorus radiopharmaceuticals in acute myocardial infarcts and other tissues. J Clin Invest 60:724-740, 1977.

9. Poliner LR, Buja LM, Parkey RW, Bonte FJ, Willerson JT: Clinicopathologic findings in 52 patients studied by technetium-99m stannous pyrophosphate myocardial scintigraphy. Circulation 59:257-267, 1979.

10. Vogel RA, Kirch D, LeFree M, Steele P: A new method of multiplanar emission tomography using a seven pinhole collimator and an Anger scintillation camera. J Nucl Med 19:648-654, 1978.

11. Holman BL, Hill TC, Wynne J, Lovett RD, Zimmerman RE, Smith EM: Single-photon transaxial emission computed tomography of the heart in normal subjects and in patients with infarction. J Nucl Med 20:736-740, 1979.

12. Keyes JW, Jr, Leonard PF, Brody SL, Svetkoff DJ, Rogers L, Lucchesi BR: Myocardial infarct quantification in the dog by single photon emission computed tomography. Circulation 58:227-232, 1978.

9. DUAL IMAGING IN ACUTE MYOCARDIAL INFARCTION

FRANS J. TH. WACKERS, ELLINOR BUSEMAN SOKOLE,
JAN VAN DER SCHOOT, GERARD SAMSON, SAMUEL LEWIS, ROBERT W.
PARKEY and JAMES T. WILLERSON

Acute myocardial infarction can be visualized by accumulation of radionuclides in the myocardium in two general ways. On one hand, the radionuclide
may be concentrated maximally in the normal myocardium and almost absent
in the region of the infarction. Thallium-201 is such an imaging agent and
the zone of infarction is demonstrated as a "cold spot" [1]. Alternatively, the
radioactive tracer may be maximally accumulated in the infarcted region. As
described in the previous chapters, ^{99m}Tc-pyrophosphate is a prototype of
imaging agents that displays the region of infarction as a "hot spot" [2].

In the present chapter, the clinical application of combined imaging with
both radiopharmaceuticals will be discussed.

Dual imaging with ^{201}Tl and ^{99m}Tc-pyrophosphate can be completed within
a 2–3 hr time period. Because of the low photon energy of ^{201}Tl this imaging
agent should be employed first. Immediately after completion of three views

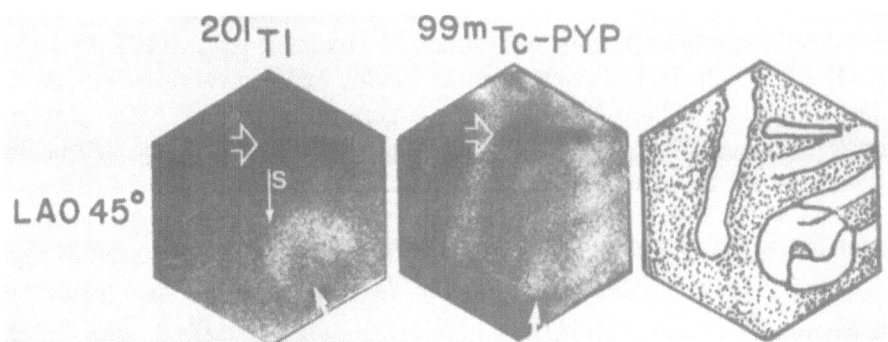

Figure 9-1. Method of determining right ventricular involvement with dual myocardial imaging.
During both studies a lead marker is taped to the chest wall within the field of view (open arrow).
This spatial reference allows accurate superimposition of schematic drawings of the images. The
^{201}Tl image (left) shows an inferoposterior defect (solid arrow) in the 45° left-anterior-oblique
(LAO) view. The site of the interventricular septum(s) separates the area of right and left
ventricle. The ^{99m}Tc-pyrophosphate image (middle) shows 3+ accumulation of the inferior wall
(solid arrow). Superimposition of schematic drawings of both images (right) shows that the
abnormal ^{99m}Tc-pyrophosphate accumulation is located lateral to the interventricular septum and
is therefore in the left ventricle. Because no uptake is seen anterior to the interventricular
septum, right ventricular involvement is not present. Reproduced with permission from
Ref. [18].

on the 80 keV X-ray peak (which usually will take 20-30 min when 2mCi of ^{201}Tl is used) ^{99m}Tc-pyrophosphate can be injected. Subsequently, imaging on the 140 keV energy peak of ^{99m}Tc can be started after $1\frac{1}{2}$ to 2 hr. Obviously there is scatter from ^{201}Tl radiation present on these images, but because of the higher photon energy of ^{99m}Tc and larger injected dose (15 mCi) the interpretation of the images is unimpaired.

By the use of a spatial marker on the chest wall the two studies can be superimposed (Figure 9-1). Berger et al. [3] compared, in a phantom study, the size of a negative image by ^{201}Tl with the size of a positive image by ^{99m}Tc-pyrophosphate of the same object. This comparative study revealed a minimal difference between the size of an area, whether visualized with ^{201}Tl or ^{99m}Tc-pyrophosphate. Thus, the imaging characteristics of the two radionuclides allow superimposition of the images.

DUAL IMAGING IN THE SUBACUTE PHASE OF INFARCTION

As outlined in the previous chapter, both imaging techniques provide different information. Each method yields its best results at a different time interval after acute myocardial infarction (Figures 8-1 and 9-2). Thallium-201 is highly sensitive during the initial acute phase, whereas ^{99m}Tc-pyrophosphate yields the best results during the subacute phase. During the subacute phase of infarction the sensitivity of both methods is not optimal. From a diagnostic viewpoint, the sensitivity to detect acute infarction may be enhanced when both imaging techniques are employed sequentially. Parkey et al. [4] studied 26 patients suspected of having acute myocardial infarcts by dual imaging. Thallium-201 imaging was performed prior to ^{99m}Tc-pyrophosphate imaging. Three views (anterior, left-anterior-oblique and left-lateral) were obtained using a single crystal camera. Of the 26 patients, 24 had acute myocardial infarcts by enzyme studies and electrocardiographic changes; 19 had transmural infarctions. The mean time of imaging after onset of chest pain was 4 days in this study. Of the 24 patients with acute myocardial infarcts all patients had abnormal ^{201}Tl scans, 22 patients (92%) had positive ^{99m}Tc-pyrophosphate scans. However, both patients with negative ^{99m}Tc-pyrophosphate scans had been positive 4 and 7 days earlier. The site of ^{201}Tl defects in all patients localized the infarcts correctly when compared to electrocardiographic location. This was also the case in 20 of the 22 patients with positive ^{99m}Tc-pyrophosphate scans. The size of the ^{201}Tl defects was grossly equal to the positive area on the ^{99m}Tc-pyrophosphate images in seven patients; in 15 patients (68%) the ^{201}Tl defect was definitely larger and in two patients the ^{201}Tl defect appeared to be slightly smaller than its ^{99m}Tc-pyrophosphate counterpart. The same investigators [5] compared the relative

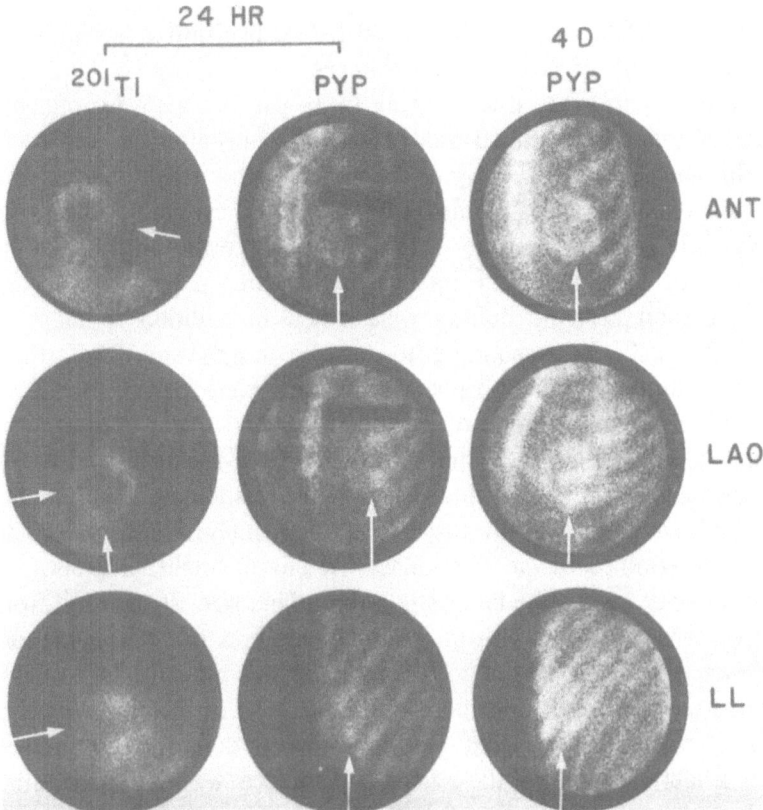

Figure 9-2. Dual imaging with ^{201}Tl and ^{99m}Tc-pyrophosphate in a patient with acute anteroseptal myocardial infarction. At 24 hr after onset of chest pain the ^{201}Tl study is clearly abnormal: defect of the anteroapical segment and diminished uptake in the septum. The ^{99m}Tc-pyrophosphate image obtained the same day is only vaguely positive. Four days after infarction the ^{99m}Tc-pyrophosphate study is markedly positive, demonstrating a "doughnut" pattern. This study clearly demonstrates that myocardial imaging with ^{201}Tl and ^{99m}Tc-pyrophosphate yields best results at different time intervals after acute infarction.

accumulation of ^{201}Tl and ^{99m}Tc-pyrophosphate at the tissue level in experimental acute myocardial infarction in dogs. Their results confirmed the almost linear relationship between myocardial blood flow and ^{201}Tl accumulation reported by others [6, 7]. On the other hand, ^{99m}Tc-pyrophosphate accumulation occurred maximally in the peripheral regions of the infarction, where residual myocardial blood flow existed. This study indicated that considerable overlap of ^{201}Tl activity with areas of intense ^{99m}Tc-pyrophosphate uptake may be present. It was postulated that passive transport of ^{201}Tl across endothelium in these areas occurred, followed by tissue sequestration in the absence of active membrane transport by myocardial cells. These findings are in agreement with our results in post mortem studies in man (chapter 6), that demonstrated the presence of residual ^{201}Tl activity in areas of necrosis. It is at present unknown if this reflects the actual tissue distribution during scintigraphy or is the result of post mortem changes.

Henning et al. [9] performed dual imaging in 35 patients with documented acute myocardial infarction within 1-5 days (earliest 22 hr) after onset of acute symptoms. In all patients three views: anterior, left-anterior-oblique and left-lateral were obtained using a single crystal gamma camera. All patients demonstrated ^{201}Tl perfusion defects; in 33 (94%) this correspondeded to the electrocardiographic location of the infarct. In the three patients with prior myocardial infarction separate defects were noted in addition to areas of decreased ^{201}Tl uptake corresponding to new Q waves and ST-T wave changes. Technetium-99m-pyrophosphate scintiscans were positive in 30 of 35 patients (86%) and the location of uptake corresponded to the electrocardiographic site of infarct in 23 of the 30 patients (77%). The five negative ^{99m}Tc-pyrophosphate scintiscans included two of four patients with nontransmural infarcts. The patients with negative ^{99m}Tc-pyrophosphate scans had biochemically (determined by creatine kinase CK curve) smaller infarcts than those with positive scans. In the latter study the infarct size, as assessed from the CK curves, was correlated with the planimetered area of ^{99m}Tc-pyrophosphate uptake on the scintiscans. A good correlation was obtained for anterior wall infarctions ($r = 0.90$) but only fair for inferior wall infarction ($r = 0.64$). The authors of this study felt that the size of ^{201}Tl defects could not be planimetered reliably. Therefore, the size of ^{201}Tl defects was expressed semiquantitatively as "small", "medium" and "large". These three groups each had significantly different mean values for CK infarct size. However, when ^{201}Tl size was compared to ^{99m}Tc-pyrophosphate size wide range of overlap among the various groups occurred. The area of decreased ^{201}Tl uptake exceeded that of myocardial ^{99m}Tc-pyrophosphate uptake in one-third of the patients. The authors concluded that ^{201}Tl imaging is more accurate than ^{99m}Tc-pyrophosphate imaging in detecting and localizing acute infarction and that ^{99m}Tc-pyrophosphate may fail to detect small infarcts.

Berger et al. [3] evaluated dual imaging with ^{201}Tl and ^{99m}Tc-pyrophosphate in 80 patients with documented acute myocardial infarction. These authors obtained two views (anterior and left-anterior-oblique) using a computerized multicrystal gamma camera. The ^{99m}Tc-pyrophosphate images were obtained 2--12 days after onset of chest pain (mean 4.5 days ± 0.3 SEM), whereas ^{201}Tl images were obtained within the first 14 days of infarction (mean 6.4 ± 0.4 days), but only two patients were studied within 24 hours of infarction . The results are shown in Figure 9-3. The combined sensitivity of ^{201}Tl and ^{99m}Tc-pyrophosphate imaging for infarct detection was 100%. However, ^{201}Tl imaging alone detected 73 of 80 patients (91%) and ^{99m}Tc-pyrophosphate imaging 76 of 80 patients (95%). All 29 patients with anterior infarction had

DUAL NUCLIDE IMAGE SENSITIVITY IN ACUTE MI

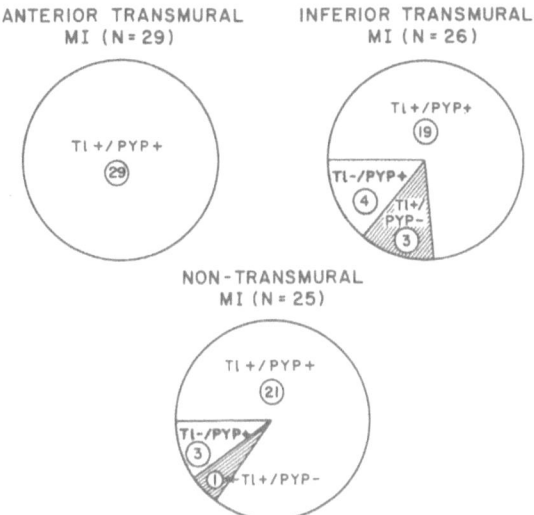

Figure 9-3. Sensitivity of ^{201}Tl and ^{99m}Tc-pyrophosphate images in patients with acute myocardial infarction. All patients had positive images with at least one of the two imaging methods. All patients with transmural anterior wall infarction had positive images by both methods. Reproduced with permission from Berger et al. [3, 20].

SIZE OF INFARCT REGION ON ^{201}Tl AND
PYP IMAGES IN TRANSMURAL MI

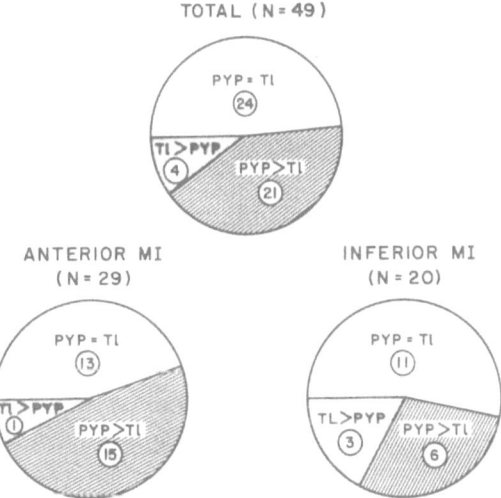

Figure 9-4. Diagrammatic display of incidence of size discordance between infarct regions on ^{201}Tl and ^{99m}Tc-pyrophosphate images in patients with transmural myocardial infarction. The predominant finding is that the area of increased ^{99m}Tc-pyrophosphate is substantially larger than the area of decreased ^{201}Tl myocardial activity. Reproduced with permission from Berger et al. [3, 20].

abnormal images by both methods. However, only 73% of 26 patients with inferior or lateral infarction and 84% of the remaining 25 patients with nontransmural infarction had dual positive images. Nine of 11 patients with false negative results by either imaging technique sustained relative small infarcts according to peak CK activity. Thallium-201 images correctly localized the site of acute transmural myocardial infarction in all patients with positive images, while ^{99m}Tc-pyrophosphate localized the site of infarction correctly in 93% of the patients with an abnormal image. Comparison of the visual impression of the size of the image infarcts revealed size discordance in

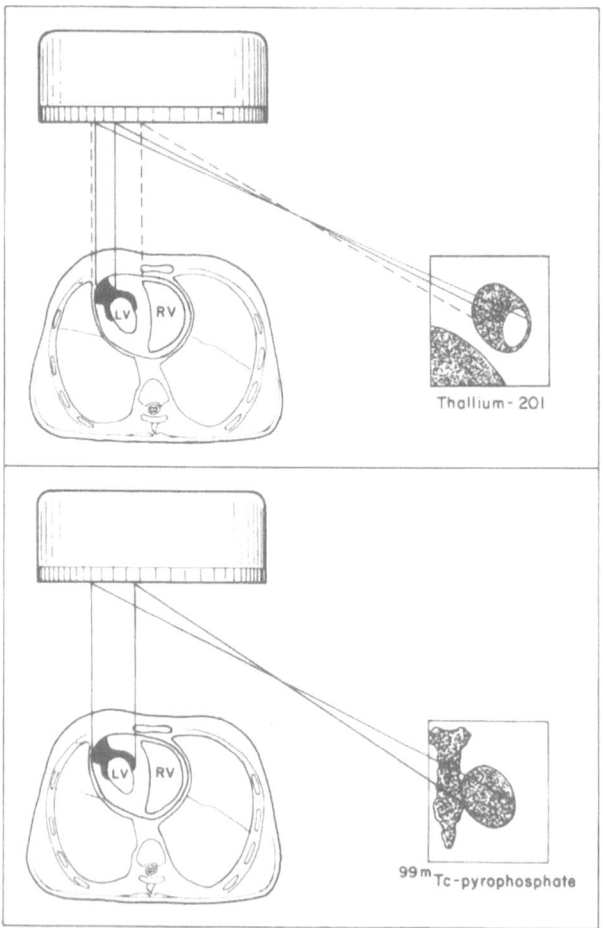

Figure 9-5. Diagrammatic explanation of reason for size discordance between ^{201}Tl and ^{99m}Tc-pyrophosphate infarct regions. Transverse section through chest at level of left ventricle is depicted with scintillation detector above and the images displayed to the right. Solid lines represent **edges** of infarct as detected by imaging; broken lines represent the outer margins of normal left ventricle as seen with ^{201}Tl. Myocardial infarction is black zone. See text. Reproduced with permission from Berger et al. [3, 20].

25 of 49 patients, who had positive images by both techniques (Figure 9-4). The ^{99m}Tc-pyrophosphate images showed larger infarcts in 21 of 49 patients. The ^{201}Tl defects were larger than the ^{99m}Tc-pyrophosphate area of uptake only in four patients with previous myocardial infarction. Since the timing of ^{201}Tl scintigraphy in this study was relatively late after infarction, no major zone of ischemia was probably present. This may explain the difference with the result of Parkey et al [4] and Henning et al. [5], who found ^{201}Tl defects frequently to be larger than the ^{99m}Tc-pyrophosphate area of uptake in patients with acute infarction. Another attractive possible explanation suggested by Berger et al. [3] is shown in Figure 9-5. At post mortem, myocardial infarction frequently displays a greater subendocardial extension than in the transmural and epicardial layers. Therefore, on the basis of the tissue distribution the same infarct will be displayed differently by ^{201}Tl than by ^{99m}Tc-pyrophosphate. The projection of the ^{201}Tl defect will appear to be relatively small, being minimized by overlying normal myocardium; whereas the projection of ^{99m}Tc-pyrophosphate accumulation appears to be larger since the subendocardial zone is projected onto the same plane.

Summarizing, during the subacute phase of infarction both imaging techniques have decreased sensitivity. Technetium-99m-pyrophosphate does not detect consistently infarcts < 3 g. Thallium-201 has limited sensitivity in small (< 5 g) and/or nontransmural infarcts. It appears that the combination of the two methods particularly in equivocal cases provides more useful information than either alone. The sensitivity to detect acute myocardial infarction will be enhanced and clinically useful information concerning the size of the infarct can be obtained.

DUAL IMAGING FOR THE DETECTION OF RIGHT VENTRICULAR INVOLVEMENT IN ACUTE INFERIOR WALL INFARCTION

Right ventricular involvement in acute myocardial infarction is an important clinical entity to recognize. The clinical syndrome of right ventricular infarction was described in 1975 by Cohn et al. [9]. The initial description of this pathophysiologic event included data on six patients with acute myocardial infarcts with hypotension and frank shock manifesting disproportionately elevated right ventricular filling pressures and a favorable therapeutic response to volume expansion.

Although right ventricular infarction was initially considered a relatively rare phenomenon [10], more recent pathologic [11–13] and clinical studies [14–18] suggest that it may be relatively common in patients with inferior wall infarcts. Erhardt et al. [11, 12] reported an overall incidence of 43% in patients who died in the coronary care unit. More recently, Isner and

Roberts[10], reviewed autopsy findings in 236 patients with acute or healed myocardial infarcts. In this obviously selected material it was noted that right ventricular infarction occurred exclusively as a complication of posterior left ventricular infarction. In none of the patients with anterior wall infarction was the right ventricle involved, whereas this occurred in 33 (24%) of 139 patients with posterior wall infarcts. Furthermore, it was noted that right ventricular infarction occurred only when there was coexistent transmural infarction involving the left ventricular posterior wall *and* septum. It is of note that in this series of patients only one patient displayed the characteristics of predominant right ventricular failure.

The first noninvasive demonstration of right ventricular dysfunction in acute inferior wall infarction by gated radionuclide cardiac blood pool imaging was reported by Rigo et al.[14]. Sharpe et al.[15] combined gated cardiac blood pool imaging with ^{99m}Tc-pyrophosphate imaging to demonstrate right ventricular involvement. Both these studies were dealing with a limited and selected group of patients. The true prevalence and clinical relevance of right ventricular involvement was not assessed by these studies.

We performed ^{201}Tl and ^{99m}Tc-pyrophosphate imaging in 78 consecutive patients with electrocardiographic evidence of acute inferior wall infarction in order to evaluate the prevalence and clinical implications of right ventricular involvement[18]. There were 58 men and 20 women, the ages ranged from 43 to 80 yr (average 55 yr). Acute inferior wall myocardial infarction was documented in all patients by characteristic rise and fall or serum enzymes and the development of diagnostic new Q waves.

All patients were studied first with ^{201}Tl shortly after admission, within 20 hr (mean 10 hr) after onset of infarction. Pyrophosphate imaging was performed at least 24 hr after infarction (mean 32 hr). For both studies, three views were obtained: anterior and 45° left-anterior-oblique, with the patient supine and a left-lateral view with the patient lying on his right side. Because the left-anterior-oblique views were obtained with the patient in supine position and with 45° angulation of the camera detector, accurate repositioning of the patient, even on two consecutive days, could be done readily. During both scintigraphic studies lead markers were taped in the same place on the chest wall of each patient. These markers were within the field of view and provided spatial reference that allowed subsequent accurate superimposition of the images (Figure 9-1).

Right ventricular involvement was determined as follows

In the 45° left-anterior-oblique images the interventricular septum, as visualized with ^{201}Tl, separates the area of the right and left ventricle. A schematic

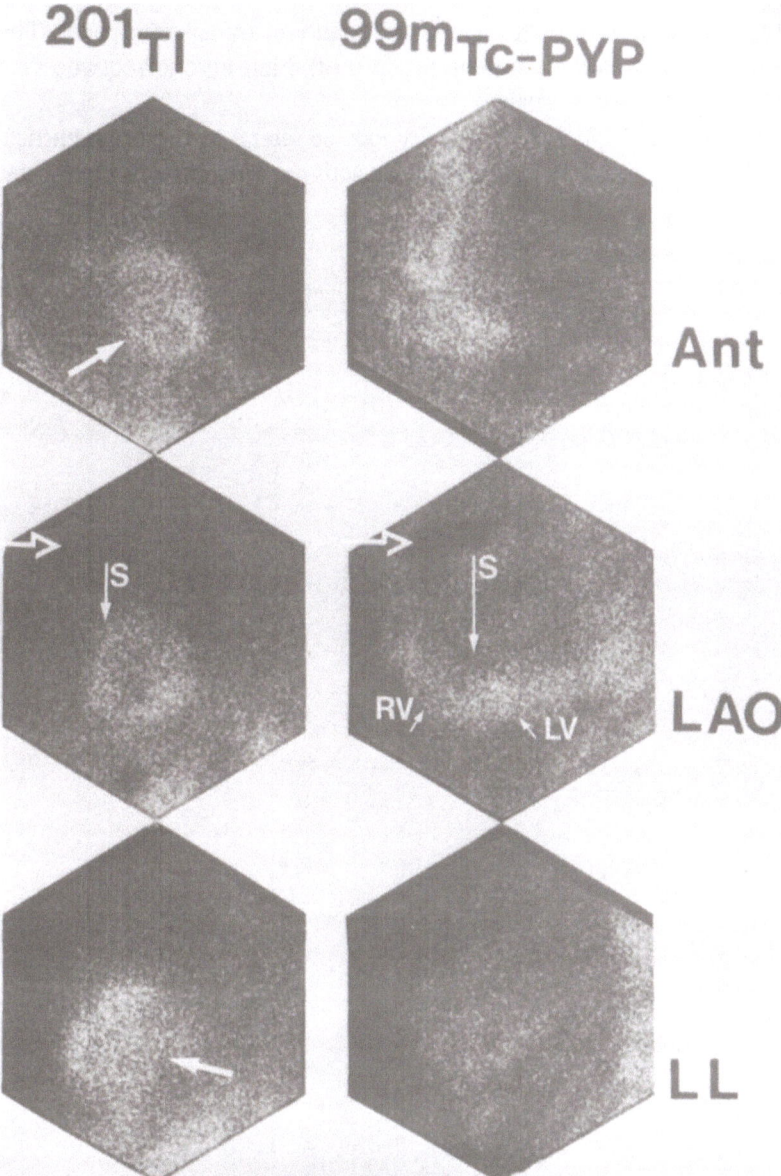

Figure 9-6. Dual imaging with ^{201}Tl and ^{99m}Tc-pyrophosphate in a patient with acute inferior wall infarction and right ventricular involvement. The patient was hemodynamically stable, without signs of right ventricular failure. The ^{201}Tl scintiscans show inferoposterior defect (arrows). The left anterior oblique (LAO) view in the ^{99m}Tc-pyrophosphate image shows typical horizontal plate-like activity of an inferior wall infarction. The spatial reference provided by the lead marker (open arrow) reveals that this activity also involves the right ventricle (RV). Abbreviations: S = septum; LV = left ventricle. Reproduced with permission from Ref. [18].

drawing of the ^{201}Tl image of the left ventricle and the position of the lead marker in the left-anterior-oblique view, was made on transparent paper. This drawing (Figure 9-1) was then superimposed on the left-anterior-oblique view of the ^{99m}Tc-pyrophosphate image.

Technetium-99m-pyrophosphate activity located lateral to the intraventricular septum was interpreted as left ventricular activity, whereas activity located

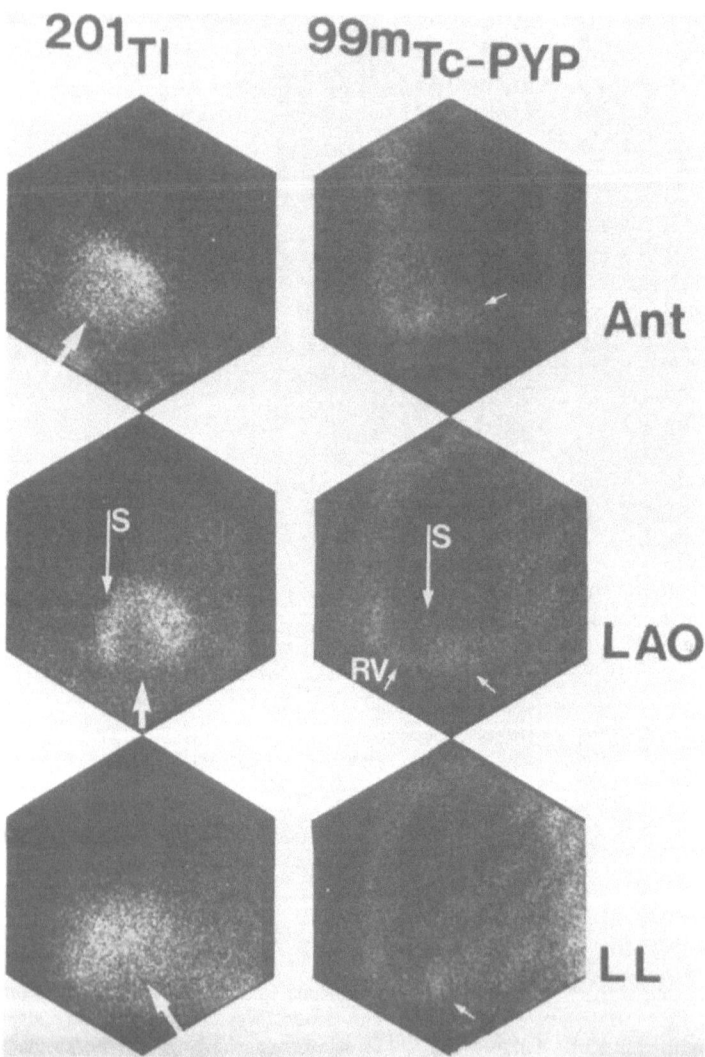

Figure 9-7. Thallium-201 and ^{99m}Tc-pyrophosphate studies in a patient with acute inferior wall infarction, without signs of right ventricular failure. A definite inferoposterior perfusion defect is visible on the ^{201}Tl scintiscans. The ^{99m}Tc-pyrophosphate left anterior oblique (LAO) image shows characteristic ω-shaped activity due to uptake in the interventricular septum (s) and in the right ventricle (rv) Reproduced with permission from Ref. [18].

anterior to the septum and adjacent to the activity of the sternum was interpreted as right ventricular activity.

Thallium-201 and ^{99m}Tc-pyrophosphate scintigraphy (Table 9-1)

All 78 patients showed inferoposterior wall perfusion defects on the ^{201}Tl scintiscans. The ^{99m}Tc-pyrophosphate scans showed abnormal focal left ventricular uptake at the inferior wall in 64 of 78 patients (82%). Superimposition of the left-anterior-oblique views with the lead markers as spatial reference points showed uptake of ^{99m}Tc-pyrophosphate in the right ventricle in 24 of

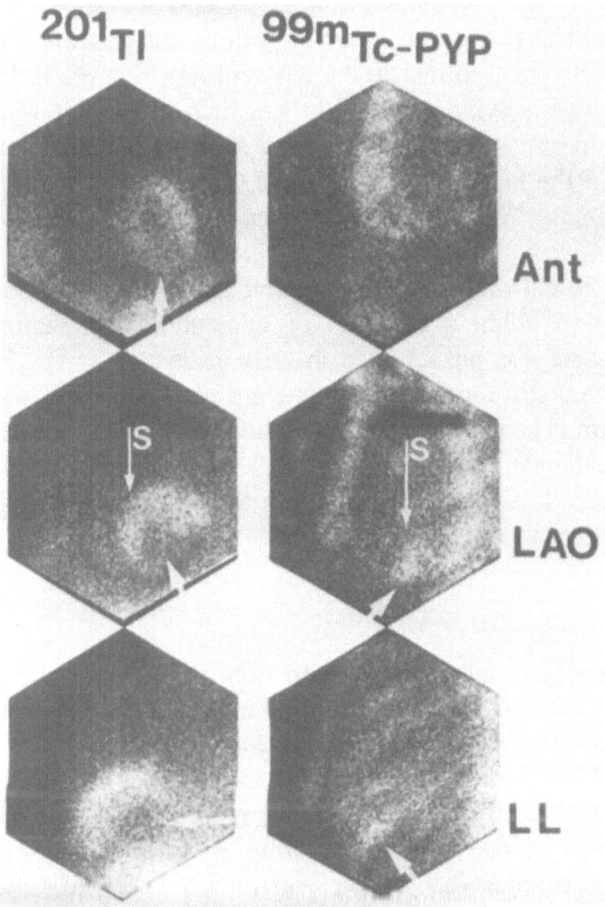

Figure 9-8. Thallium-201 and ^{99m}Tc-pyrophosphate studies in a patient with acute inferoposterior wall infarction. The ^{201}Tl study shows an extensive inferoposterior wall defect. The ^{99m}Tc-pyrophosphate scans demonstrate accumulation at the inferior wall, without right ventricular involvement.

Table 9-1. Results in 78 consecutive patients with acute inferior infarction [18] ·

Thallium-201 positive	Technetium-^{99m}Tc-pyrophosphate	
	Positive ($\geq ++$)	Negative
78/78	64/78	14/78
	LV+RV− LV+RV−	
	40/64 24/64	

LV+RV+ = abnormal accumulation of ^{99m}Tc-pyrophosphate in both the left and right ventricles. LV+RV− = abnormal ^{99m}Tc-pyrophosphate accumulation in the left but not the right ventricle

64 patients (37.5%) (group A). Examples of these patients are shown in Figures 9-6 and 9-7. Thirteen patients in group A showed right ventricular ^{99m}Tc-pyrophosphate activity equal to that in the left ventricle, whereas in 11 patients ^{99m}Tc-pyrophosphate activity was slightly less than in the left ventricle. In 40 patients with positive ^{99m}Tc-pyrophosphate scans *no* accumulation was present in the area of the right ventricle (group B (Figure 9-8). Fourteen of the 78 patients had negative ^{99m}Tc-pyrophosphate scans (group C). In seven of these 14 patients there was only 1+ and diffuse uptake; in seven other patients no activity was present. In these 14 patients, imaging was performed at a mean time interval of 28 hr after onset of infarction. Technetium-99m-pyrosphosphate imaging was not repeated in these patients.

In 25 of 78 patients, the defect on the ^{201}Tl scintiscans also partly involved the interventricular septum. The prevalence of septal involvement was greater in group A (12 of 23 patients) than in group B (10 of 40 patients). This difference is significant ($P = 0.03$) when verified with the Fisher Exact test.

Incidence of congestive heart failure (Table 9-2)

The presence of congestive heart failure was judged from the physical examination. Hemodynamic monitoring (arterial pressure line, Swan-Ganz catheter) was only performed in patients with severe pump failure. Left-sided congestive heart failure occured in 18 of 78 patients. The incidence of congestive heart failure was not significantly different among groups A, B and C. Cardiogenic shock occurred in two patients in group A, three patients in group B and two patients in group C.

Only one patient in this study showed signs of moderate right-sided congestive heart failure. This patient had "2+" ^{99m}Tc-pyrophosphate uptake in the right ventricle. The clinical course in this patient was uneventful after conventional treatment with diuretics and digitalis.

Table 9-2. Relation between results of ^{99m}Tc-pyrophosphate imaging and incidence of congestive heart failure and cause of death [18]

Group	PYP$_{LV}$	PYP$_{RV}$	LCHF class I	II	III	IV	RCHF	Cause of death CR	CS
Group A (24 pts)	≥++	≥++	18	3		2	1	1	2
Group B (40 pts)	≥++	—	30	6	1	3			3
Group C (14 pts)	+	—	6	1					
	—	—	5			2			2

CR = cardiac rupture; CS = cardiogenic shock; LCHF class = Killip's classification for left-sided congestive heart failure; PYP$_{LV}$ = ^{99m}Tc-pyrophosphate uptake in the left ventricle; PYP$_{RV}$ = ^{99m}Tc-pyrophosphate uptake in the right ventricle; RCHF = right-sided congestive heart failure
++, + and − = grading for ^{99m}Tc-pyrophosphate uptake

Clinical implications

Our data demonstrate the feasibility of noninvasive detection of right ventricular involvement in patients with acute inferior wall infarction by simple static imaging with ^{201}Tl and ^{99m}Tc-pyrophosphate. The external spatial reference markers allow superimposition of the images. In this study myocardial imaging with ^{99m}Tc-pyrophosphate was less sensitive than ^{201}Tl imaging to detect left ventricular infarcts, although not significantly lower than reported by others [6]. It is conceivable that more positive results would be obtained with ^{99m}Tc-pyrophosphate if repeated imaging was performed.

Assuming that accumulation of ^{99m}Tc-pyrophosphate accumulation indicates myocardial damage, 37.5% of the patients with acute inferior wall had right ventricular involvement. Sharpe et al. [15] reported that ^{99m}Tc-pyrophosphate uptake in the right ventricle correlated with right ventricular dysfunction as judged from gated cardiac blood pool imaging. Since the original description by Cohn et al. [9] of the clinical findings in patients with right ventricular infarction, four other clinical studies in relatively small series of patients suggested a relative high frequency of right ventricular involvement in acute inferior wall infarction. Rigo et al. [14] and Sharpe et al. [15] used gated cardiac blood pool imaging to visualize right ventricular dysfunction. Their studies indicated a prevalence of 43 and 40% respectively. Recently Reduto et al. [17] and Tobinick et al. [16] reported abnormal right ventricular ejection fraction as assessed by radionuclide first-pass method in 50% and 37%, respectively of patients with acute inferior wall infarcts.

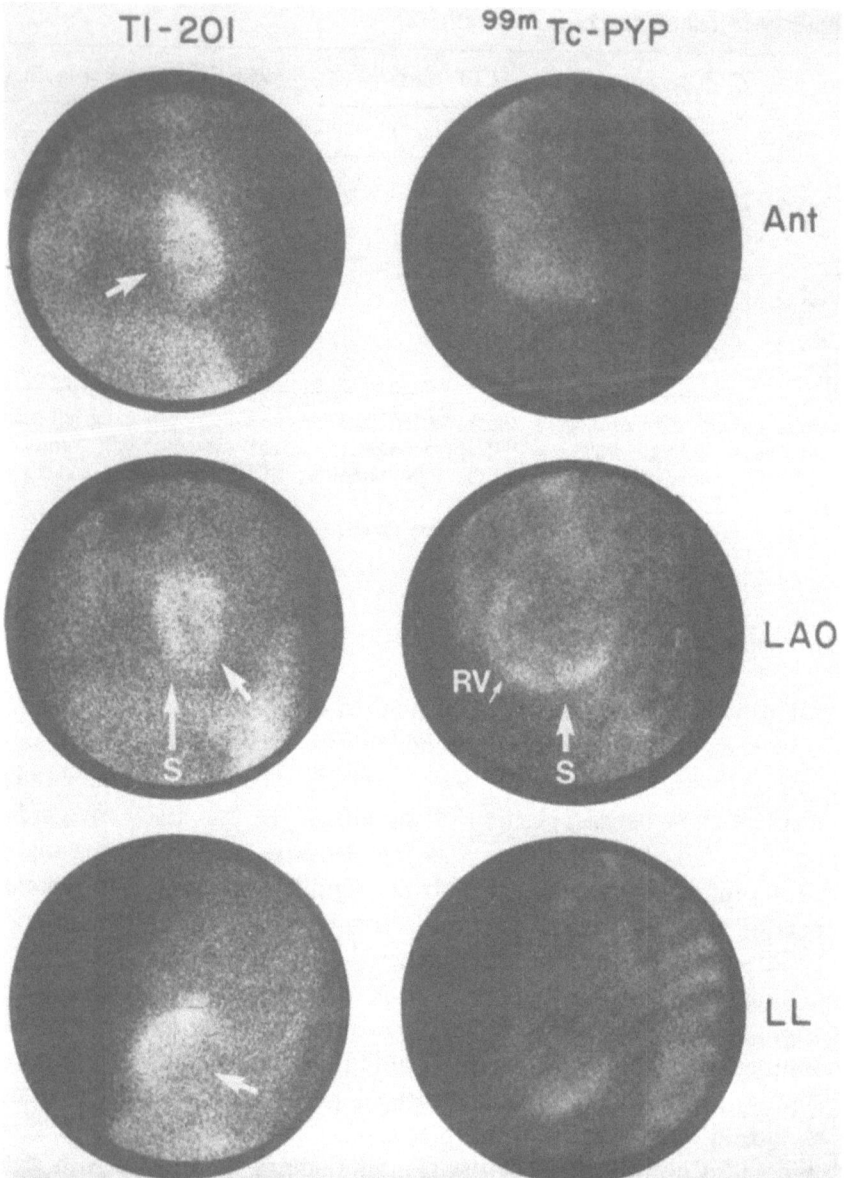

Figure 9-9. A: Dual imaging with ^{201}Tl and ^{99m}Tc-pyrophosphate in a patient with acute inferior wall infarction and right ventricular involvement and the classic clinical symptoms of severe right ventricular failure. Note that the amount of ^{99m}Tc-pyrophosphate accumulation in the right ventricle is more impressive than in the images in Figures 9–7 and 9–8, rv = right ventricle, s = septum. *B:* Electrocardiogram of the patient in Figure 9-9A, ST segment elevation is present in leads II, III, aVF and right precordial leads $V_3R - V_6R$. The electrocardiographic changes in the right precordial leads occur often in right ventricular infarction [21].

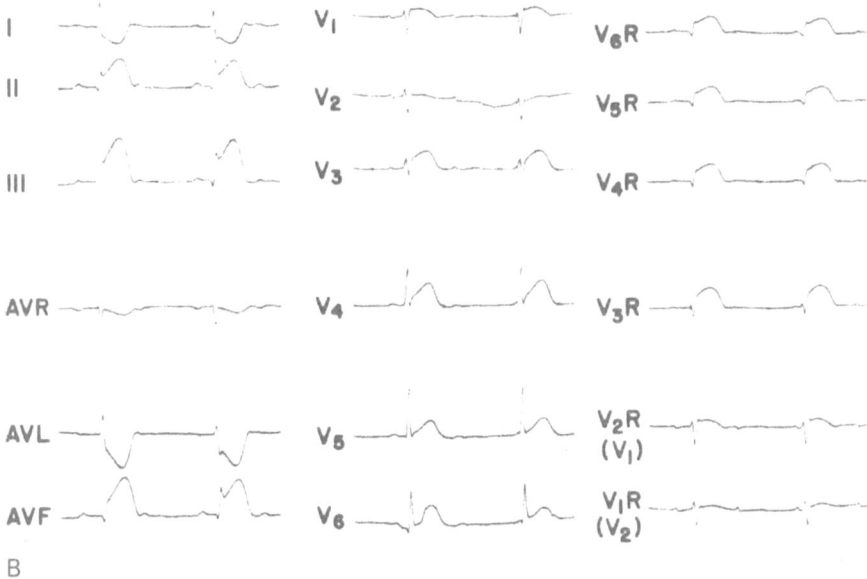

B

One of the intriguing aspects of right ventricular infarction is that it may lead to right ventricular failure and cardiogenic schock, but more often does not do so. None of the patients in the consecutive series described above, who had right ventricular involvement demonstrated severe right ventricular failure. Only one patient with positive ^{99m}Tc-pyrophosphate uptake in the right ventricle showed moderate evidence of elevated central venous pressure and systemic venous engorgement. The incidence of cardiogenic shock was not different in the group with and without right ventricular involvement. These patients showed right ventricular filling pressures within normal limits and significantly elevated pulmonary wedge pressures consistent with severe left ventricular failure. After completion of the above described study in a consecutive series of patients, we studied five separate patients (over a 2 yr period), who presented with the classic clinical findings of right ventricular infarction as described by Cohn et al. [9]. These patients all showed more impressive ^{99m}Tc-pyrophosphate uptake in the right ventricle (Figures 9-9 and 9-10) than the patients with subclinical right ventricular involvement in the consecutive series. This finding would suggest that the extent of right ventricular damage determines the presence or absence of typical clinical symptoms. However, the data reported by Isner and Roberts [13] do not support this thesis. The autopsy data suggested that right ventricular dilatation (= dysfunction?) was not simply a function of the anatomic extent of the right ventricular infarct. These investigators proposed that the extent of septal involvement was more likely to be a determinant factor.

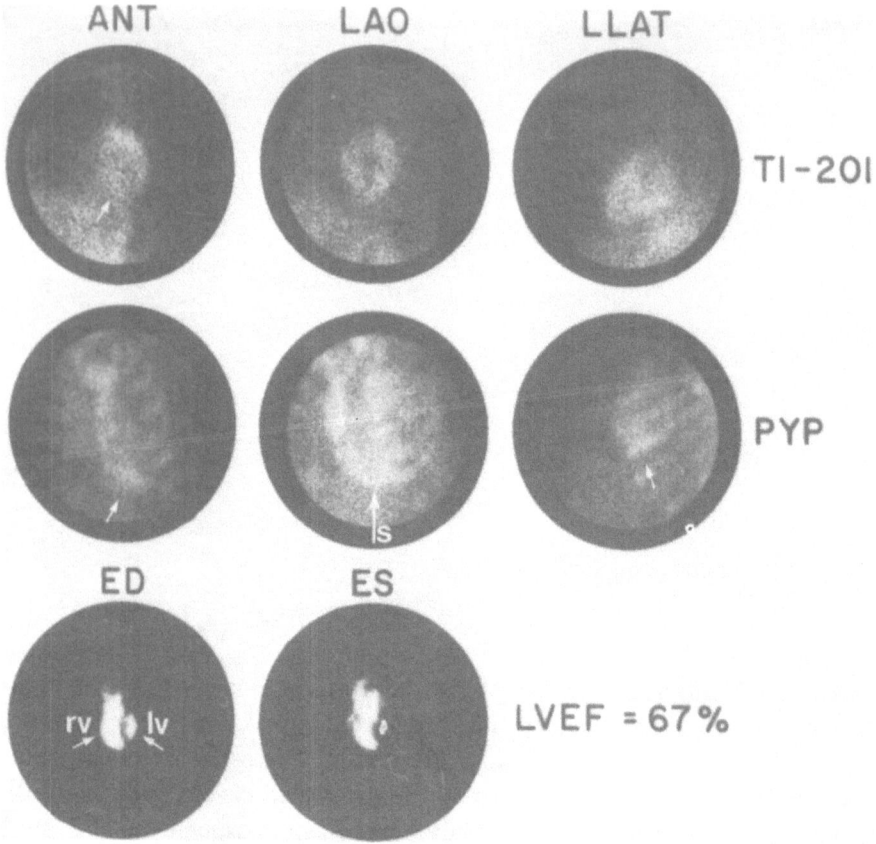

Figure 9-10. Myocardial imaging with ^{201}Tl and ^{99m}Tc-pyrophosphate, and multiple ECG-gated cardiac blood pool imaging in a patient with acute inferior wall infarction and cardiogenic shock. The ^{201}Tl scintiscans, show a normal size of the left ventricle and a small perfusion defect only visible on the anterior view (arrow). The ^{99m}Tc-pyrophosphate scintiscans show accumulation in the inferior wall of the left ventricle, but also extensive uptake in the right ventricle (rv). The multiple ECG-gated blood pool study shows a markedly enlarged akinetic right ventricle and a normally sized, well contracting left ventricle. Left ventricular ejection fraction is 67% (normal). These data are diagnostic for right ventricular infarction.

Septal involvement was clearly present in approximately half of the patients in our series with subclinical right ventricular involvement. The example of a patient with the clinical right ventricular infarction shown in Figure 9-9 demonstrates that although some septal involvement is present, this is not the predominant feature of the image.

Cohn[19] reviewing the accumulated information on right ventricular infarction, felt that many other factors may contribute possibly to the development of right ventricular pump failure, including the severity of ischemia and infarction of the left ventricle and its compliance, the pulmonary vascular resistance, the site and density of the right ventricular infarct, the systolic movement of the septum and the function of the tricuspid and mitral valves.

The recognition of right ventricular dysfunction is important since not only the *appropriate* therapy should be instituted but also *inappropriate* therapy should be avoided. Volume loading will result in striking improvement of cardiac output and clinical survival, whereas administration of diuretics is relatively contraindicated [14, 19]. Dual imaging with ^{201}Tl and ^{99m}Tc-pyrophosphate provides a simple and noninvasive method of recognizing the subgroup of patients, who may have hemodynamic deterioration due to major right ventricular involvement. Appreciation of the condition and subsequent appropriate treatment may be life-saving in this group.

DIFFERENTIATION OF OLD AND ACUTE INFARCTION

In patients who are admitted relatively late (2–3 days) after an acute episode of chest pain, the electrocardiogram may show pathologic Q waves or nonspecific stable ST-T segment changes. Serial enzyme determinations may fail to show the typical rise and fall suggesting acute infarction. In these patients it may be clinically relevant to determine with more certainty whether the infarct is old or new.

Although imaging with ^{99m}Tc-pyrophosphate imaging alone would be sufficient when positive, dual imaging will provide additional information. A large or moderate ^{201}Tl defect combined with a negative ^{99m}Tc-pyrophosphate scan is very likely to indicate prior infarction. The ^{201}Tl study provides information about size of the left ventricle and size of infarction. A small ^{201}Tl defect and negative ^{99m}Tc-pyrophosphate scan may represent old myocardial infarction. However, since ^{99m}Tc-pyrophosphate scans are less sensitive in detecting small infarcts and timing after the acute event is critical, there still may exist the possibility of a small amount (< 3 g) of acute myocardial necrosis. A negative ^{201}Tl study combined with a definite positive ^{99m}Tc-pyrophosphate is diagnostic for acute myocardial infarction and is very suggestive of a subendocardial infarct. Table 9-3 lists schematically the various combinations that may occur and the most likely interpretation.

It is worthwhile to emphasize that the value of the information obtained by each imaging method is importantly related to the appropriate timing of the study after the acute event. Furthermore, for the correct interpretation of the ^{99m}Tc-pyrophosphate images the possibility of accumulation in the presence of acute myocardial necrosis not caused by acute myocardial infarction (unstable angina, external DC counter shock and persistent positivity after previous myocardial infarct) should be considered.

Table 9-3. Myocardial imaging with ^{201}Tl and ^{99m}Tc-pyrophosphate in patients with question of prior myocardial infarction *

Thallium-201	^{99m}Tc-pyrophosphate	Interpretation
+ +	+ +	Acute MI
+ +	−	Prior MI
+	−	Uncertain; possibly acute ischemia
−	−	No MI
±	±	Uncertain
−	+	Acute MI
−	+ +	New, nontransmural MI

* Assuming that dual imaging is performed on the 2nd or 3rd day after onset of symptoms
MI = myocardial infarction + + = definitely positive; + = positive; ± = questionable; − = normal

In summary, in certain circumstances there clearly is a place for dual myocardial imaging. The combined techniques will provide the clinician with more useful information than each method alone. It will allow one to detect acute myocardial infarction more reliably and to evaluate the overall extent of myocardial damage more completely.

We would recommend dual imaging a) during the subacute phase after an episode of acute chest pain if the correct diagnosis is still in doubt; b) in patients with probably small infarctions; c) in patients with acute inferior wall infarction in cardiogenic shock in whom right ventricular infarction is suspected; and d) for the differentiation between old and new infarction.

REFERENCES

1. Wackers FJTh, Busemann Sokole E, Samson G, van der Schoot JB, Lie KI, Liem KL, Wellens HJJ: Value and limitations of thallium-201 scintigraphy in the acute phase of myocardial infarction. N Engl J Med 295:1-5, 1976.
2. Parkey RW, Bonte FJ, Meyer SL, Atkins JM, Curry GL, Stokely EM, Willerson JT: A new method for radionuclide imaging of acute myocardial infarction in humans. Circulation 50:540-546, 1974.
3. Berger HJ, Gottschalk A, Zaret BL: Dual radionuclide study of acute myocardial infarction: comparison of thallium-201 and technetium-99m stannous pyrophosphate imaging in man. Ann Intern Med 88:145-154, 1978.
4. Parkey RW, Bonte RJ, Stokely EM, Lewis SE, Graham KD, Buja LM, Willerson JT: Acute myocardial infarction imaged with ^{99m}Tc-stannous pyrophosphate and ^{201}Tl: a clinical evaluation. J. Nucl Med 17:771-779, 1976.
5. Buja LM, Parkey RW, Stokely EM, Bonte FJ, Willerson JT: Pathophysiology of technetium-99m stannous pyrophosphate and thallium-201 scintigraphy of acute anterior myocardial infarcts in dogs. J Clin Invest 57:1508-1522, 1976.
6. Strauss HW, Harrison K, Langan JK, Lebowitz E, Pitt B: Thallium-201 for myocardial imaging: relation of thallium-201 to regional myocardial perfusion. Circulation 51:641-645, 1975.
7. DiCola VC, Downing SE, Donabedian RK, Zaret BL: Pathophysiological correlates of thallium-201 myocardial uptake in experimental infarction. Cardiovasc Res XI:141-146, 1977.

8. Henning H, Schelbert HR, Righetti A, Ashburn WL, O'Rourke R: Dual myocardial imaging with technetium-99m pyrophosphate and thallium-201 for detecting, localizing and sizing acute myocardial infarction. Am J Cardiol 40:147-155, 1977.

9. Cohn JN, Guiha NH, Broder MI, Limas, CJ: Right ventricular infarction: clinical and hemodynamic features. Am J Cardiol 33:209-214, 1974.

10. Appelbaum E, Nicholson RNB: Occlusive disease of the coronary arteries, Am Med J 10:662-680, 1934.

11. Erhardt LR: Clinical and pathological observations in different types of acute infarction. Acta Med Scand suppl:560, 1974.

12. Erhardt LR: Right ventricular involvement in acute myocardial infarction. Eur J Cardiol 4:411-418, 1976.

13. Isner JM, Roberts WC: Right ventricular infarction complicating left ventricular infarction secondary to coronary heart disease. Am J Cardiol 42:885-894, 1978.

14. Rigo P, Murray M, Taylor DR, Weisfeldt ML, Kelly DT, Strauss HW, Pitt B: Right ventricular dysfunction detected by gated scintiphotography in patients with acute inferior myocardial infarction. Circulation 52:268-274, 1975.

15. Sharpe DN, Botvinick EH, Shames DM, Schiller NB, Massie BM, Chatterjee K, Parmley WW: The noninvasive diagnosis of right ventricular infarction. Circulation 57:483-490, 1978.

16. Tobinick E, Schelbert HR, Henning H, LeWinter M, Taylor A, Ashburn WL, Karliner JS: Right ventricular ejection fraction in patients with acute anterior and inferior myocardial infarction assessed by radionuclide angiography. Circulation 57:1078-1084, 1978.

17. Reduto LA, Berger HJ, Cohen LS, Gottschalk A, Zaret BL: Sequential radionuclide assessment of left and right ventricular performance after acute transmural myocardial infarction. Ann Intern Med 89:441-447, 1978.

18. Wackers FJTh, Lie KI, Busemann Sokole E, Res J, van der Schoot JB, Durrer D: Prevalence of right ventricular involvement in inferior wall infarction assessed with myocardial imaging with thallium-201 and technetium-99m pyrophosphate. Am J Cardiol 42: 358-362, 1978.

19. Cohn JN: Right ventricular infarction revisted. Am J Cardiol 43:666-668, 1979.

20. Zaret BL, Berger HJ: Dual radionuclide imaging of myocardial infarction. In: Cardiovascular nuclear medicine (2nd edition, pp 281-304. Strauss HW, Pitt B, eds. St. Louis: Mosby, 1979.

21. Erhardt R, Sjogren A, Wahlberg I: Single right-sided precordial lead in the diagnosis of right ventricular involvement in inferior myocardial infarction. Am Heart J 91:571-576, 1976.

UNSTABLE ANGINA PECTORIS

10. THALLIUM-201 MYOCARDIAL IMAGING IN UNSTABLE AGINA AND VARIANT ANGINA

FRANS J. TH. WACKERS, K.I. LIE, KOEN L. LIEM, ELLINOR BUSEMANN SOKOLE and JAN B. VAN DER SCHOOT

Scintigraphic myocardial perfusion defects with ^{201}Tl may represent either myocardial infarction or a region of transient ischemia. The results of repeated imaging in patients with acute myocardial infarction suggested that during the initial acute phase, in addition to necrotic tissue, surrounding transient ischemic tissue may be visualized [1]. Moreover, scintigraphic defects, indistinguishable from those seen in (acute) myocardial infarction can be obtained following exercise induced ischemia [2–6] or ischemia resulting from coronary spasm in variant angina [19]. An important portion of coronary care unit admissions includes patients who have repeated episodes of myocardial ischemia, i.e., patients with unstable angina. Therefore, it is of clinical relevance in the coronary care unit to evaluate the potential role of ^{201}Tl scintigraphy in patients with unstable angina. In the present chapter we will discuss 1) the pattern of ^{201}Tl scintigraphy in patients with unstable angina; and 2) the potential predictive value of ^{201}Tl scintigraphy in identifying patients with unstable angina who have a poorer prognosis or greater tendency to subsequently develop acute myocardial infarction.   All patients with unstable angina pectoris were purposely studied during the pain free period. It seemed conceivable that injecting ^{201}Tl during an anginal attack would result in a high percentage of scintigraphic defects and probably diminish a potential discriminative value of the method. Moreover, in clinical practice the majority of patients arrive at the coronary care unit some time after the last anginal attack. If a diagnostic test performed at this time could distinguish high and low risk patients, important therapeutic decisions might be made at the earliest possible times.

We have studied 98 patients with unstable agina with ^{201}Tl scintigraphy within 18 hr of the last anginal attack [7]. For this particular study, patients with a history or electrocardiographic evidence of previous myocardial infarcts were excluded, because ^{201}Tl defects in these patients could be due either to the previous infarction or myocardial ischemia. Patients with left bundle branch block or electrocardiographic signs of left ventricular hypertrophy were also excluded, because these pre-existing abnormalities might obscure electrocardiographic signs of ischemia.

Unstable angina was defined as a history of typical angina pectoris with increasing frequency and severity of the chest pain within a short time period (within 7–10 days), frequently with progression to angina at rest and/or during the night. In 84 patients this clinical syndrome occurred without previous angina, while in 14 patients previously stable angina had been present. All patients were, after admission to the coronary care unit treated with bedrest, sedation, nitrates and propanolol.

Thallium-201 scintigraphy

Of the 98 patients, 39 (40%) had positive scintiscans, 27 (27%) had questionable scans and 32 (33%) had normal scans. For further analysis the questionable scans are considered negative, since interobserver variability is greater in these borderline studies [8]. Of the patients with positive scintiscans the size of the defects was classified by observer's estimation as small (<25% of visualized left ventricle on three views), medium (25–40%) or large (>40%) and accordingly a score of 1, 2, or 3 was given. In addition, to appreciate the difference between defects with residual activity and those with virtually no residual activity as compared to background activity, a score of 1 or 2 respectively, was given. Thus, a maximum score of 5 was given for a large

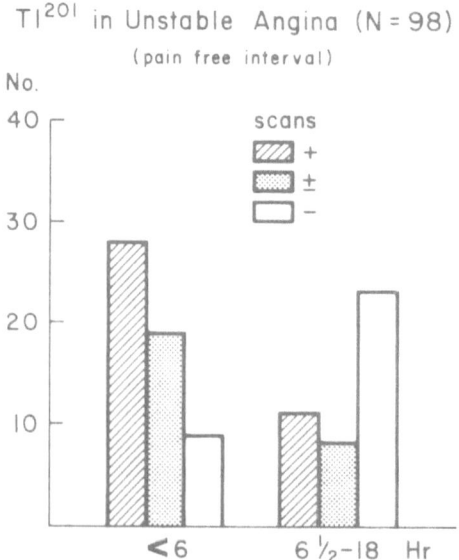

Figure 10-1. Relationship between results of ^{201}Tl scintigraphy and the time of scintigraphy after last anginal episode. + = positive scintiscans; ± = questionable scintiscans; − = normal scintiscans.

defect with no residual activity and a minimum score of 2 for a small defect with residual activity. Of the 39 patients with positive scintiscans, the defect was estimated to be "small" in 19 patients, "medium" in eight patients and "large" in 12 patients. In 20 of 39 patients no residual activity was present and in 19 patients residual activity was present. The score for the size of defects was 2 in 10 patients, 3 in 14 patients, 4 in six patients and 5 in nine patients.

Results of scintigraphy and time of imaging after angina

In patients with unstable angina, a definite relationship was apparent between the results of scintigraphy and the time interval after the last anginal attack (Figure 10-1). This is similar to our findings in patients with acute myocardial infarction [1].

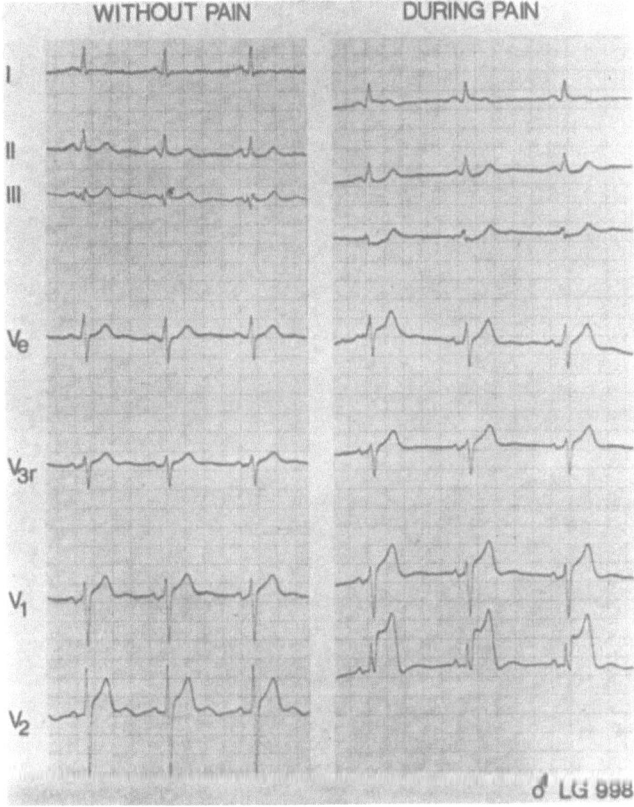

Figure 10-2. Electrocardiogram during the pain free period and during pain in a patient with unstable angina. During angina impressive ST segment elevation occurred in leads I, aVL and V_{2-6}. Thallium-201 scintiscans of this patient are shown in Figure 10-3.

Fifty-six of 98 patients were studied within 6 hr, and 42 patients were studied between $6\frac{1}{2}$ and 18 hr after the last anginal attack. Twenty-eight of 56 patients (50%) studied within 6 hr after the last anginal attack had positive ^{201}Tl scans, compared to 11 of 42 patients (26%) studied later ($P<0.05$). Examples of transient perfusion defects are shown in Figures 10-3 and 10-4. Figure 10-3 displays ^{201}Tl scintiscans of a patient with a typical history of unstable angina or recent onset. The attacks of angina at rest were associated with electrocardiographic ST-segment elevations in leads I, aVL and $V_2 - V_6$, returning to baseline after reflief of pain by sublingual nitroglycerin (Figure 10-2). For the first study (4-2-1976) ^{201}Tl was injected $3\frac{1}{2}$ hr after such an attack. The patient was free of pain and the electrocardiogram was normal at

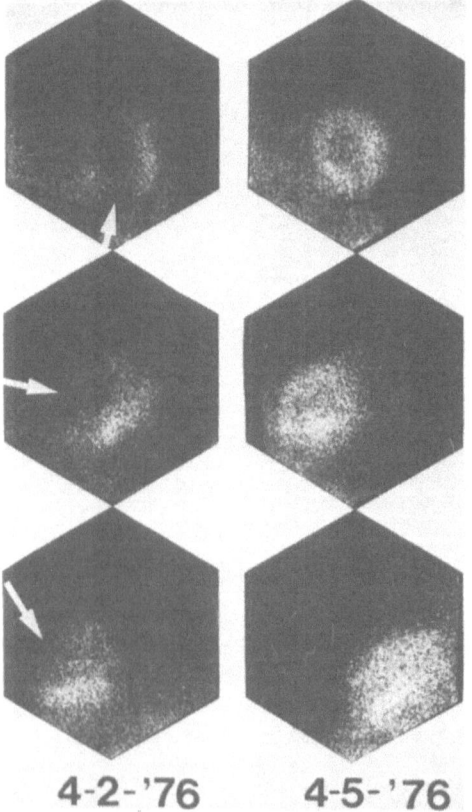

4-2-'76   4-5-'76

Figure 10-3. Repeated ^{201}Tl scintigraphy of the patient whose electrocardiogram is shown in Figure 10-2. On April 2, ^{201}Tl was injected $3\frac{1}{2}$ hr after an anginal episode, which was associated with electrocardiographic changes as shown in Figure 10-2. The ^{201}Tl study shows an anteroseptal perfusion defect (arrows). On April 5, the study was repeated after a new injection of ^{201}Tl. The patient had no recurrent anginal attacks for more than 24 hr being treated with propranolol. The scintiscans show a nearly normal accumulation of ^{201}Tl in the left ventricle. Reproduced with permission from Ref. [7].

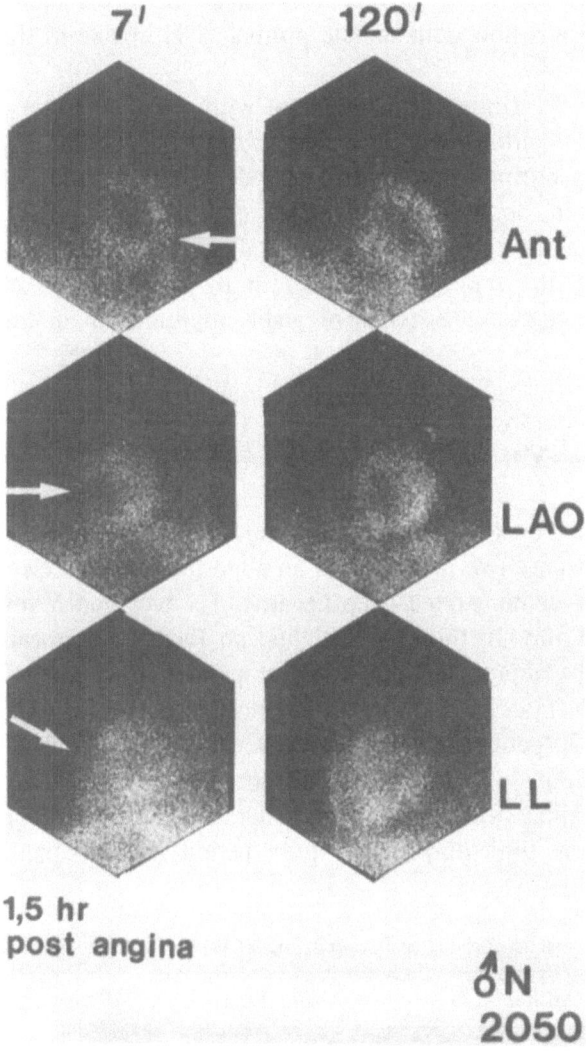

7' 120'

Ant

LAO

LL

1,5 hr
post angina

♂N
2050

Figure 10-4. Serial myocardial imaging after a single dose of ²⁰¹Tl in a patient with unstable angina. Left, scintiscans 1½ hr after last anginal attack, 7 min after injection. The scintiscans show an anteroseptal defect (arrows). Right, scintiscans obtained 120 min after injection. The scintiscans show a nearly normal image of the left ventricle. Reproduced with permission from Ref. [7].

the time of injection. The ²⁰¹Tl scintiscans show a definite anteroseptal perfusion defect. Cardiac serum enzymes (CK, SGOT, LDH), obtained serially for each 6 hr subsequently remained normal and the electrocardiogram also failed to show evidence of myocardial infarction. The patient was treated with propanolol 240 mg/day and nitrates. The patient responded well to this treatment and sustained no recurrent attacks of agina. Three days later

(4-5-1976) ^{201}Tl scintigraphy was repeated *after a new injection* of the radio-pharmaceutical. The scintiscans now demonstrate normal ^{201}Tl uptake in the left ventricle on all three views.

Figure 10-4 shows the ^{201}Tl scintiscans in a patient with a similar history. However, serial imaging was performed after a *single dose* of [201]Tl. The first set of images was obtained during the pain free period, $1\frac{1}{2}$ hr after the last anginal attack. The scintiscans show a definite anteroseptal perfusion defect. Two hours later a new series of delayed images is obtained, showing almost normal images. Apparently the septal defect filled in by redistribution of [201]Tl. This suggests severe transient ischemia of viable myocardium in the septal region.

Relationship between thallium-201 scintigraphy and electrocardiogram

During the pain free periods 76 or 98 patients had a normal baseline electro-cardiogram (Table 10-1). Twenty-two patients had an abnormal baseline elec-trocardiogram, of whom 15 demonstrated deep negative T-waves and seven ST-segment depression >1 mm. In these 22 patients, no further electrocar-diographic changes could be appreciated during chest pain. During anginal attacks (Table 10-1) the electrocardiogram remained normal in 46 patients, but changed transiently in 30 patients (ST-segment depression >1 mm in 12 patients; ST-segment elevation >2 mm in 18 patients, Table 10-2). Thus, ST-segment changes compatible with myocardial ischemia were present on the electrocardiogram at any time during the study period in 52 patients (53%).

Table 10-1. Relationship between results of ^{201}Tl scintigraphy and ECG [7]

Scintiscans	(No. pts)	Pain free ECG		Angina ECG		Total Abn. ECG
		N	Abn.	N	Trans. Abn.	
Positive	(39)	26	13	7	19	32
Questionable	(27)	19	8	10	9	17
Normal	(32)	31	1	29	2	3
Total	(98)	76	22	46	30	52

Abbreviations: Abn. = abnormal; N = normal; Trans. = transient

Of the 39 patients with positive scintiscans, 13 patients (33%) showed electrocardiographic abnormalities at the time of scintigraphy. During an attack of chest pain 19 additional patients showed transient electrocardiogra-phic abnormalities. Thus, a total of 32 (82%) patients with positive scintiscans

Table 10-2. Results of ^{201}Tl scintigraphy in relation to ECG changes [7]

Scintiscans	ECG				Total
	N.	Neg-T	ST↓	ST↑	
Positive	7	(8)*	6(+5)	13	39
Questionable	10	(6)	5(+2)	4	27
Normal	29	(1)	1	1	32
Total	46	(15)	12(+7)	18	98

* Figures in parentheses indicate ECG abnormalities present during pain free period
Abbreviations: N = normal ECG; Neg-T = deep negative T waves developing during the observation period; ST ↑↓ = direction of ST-segment shift

showed an abnormal electrocardiogram either during pain or during the pain free period. Of the 32 patients with normal ^{201}Tl scintiscans, only one demonstrated electrocardiographic abnormalities at the time of scintigraphy. During an attack of chest pain, two additional patients showed transient electrocardiographic abnormalities.

Table 10-2 shows the relationship between the results of ^{201}Tl scintigraphy and specific electrocardiographic changes at any time during the study period. ST-segment elevations were all transient and occurred in 18 patients, 13 (72%) of whom had positive ^{201}Tl scintiscans. ST-segment depression occurred in 19 patients; in 12 patients these ST-segments depressions were present only transiently during angina. Eleven (58%) of the 19 patients with ST-segment depression has positive scans. Deep inverted T-waves developed during the observation period in 15 patients, eight (53%) of whom had positive scans.

Clinical course

None of the 38 patients had enzyme level rises at the time of scintigraphy or during the following 12 hr. Eighty-one (83%) patients responded favorably to medical treatment and their angina became clinically stable. Following admission, 17 patients (17%) had a complicated course. Six patients had a new attack of chest pain within 48 hr (mean 22 hr) after scintigraphy and sustained acute transmural myocardial infarction, documented by typical cardiac enzyme elevations and the development of pathologic Q-waves on the electrocardiogram. The 11 remaining patients continued to have chest pain despite maximal medical treatment with propanolol and nitrates. These patients underwent coronary angiography and subsequently all had coronary bypass surgery. There was no perioperative myocardial infarcts identified in these patients.

Comparison of value of thallium-201 scintigraphy with electrocardiogram

The relationship between the scintigraphic results and specific electrocardiographic changes in the 17 patients with complicated courses is shown in Table 10-3. Of these 17 patients who had complicated courses, 13 (76%) had positive scintiscans, whereas only one (12%) had abnormal electrocardiagrams at the time of scintigraphy during the pain free period. However, during an attack of angina 12 of the remaining 15 patients showed transient electrocardiographic changes. In contrast, of the 81 patients with uncomplicated courses, 26 (32%) had positive scintiscans ($P < 0.01$), while 20 (25%) had abnormal electrocardiograms at the time of scintigraphy. During an attack of angina 18 additional patients showed transient electrocardiographic changes. Thus, during the pain free period in the same patient group, more patients had abnormal ^{201}Tl scans than abnormal electrocardiograms (39 versus 22, $P < 0.01$).

Table 10-3. Results of ^{201}Tl scintigraphy in relation to ECG changes in 17 patients with unstable angina and complicated subsequent course [7]

Scintiscans	AMI				Total	CBS				Total
ECG	N	Neg T	ST↓	ST↑		N	Neg T	ST↓	ST↑	
Positive	1	2 (+1)*			4	1		1	7	9
Questionable	1			1	2		(1)	1		2
Normal					0					0
Total	2	2 (+1)	1		6	1	(1)	2	7	11

* Figures in parentheses indicate ECG abnormalities present during pain free period.
Abbreviations: N = normal ECG; Neg T = deep negative T waves developing during the observation period; ST↓↑ = direction of ST-segment shift; AMI = acute myocardial infarction; CBS = coronary bypass surgery

From these data the sensitivity, specificity and predictive accuracy* in identifying patients with complicated course can be determined for ^{201}Tl scintigraphy, electrocardiography, and the combination of the two (Table 10-4).

The *sensitivity* for an abnormal baseline electrocardiogram to identify patients with complicated courses was 11%, for transient electrocardiographic changes during angina 70%, for positive scintiscans during the pain free period 76%, for the combination of an abnormal baseline electrocardiogram and transient electrocardiographic abnormalities 82%, for the combination of positive ^{201}Tl scintiscans and/or transient electrocardiographic abnormalities 88% and for the combination of positive scans with any electrocardiographic

---

* Sensitivity, specificity and predictive accuracy are defined in chapter 6, p. 152.

Table 10-4. Diagnostic value of ^{201}Tl scintigraphy and ECG in patients with unstable angina [7]

	Sensitivity	Specificity	Predictive accuracy
Abn. ECG, baseline	11%	75%	9%
Abn. ECG, transient	70%	77%	40%
Positive scans	76%	67%	33%
Abn. ECG, baseline and Abn. ECG, transient	82%	53%	26%
Positive scans and Abn. ECG, baseline	82%	58%	29%
Positive scans and Abn. ECG, transient	88%	56%	30%
Positive scans and ABN. ECG, baseline and Abn. ECG, transient	94%	46%	27%

abnormality at any time 94%. The *specificity* of electrocardiographic abnormalities (baseline or transient) was only slightly higher than for positive ^{201}Tl scans (75% and 77%, versus 67%, respectively). The *predictive value* of transient electrocardiographic changes was 40% and of positive scintiscans 33%, while the other tests or combinations had somewhat lower predictive values.

Clinical implications

The group of patients with unstable angina described in this study, probably is representative of patients with unstable angina routinely seen in coronary care units. Other than prior myocardial infarction and electrocardiographic conduction abnormalities, no exclusion criteria were applied.

This study demonstrates clearly that positive ^{201}Tl scintiscans do not necessarily imply sustained myocardial infarction. Our findings indicate that in patients with unstable angina the results of myocardial ischemia, as assessed by ^{201}Tl uptake persists longer than can be judged from observation of the patient's clinical status and electrocardiogram. Figure 10-3 suggests clearly that a dynamic transport mechanism must play a role in ^{201}Tl uptake. Although the degree of the coronary artery stenosis during the pain free period must have been unaltered, the myocardial uptake of ^{201}Tl was different during the unstable phase (shortly after angina) as compared to 3 days later when the patient had stabilized. Also serial imaging after a single dose suggests delayed uptake of ^{201}Tl in a previously ischemic area.

Recently, Gewirtz et al. [9] demonstrated that transient perfusion defects on resting ^{201}Tl scintiscans can also be obtained in patients with severe but stable angina pectoris. This was noted in a highly selected group of patients with severe coronary artery disease. Thallium-201 scintigraphy was performed at rest in 20 patients. In these patients perfusion defects were present in 43 of 120 segments. In 23 segments the defect appeared transient and filled in at delayed imaging; 20 of these segments were located in the distribution of 90–99% stenotic coronary arteries. Almost all these patients showed cineangiographic wall motion abnormalities in the same area; although no previous myocardial infarction was present. It was felt that in these patients significantly decreased resting myocardial blood flow existed distal to the site of the stenosis in the coronary artery.

Recently, Berger et al. [10] reported similar findings again in a highly selected group of patients. It is unfortunate that although the observation is correct, these reports suggest that defects on resting ^{201}Tl scintiscans, in the absence of prior infarction, occur frequently. In our experience, this is not the case and in fact this occurs only rarely.

Although reduced resting myocardial blood flow may be responsible in part for our findings in patients with unstable agina, it seems likely that (in addition) a more dynamic mechanism plays a role. First, we observed a definite time relationship between the presence of ^{201}Tl defects and the time of imaging after the last anginal attack (Figure 10-1). Secondly, the patient study in Figure 10-3 demonstrates that the initial distribution of ^{201}Tl shortly after injection may be different depending on the clinical status in patients with unstable angina. Therefore, decreased uptake of ^{201}Tl in patients with unstable angina probably is not just a simple hemodynamic phenomenon due to decreased resting regional blood flow, but rather related to a persisting effect of severe ischemia on the active transmembrane transport, after subjective relief of angina. Weich et al. [11] demonstrated a prolonged effect of myocardial hypoxia, which persisted after recovery, on ^{201}Tl myocardial extraction fraction (see chapter 2).

The sensitivity of ^{201}Tl scintigraphy to detect patients at risk for a complicated course appeared to be considerably higher than the specificity and predictive accuracy. However, in patients with unstable angina a sensitive test is more important than a specific test, because false negative results are less desirable than false positive ones. The patients who subsequently had a complicated clinical course had significantly more positive scans than those who responded favorably to medical treatment (70% versus 32%, $P < 0.01$). These patients with a complicated course also had larger defects than the remaining patients. Positive ^{201}Tl scintigraphy in patients with unstable angina provides additional information that acute coronary insufficiency is present and indicates a potential high risk group. One third of these patients may be at risk for complicated courses, failure to respond to medical treatment and development of acute infarction during the first 24 hr.

Wilson et al. [12] and Prinzmetal et al. [13] were the first to recognize a variant form of angina pectoris. In contrast to angina on effort it occurred almost exclusively at rest, was associated with impressive ST-segment elevation and was frequently accompanied by complete atrioventricular block of ventricular arrhythmias. Coronary vasospasm was postulated as a possible explanation and more recently coronary spasm has been demonstrated as a cause of *variant agina* in patients with normal coronary arteries [14], in patients with hemodynamically insignificant coronary lesions and also in patients with significant fixed coronary obstructions [15]. Thus, the anatomic substrate of variant angina varies from normal to severely stenotic coronary arteries. A thus far unproved speculation is that platelets aggregates may play a role either primarily, possibly with subsequent vasospasm as a result of release of platelet vasoactive substances (thromboxane A_2), or secondary due to hypoxia occuring during spasm.

Recently, important progress has been made in understanding the mechanisms involved in angina at rest [16–22]. It has been demonstrated that attacks of agina at rest were not preceded by any detectable increase of hemodynamic indices determining myocardial oxygen consumption [16, 18]. Thus, the balance between myocardial supply and demand was not disturbed prior to the attack. Regional myocardial perfusion during anginal attacks was studied by Maseri et al. [22] in 32 patients by injecting ^{201}Tl at the time electrocardiographic changes were present. In 25 of 26 patients with ST-segment elevation during the ischemic episode, ^{201}Tl scintigraphy revealed a massive myocardial perfusion defect corresponding to the electrocardiographic location of ischemic changes. In the patient with a negative ^{201}Tl study, the attack subsided about 1 min after injection and scintigraphy was performed 10 min later. In four patients pseudonormalization of T waves was observed during chest pain; all patients demonstrated massive myocardial perfusion defects. In two patients with ST-segment depression during angina myocardial perfusion defects were also noted. These studies demonstrate that some patients develop angina at rest as a consequence of primarily reduced coronary blood flow [22].

Although coronary vasospasm generally occurs at rest, a number of patients have now been reported with exertion related angina due to spasm [23–27]. McLaughlin et al. [23] described a patient with typical angina pectoris which occurred invariably 3–4 min *after* exertion. This patient had normal coronary arteries and chest pain could be provoked by intravenous administration of ergonovine maleate. Thallium-201 imaging during pain, after exercise reproducibly demonstrated a perfusion defect in the region supplied by the artery with documented vasospasm. Waters et al. [25] reported exertional angina with ST-segment elevations in seven patients and ^{201}Tl defects could be demonstrated, although none of these patients had significant coronary artery disease. We studied a group of 11 patients with chest pain and angiographically documented normal or insignificantly stenotic (<40%) coronary arteries. In these patients ergonovine maleate was injected as small boluses of increasing strength. The maximal injected total dose ranged from 0.4 to 0.6 mg. In four of 11 patients severe episodes of chest pain, associated with ST-segment elevation (Figure 10-5) could be provoked. The remaining seven patients had a negative response. In all patients with provocable chest pain, ^{201}Tl perfusion defects were obtained when ^{201}Tl was injected during electrocardiographic ST-segment elevation (Figures 10-6, 10-7 and 10-9). In none of the patients with negative ergonovine response were abnormal ^{201}Tl scintiscans obtained.

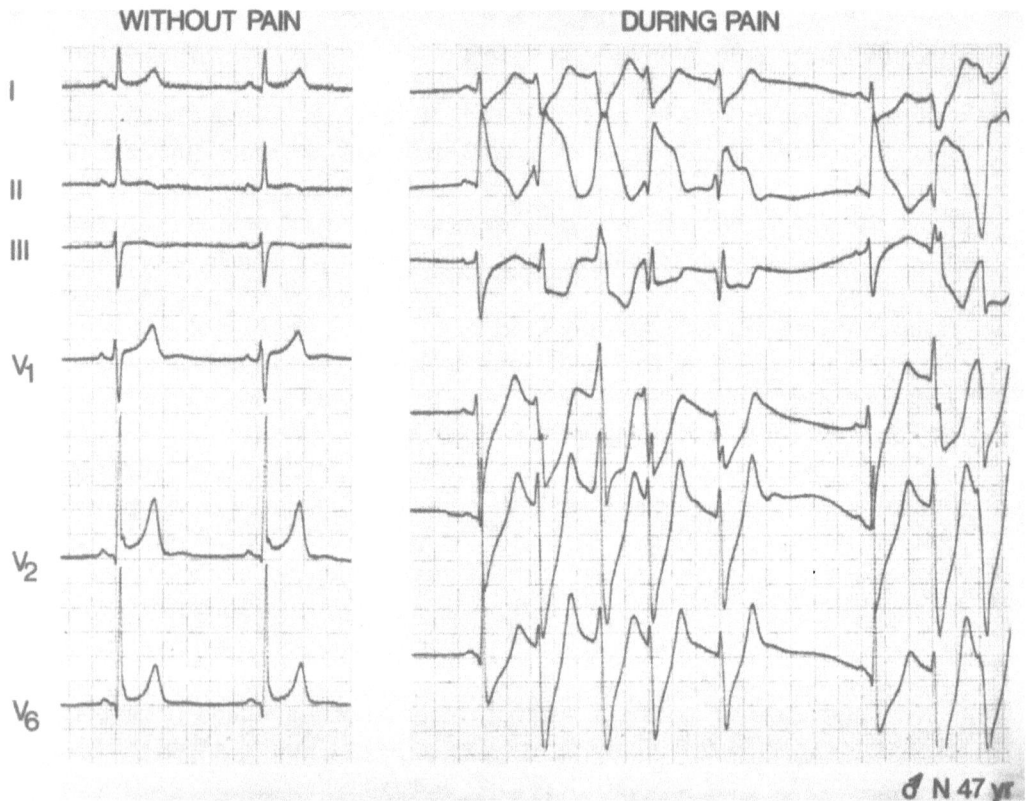

Figure 10-5. Electrocardiograms of a patient with angiographically normal coronary arteries and vasospasm of the right coronary artery. Left, baseline electrocardiogram showing early repolarization, but otherwise normal. Right, electrocardiogram during coronary spasm. A shift of the electrical axis to the right occurred. Marked ST segment elevation is present in lead II, With reciprocal changes in the other leads. The first and sixth beat are normally conducted. The second to fifth beat represents a short burst of (probably) ventricular tachycardia.

In the patients with normal coronary arteries the appropriate timing of the ^{201}Tl administration is important. In one patient, ^{201}Tl was injected when the patient reported feeling the peripheral effects of ergonovine (numbness and tingling of the extremities). Only 2–3 min later the typical chest pain and electrocardiographic changes occurred (Figure 10-5). The ^{201}Tl scans obtained at this occasion were completely normal. On another day ^{201}Tl was injected

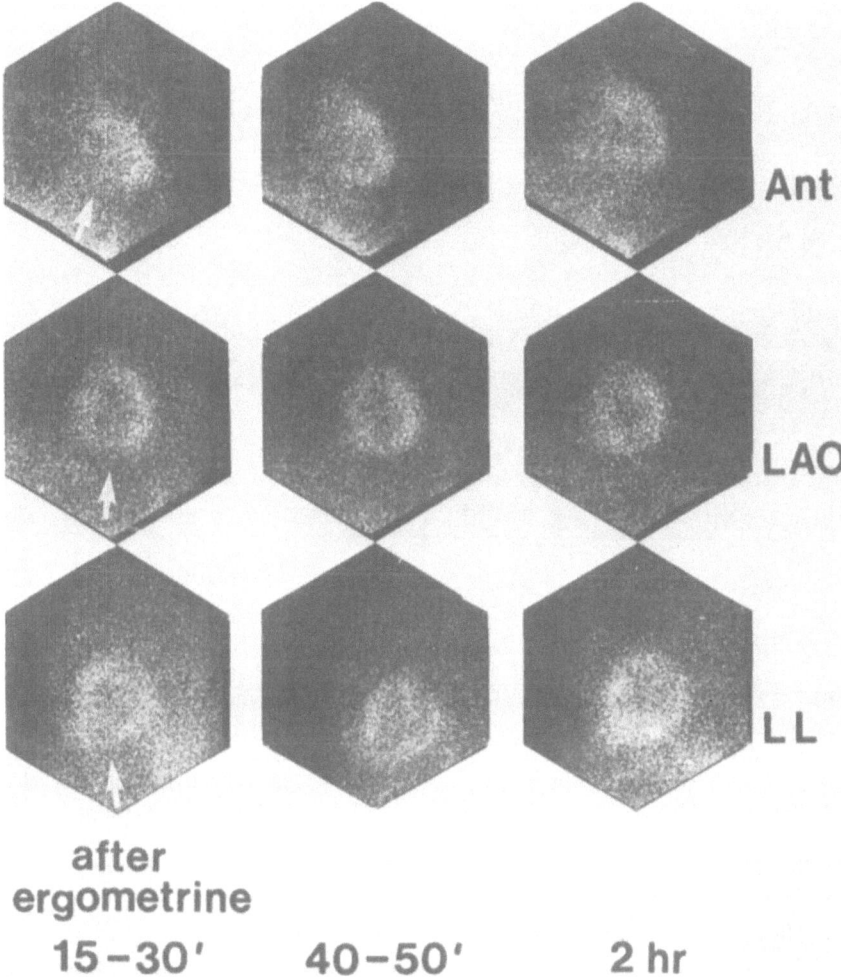

after ergometrine

15–30'   40–50'   2 hr

Figure 10-6. Serial ^{201}Tl scintigraphy in the same patient as in Figure 10-5 after provocation of coronary spasm with intravenous ergometrine. Thallium-201 was injected during appearance of ST segment elevation on the electrocardiogram.

Myocardial imaging performed from 15 to 30 min after injection of ^{201}Tl (left) demonstrates a discrete inferior wall perfusion defect (arrows), which subsequently fills in rapidly by redistribution. Middle, the images are nearly normal; 2 h after injection (right) no perfusion defect is present.

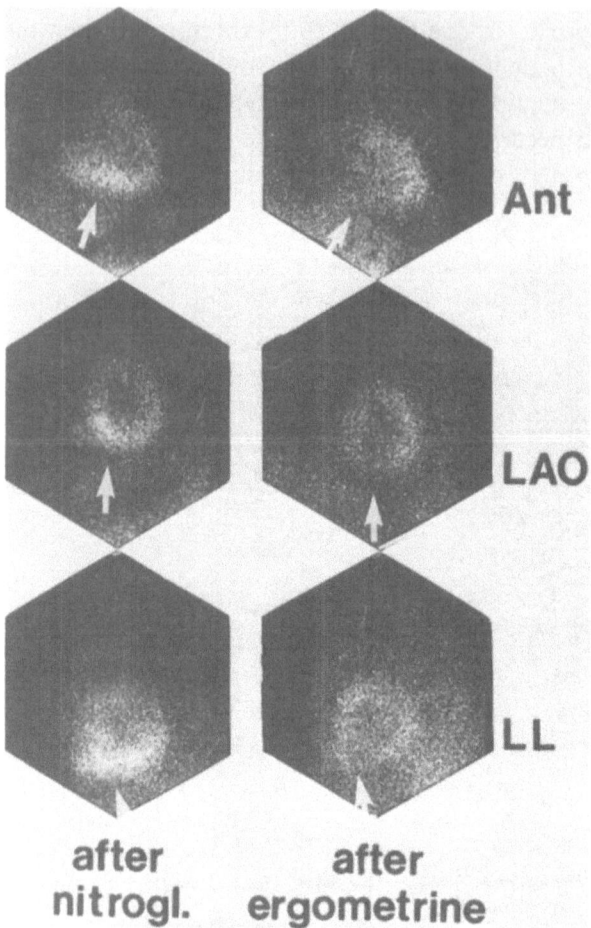

Ant

LAO

LL

after
nitrogl.

after
ergometrine

Figure 10-7. Thallium-201 images in the same patient as in Figures 10-5 and 10-6. Right, ^{201}Tl scintiscans obtained shortly after provocation of coronary spasm. An inferior wall perfusion defect is present (arrows). Left, ^{201}Tl scintiscans obtained shortly after relief of a spontaneous attack of chest pain by sublingual nitroglycerin. Thalium-201 was injected approximately 1 min after relief of pain. The scintiscans show *increased* uptake of ^{201}Tl in the inferior wall. See text.

during the presence of ST-segment elevation on the electrocardiogram. This time an inferior wall perfusion defect was present on the first series of images (Figure 10-6). Rapid filling-in if this defect could be observed within 60 min. On another occasion ^{201}Tl was injected in the same patient shortly after relief of a spontaneous attack of chest pain by sublinguinal nitroglycerin. This time no defect was present but relatively increased uptake in the inferior wall was noted (Figure 10-7). It seems conceivable that since ^{201}Tl was injected within 2 min after relief of pain by nitroglycerin, reactive reperfusion hyperemia after occlusive vasospasm is visualized. Coronary angiography in this patient demonstrated normal coronary arteries in the absence of chest pain. However,

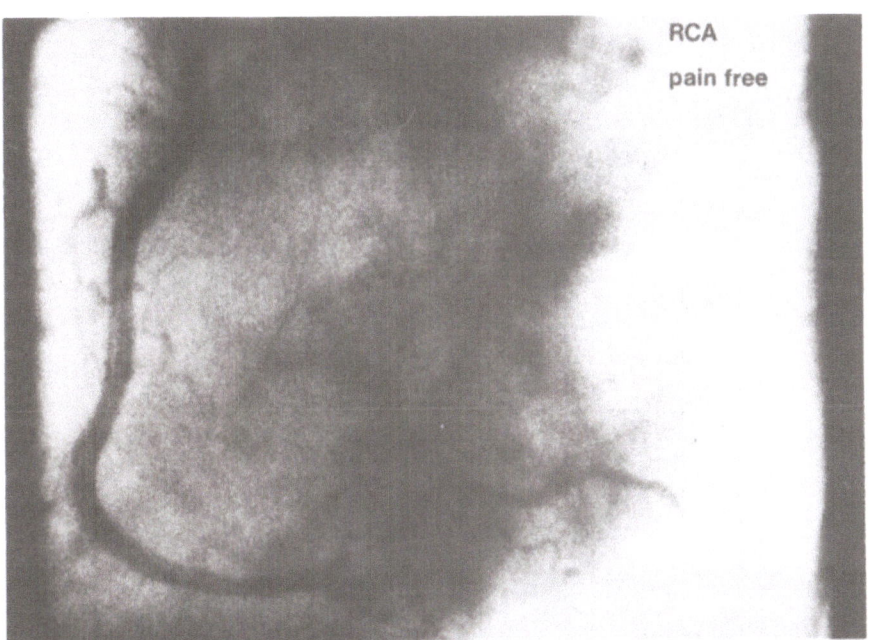

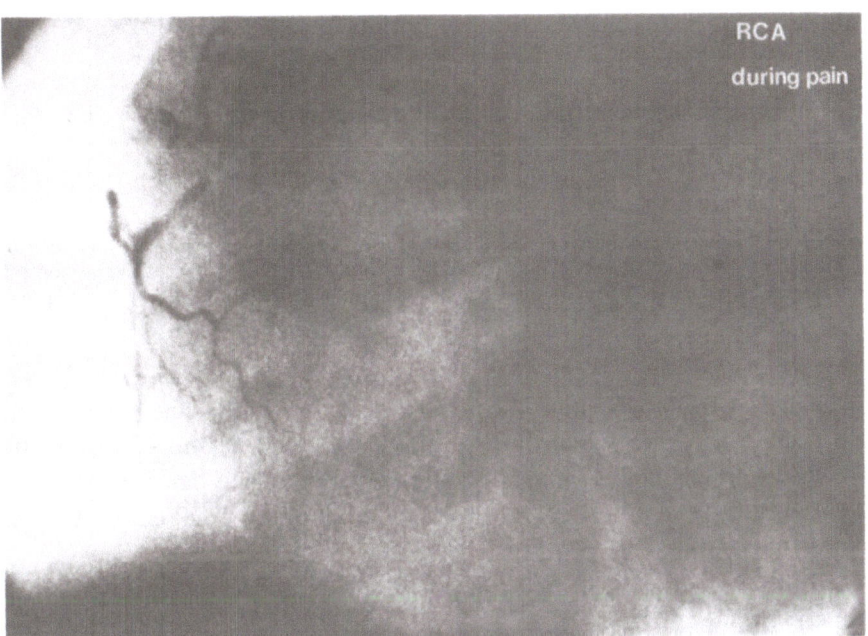

Figure 10-8. Coronary angiography in left anterior oblique projection of the same patient as in Figures 10-5, 10-6 and 10-7. (A) Angiogram of the right coronary artery during pain free period. No lesions are present. (B) Angiogram of the right coronary artery during ergonovine provoked vasospasm. The right coronary artery is almost completely occluded.

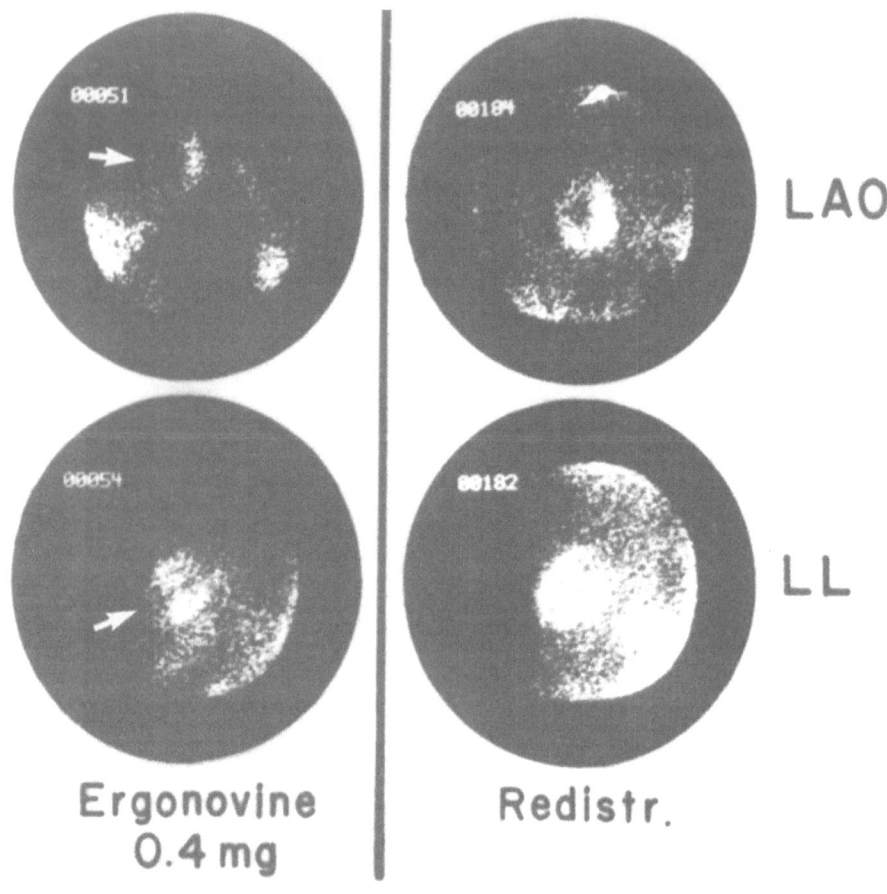

Figure 10-9. Thallium-201 scintiscans in a patient with insignificant (approximately 40% narrowing) disease of the proximal left anterior descending coronary artery. Left, positive response to provocation of spasm with 0.4 mg of ergonovine: a definite anteroseptal perfusion defect (arrows) is present. Right, after 4 hr of redistribution the ^{201}Tl scans are completely normal.

immediately after provocation of coronary spasm by ergonovine, almost complete occlusion of the right coronary artery occurred (Figure 10-8). Figure 10-9 shows an example of a severe anteroseptal perfusion defect after provocation of spasm in a patient with insignificant (40%) disease of the left anterior descending coronary artery.

In three of four patients with documented normal coronary arteries and coronary spasm, we injected ^{201}Tl 45-60 min after the last attack of chest pain. In all three patients the ^{201}Tl scintiscans were normal at this time. This is in contrast to our findings in patients with unstable agina and significant fixed coronary artery disease, in whom abnormal ^{201}Tl scintiscans were obtained several hours after the last anginal attack.

Clinical implications

Thallium-201 scintigraphy may be of clinical importance in patients with coronary vasospasm.

Although coronary angiography in most instances is indicated in patients with recurrent ST-segment elevations during angina, the temporal characteristics of ^{201}Tl imaging might be of help in differentiating between patients with normal coronary arteries and those with significant coronary artery disease. A normal ^{201}Tl study shortly after an attack of variant angina is suggestive of normal coronary anatomy [28]. Moreover, ^{201}Tl scintigraphy may provide insight in the pathophysiologic mechanism responsible for angina in these patients. The site of the ^{201}Tl perfusion defects provide an indication of the possible site of coronary vasospasm.

Presently, patients with documented coronary spasm are commonly followed on medical treatment (mostly calcium antagonists, such as nefidipine or verapamil). Thallium-201 scintigraphy combined with ergonovine provocation might be a noninvasive means to evaluate the efficacy of this treatment. As described above, the correct timing of ^{201}Tl administration during the provocation may be crucial to avoid false negative results.

REFERENCES

1. Wackers FJTh, Busemann Sokole E, Samson G, van der Schoot JB, Lie KI, Liem KL, Wellens HJJ: Value and limitations of thallium-201 scintigraphy in the acute phase of myocardial infarction. N Engl J Med 295:1-5, 1976.
2. Bailey IK, Griffith LSC, Rouleau J, Strauss HW, Pitt B: Thallium-201 myocardial perfusion imaging at rest and during exercise. Circulation 55:79-87, 1977.
3. Ritchie JL, Trobaugh GB, Hamilton GW, Gould KL, Narahara KA, Murray JA, Williams DL: Myocardial imaging with thallium-201 at rest and during exercise: comparison with coronary arteriography and resting and stress electrocardiography. Circulation 56:66-71, 1977.
4. Lenaers A, Block P, van Thiel E, Lebedele M, Becquevort P, Erbsmann F, Ermans AM: Segmental analysis of Tl-201 stress myocardial scintigraphy. J Nucl Med 18:509-516, 1977.
5. Ritchie JL, Zaret BL, Strauss HW, Pitt B, Berman DS, Schelbert HR, Ashburn WL, Berger HJ, Hamilton GW: Myocardial imaging with thallium-201: a multicenter study in patients with angina pectoris or acute myocardial infarction. Am J Cardiol 42:345-350, 1978.
6. Botvinick EH, Taradash MR, Shames DM, Parmley WW: Thallium-201 myocardial perfusion scintigraphy for the clinical clarification of normal, abnormal and equivocal electrocardiographic stress tests. Am J Cardiol 41:43-51, 1978.
7. Wackers FJTh, Lie Ki, Liem KI., Busemann Sokole E, Samson G, van der Schoot JB, Durrer D: Thallium-201 scintigraphy in unstable angina pectoris. Circulation 57:738-742, 1978.
8. Trobaugh GB, Wackers FJTh, Busemann Sokole E, DeRouen TA, Ritchie JL, Hamilton GW: Thallium-201 myocardial imaging: an interinstitutional study of observer variability. J Nucl Med 19:359-363, 1978.
9. Gewirtz H, Beller GA, Strauss HW, Dinsmore RE, Zir LM, McKusick KA, Pohost GM: Transient defects of resting thallium scans in patients with coronary artery disease. Circulation 59:707-713, 1979.

10. Berger BC, Watson DD, Burwell LR, Crosby IK, Wellons HA, Teates CD, Beller GA: Redistribution of thallium at rest in patients with stable and unstable angina and the effect of coronary artery bypass surgery. Circulation 60:1114-1125, 1979.

11. Weich HF, Strauss HW, Pitt B: The extraction of thallium-201 by the myocardium. Circulation 56:188-191, 1977.

12. Wilson FN. Johnston FD: The occurrence in angina pectoris of electrocardiographic changes similar in magnitude and in kind to those produced by myocardial infarction. Am Heart J 22:64-74, 1941.

13. Prinzmetal M, Kennamer R, Merliss R, Wada T, Bor N: Angina pectoris – I. A Variant form of angina pectoris. Am J Med 27:375-388, 1959.

14. Oliva PB, Potts DE, Pluss G: Coronary arterial spasm in Prinzmetal angina. N Engl J Med 288:745-751, 1973.

15. Wiener L, Kasparian H, Duca PB, Walinsky P, Gottlieb RS, Hanckel F, Brest AN: Spectrum of coronary arterial spasm. Clinical, angiographic and myocardial metabolic experience in 29 cases. Am J Cardiol 38:945-955, 1976.

16. Cuazzi M, Polese A, Florentini C, Magrini F, Olivari MT, Bartorelli C: Left and right heart hemodynamics during spontaneous angina pectoris. Comparison between angina with ST-segment depression and angina with ST-segment elevation. Br Heart J 37:401-413, 1975.

17. Maseri A, Mimmo R, Chierchia S, Marchesi C, Pesola A, L'Abbate A: Coronary spasm as a cause of acute myocardial ischemia in man. Chest 68: 625-633, 1975.

18. Figueras J, Singh BH, Phil D, Ganz. W, Charuzi Y, Swan HFC: Mechanism of rest and nocturnal angina: observations during continuous hemodynamic and electrocardiographic monitoring. Circulation 59:955-968, 1979.

19. Maseri A, Parodi O, Severi S. Pesola A: Transient transmural reduction of myocardial blood flow, demonstrated by thallium-201 scintigraphy, as a cause of variant angina. Circulation 54:280-288, 1976.

20. Maseri A, Pesola A, Marzilli M, Severi S, Parodi O, L'Abbate A, Ballestra AM, Maltinti G, DeNes DM, Biagini A: Coronary vasospasm in angina pectoris. The Lancet: 713-717, April 2, 1977.

21. Maseri A, L'Abbate A, Baroldi G, Chierchia S, Marzilli M Ballestra AM, Severi S, Parodi O, Biagini A, Distante A, Pesola A: Coronary Vasospasm as a possible cause of myocardial infarction: a conclusion derived from the study of « preinfarction" angina. N Engl J Med 229:1271-1277, 1978.

22. Maseri A, Severi S, DeNes M, L'Abbate A, Chierchia S, Marzilli M, Ballestra AM, Parodi O, Biagini A, Distante A: "Variant" angina: one aspect of a continuous spectrum of vasospastic myocardial ischemia. Am J Cardiol 42:1019-1035, 1978.

23. McLaughlin PR, Doherty PW, Martin RP, Goris ML, Harrison DC: Myocardial imaging in a patient with reproducible variant angina. Am J Cardiol 39:126-129, 1977.

24. Yasue H, Omote S, Takizawa A, Nagao M, Miwa K, Tanaka S: Exertional angina pectoris caused by coronary arterial spasm: effects of various drugs. Am J Cardiol 43:647-652, 1979.

25. Waters DD, Chaitman BR, Dupras G., Theroux P, Mizgala HF: Coronary artery spasm during exercise in patients with variant angina. Circulation 58:580-585, 1979.

26. Yasue H, Omote S, Takizawa A, Nagao M, Miwa K, Tanaka S: Circadian variation of exercise capacity in patients with Prinzmetal's variant angina: role of exercise-induced coronary arterial spasm. Circulation 59:938-948, 1979.

27. Specchia, G. DeServi S. Falcone C. Bramucci E, Angoli L, Mussini A, Marinoni GP, Montemartini C, Bobba P Coronary arterial spasm as a cause of exercise-induced ST-segment elevation in patients with variant angina. Circulation 59:948-953, 1979.

28. Lie KI, Wackers F, Liem K, David G, Busemann Sokole E, Samson G, van der Schoot J, Durrer D: Thallium-201 scintigraphy for differentiation between variant angina and intermediate coronary syndrome. Circulation 56, suppl II, III 229, 1977.

11. TECHNETIUM-99m-PYROPHOSPHATE MYOCARDIAL IMAGING IN UNSTABLE ANGINA

JAMES T. WILLERSON, ROBERT W. PARKEY, FREDERICK J. BONTE, SAMUEL E. LEWIS and L. MAXIMILIAN BUJA

Technetium-99m-pyrophosphate myocardial scintigrams may be abnormal in patients with unstable angina pectoris even if serum enzymes are normal and the electrocardiogram is either normal or nonspecifically abnormal and demonstrates ST-T wave changes [1–3]. Abnormal ^{99m}Tc-pyrophosphate scintigrams in these patients often demonstrate faint (" 2 + ") and poorly localized increased ^{99m}Tc-pyrophosphate uptake (Figures 11-1, 11-2 and 11-3).

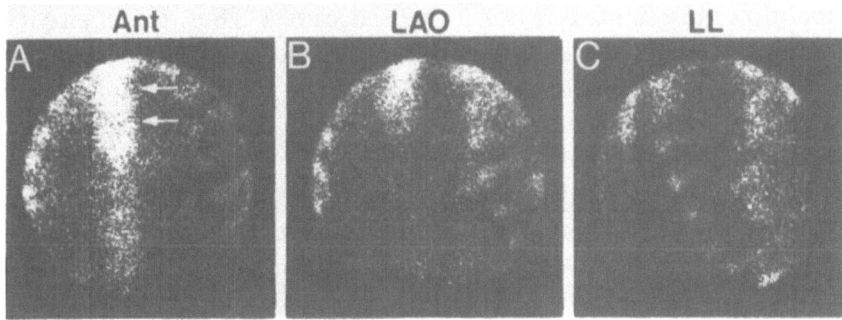

Figure 11-1. A negative ^{99m}Tc-pyrophosphate myocardial scintigram is shown in the anterior (panel A), left anterior oblique (panel B), and left lateral (panel C) imaging projections. The closed arrows mark the radionuclide uptake in the sternum.

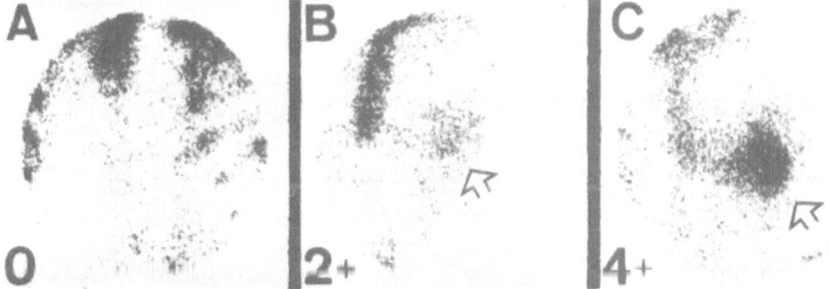

Figure 11-2. The grading scheme utilized for the interpretation of ^{99m}Tc-pyrophosphate myocardial scintigrams at our institution is shown. We regard ^{99m}Tc-pyrophosphate myocardial scintigrams that are "2+–4+" in intensity as being abnormal and reflecting acute myocardial necrosis.

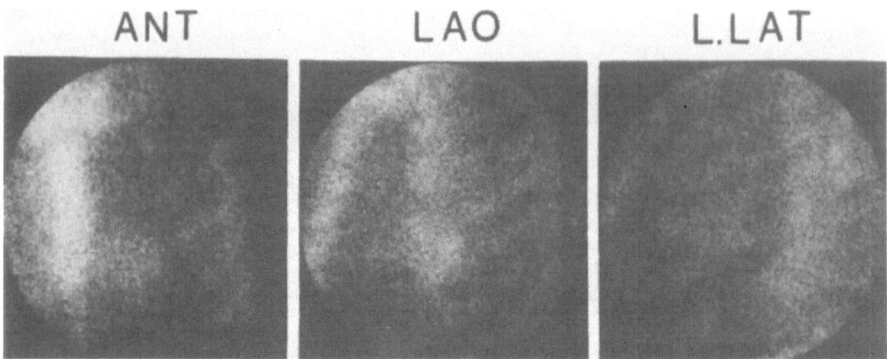

ANT   LAO   L.LAT

Figure 11-3. An acute nontransmural (subendocardial) myocardial infarct as demonstrated by ^{99m}Tc-pyrophosphate myocardial imaging is shown. Note that the ^{99m}Tc-pyrophosphate uptake is fainter and less well localized than occurs with acute transmural myocardial infarcts.

The major problem with using enzymes and electrocardiograms to confirm or deny the presence of acute myocardial necrosis in patients with unstable angina pectoris is that such individuals have often had pain for days to weeks and the myocardial damage is usually subendocardial. Thus, serum enzymes may be normal simply because acute myocardial necrosis has occurred prior to or after enzyme testing is performed. In addition, the electrocardiogram is not capable of detecting acute subendocardial myocardial infarcts with certainty but may only demonstrate ST depression and T wave inversion consistent with either subendocardial ischemia or infarction. It has been known for many years that a certain percentage of patients with acute myocardial infarcts do not have these lesions detected by enzyme testing and electrocardiographic analysis [3–6].

We have found that appriximately one third of patients with the syndrome of unstable angina pectoris have abnormal ^{99m}Tc-pyrophosphate myocardial scintigrams even in the absence of abnormal enzymes and electrocardiographic confirmation of the presence of acute myocardial necrosis [1–3]. In patients in whom we have had the opportunity to make autopsy clinicopathologic correlates between the results of ^{99m}Tc-pyrophosphate myocardial scintigraphy and the presence or absence of acute myocardial necrosis, we have ordinarily found that the " 2 + " and " poorly localized " abnormal scintigrams correlate with the presence of multicellular damage located in the subendocardial region (Figure 11-3). Others have also shown a close correlation between abnormal ^{99m}Tc-pyrophosphate myocardial scintigram and elevated creatinekinase-MB isoenzyme values when serial and frequent enzyme testing is used in patients with unstable angina pectoris [7].

Thus, ^{99m}Tc-pyrophosphate myocardial imaging technique appears to represent a sensitive means to detect acute multicellular injury associated with the clinical syndrome of unstable angina pectoris even when cardiac enzymes are normal and the electrocardiogram does not definitively document the presence of acute myocardial necrosis. This is of clinical use because it allows one to determine the presence of heart muscle injury and then proceed in the most appropriate manner for an individual patient. The major unresolved question presently concerning patients with unstable pectoris and abnormal ^{99m}Tc-pyrophosphate myocardial scintigrams is whether they are the patients most in need or least in need of coronary artery revascularization. Empirically, we have found that many of the abnormal ^{99m}Tc-pyrophosphate myocardial scintigrams become normal following revascularization in patients in this subgroup. Broad comparisons between individuals in this setting that have abnormal or normal ^{99m}Tc-pyrophosphate myocardial scintigrams with subsequent clinical course are still needed.

REFERENCES

1. Buja LM, Poliner L, Parkey RW, et al.: Clinicopathologic findings in patients with persistently positive technetium-99m stannous pyrophosphate myocardial scintigrams and myocytolytic degeneration after acute myocardial infarction. Circulation 56:1016, 1977.
2. Donsky MS, Curry GC, Parkey RW, et al.: Unstable angina pectoris: Clinical, angiographic, and myocardial scintigraphic observations. Br Heart J 38:257, 1976.
3. Poliner LR, Buja LM, Parkey RW, Bonte FJ, Willerson JT: Clinicopathologic findings in 52 patients studied by technetium-99m stannous pyrophosphate myocardial scintigrams. Circulation 59:257, 1979.
4. Roberts WC: The coronary arteries and left ventricle in clinically isolated angina pectoris. A necropsy analysis. Circulation 54:388, 1976.
5. Alison HW, Moraski RE, Mantle JA, et al.: Coronary anatomy and arteriography in patients with unstable angina pectoris. Am J Cardiol 35:118, 1975.
6. Eliot RS, and Edwards JE: Pathology of coronary atherosclerosis and its complications. In: The Heart, 3rd edition, p 1003, Hurst JW, ed. New York: McGraw-Hill, 1974.
7. Jaffe AS, Klein MS, Patel BR, et al.: Abnormal technetium-99m pyrophosphate images in unstable angina: ischemia versus infarction? Am J Cardiol 44:1035, 1979.

MYOCARDIAL IMAGING IN PATIENTS
WITH ATYPICAL CHEST PAIN

12. THALLIUM-201 MYOCARDIAL IMAGING AS A SELECTION METHOD FOR THE CORONARY CARE UNIT

FRANS J. TH. WACKERS, K.I. LIE, ELLINOR BUSEMANN SOKOLE, GERARD SAMSON and JAN B. VAN DER SCHOOT

In many patients admitted to the coronary care unit, the diagnosis of acute myocardial infarction is evident at the time of arrival at the hospital. However, among the patients referred to a coronary care unit a significant number has complaints which are determined later not to be caused by acute coronary artery insufficiency. In many of these patients, the history and the initial electrocardiogram will provide sufficient information to recognize the noncardiac etiology of the complaints. Nevertheless, a substantial group of patients still remains in whom initial evaluation provides a questionable history and a nondiagnostic electrocardiogram: in these patients admission and further observation for at least 24 hours in the coronary care unit seems unavoidable to rule out acute myocardial infarction or ischemia. In order to maximize efficient management and use of the coronary care unit, early and proper characterization of patients in whom the diagnosis remains in question is essential.

In the previous chapters we have demonstrated that ^{201}Tl scinigraphy is a highly sensitive technique for the detection of acute myocardial infarction, especially during the first hours after onset of symptoms of chest pain [1]. In addition, we reported that a considerable number of patients with unstable angina may have abnormal ^{201}Tl scintiscans during the pain free period after an anginal attack [2].

These results suggested that ^{201}Tl scintigraphy may have potential value to serve as a more appropriate means of selecting patients for admission to the coronary care unit. In order to evaluate this possibility, we performed a prospective study from September 1975 to September 1976 [3]. During this period, 1861 patients were referred to the coronary care unit because of presumed acute myocardial infarction. The admission policy for these patients is shown in Figure 12-1. There were 1212 patients (65%) who were directly admitted because of evident acute cardiac disease based on history and/or electrocardiogram. In 338 patients (18%) cardiac disease could be ruled out by history, symptoms, further examination and electrocardiogram. These patients were either transferred to other departments or were allowed to return home. A diagnostic problem was posed by 311 (17%) patients because of atypical

224

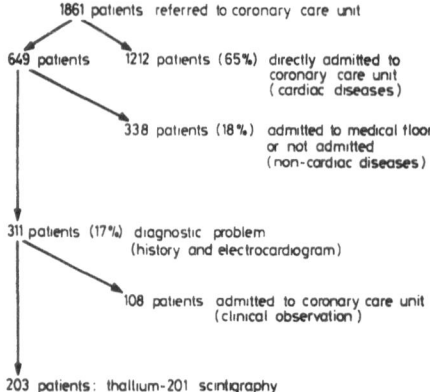

1861 patients referred to coronary care unit

649 patients   1212 patients (65%) directly admitted to
                                      coronary care unit
                                      (cardiac diseases)

                338 patients (18%) admitted to medical floor
                                      or not admitted
                                      (non-cardiac diseases)

311 patients (17%) diagnostic problem
                   (history and electrocardiogram)

                108 patients admitted to coronary care unit
                            (clinical observation)

203 patients: thallium-201 scintigraphy

Figure 12-1. Admission policy in 1861 patients referred to the coronary care unit. In 203 patients [201]Tl Scintigraphy was evaluated as a potential selection method. See text. Reproduced with permission from Ref. [3].

history and/or nondiagnostic electrocardiogram. Such patients are usually admitted to the coronary care unit for further evaluation over a period of at least 24 hr to rule out acute myocardial infarction. In 203 of the 311 patients ^{201}Tl scintigraphy was performed on arrival in the coronary care unit. In these patients the time interval between the last episode of chest pain and scintigraphy did not exceed 10 hr. Entry into this study of these 203 patients in whom the diagnosis initially was unclear, was determined only by the availability of the radiopharmaceutical and the gamma camera.

THALLIUM-201 SCINTIGRAPHY AND ELECTROCARDIOGRAM

Thallium-201 scintigraphy was performed in the 203 patients as soon as possible after arrival at the hospital. Imaging and analysis of the scintiscans was performed as described in previous chapters. Of the 203 patients, 49 had positive, 47 had questionable and 107 had normal ^{201}Tl scintiscans. It should

Table 12-1. Relation between results of ^{201}Tl scintigraphy and electrocardiograms in 203 patients [3]

Scintigraphy	Electrocardiogram		Total
	Normal	Nonspecific ST-T segment changes	
Defect	12	37	49
Questionable	17	30	47
Normal	49	58	107

be emphasized that in none of these patients was the diagnosis clear by either history or electrocardiogram. Except for one patient, who had complete left bundle branch block, all patients showed a normal initial ventricular activation pattern on the electrocardiogram at the time of scintigraphy. The electrocardiogram was normal in 78 patients and showed non-specific ST-segment changes in 125 patients. The relationship between scintigraphic results and electrocardiographic findings is shown in Table 12-1.

FINAL DIAGNOSIS

The final diagnosis in these patients was based upon the results of serial enzyme determinations (SGOT, SGPT, LDH and CKMB), the development of electrocardiographic changes and the impression obtained after further clinical evaluation.

The following diagnostic criteria were used:

Acute myocardial infarction

(1) Enzyme levels showing typical rise and fall after admission; (2) electrocardiographic development of diagnostic Q waves of more than 0.03 s in duration, loss of R waves or T wave inversion.

Unstable angina progressing to acute myocardial infarction

(1) Normal enzyme levels at the time of scintigraphy; and (2) occurrence of a new severe attack of chest pain within 24 h after admission to the hospital, followed by electrocardiographic development of diagnostic Q waves, loss of R waves, or T wave inversion, and typical rise and fall of enzyme levels.

Unstable angina

(1) Normal enzyme levels during the observation period; (2) upon further questioning a history suggesting angina pectoris increasing in severity and frequency within a period of approximately 10 days before admission; and (3) transient electrocardiographic changes were not required. Note: Since all the patients included in this study had atypical history on admission, the term "unstable angina" is defined more liberally than usual.

Previous myocardial infarction

(1) Diagnostic Q wave on the electrocardiogram; and (2) normal enzyme levels during the observation period.

Stable angina pectoris

(1) Normal enzyme levels; and (2) history of chest pain occuring on exertion and disappearing at rest, relieved by nitroglycerin.

Atypical complaints

(1) Normal enzyme levels; and (2) after further questioning, it was felt that the complaints were atypical for angina pectoris and, most likely of noncardiac origin.

On the basis of serum enzyme determination, *34 patients (17%) had acute myocardial infarcts at the time of scintigraphy.* Fourteen of these patients evolved electrocardiographic transmural infarcts with peak SGOT rise of more than 4 times the upper limit of normal. Of these patients two had recurrent myocardial infarcts. Twenty patients had electrocardiographic nontransmural or biochemically small infarcts (SGOT rise less than 4 times upper limit of normal). *Forty-seven patients (23%) had "unstable angina"* at the time of ^{201}Tl scintigraphy; in seven of these this progressed to acute myocardial infarction within 24 hours after admission, and four of these seven patients had electrocardiographic evidence of transmural infarcts. The remaining 40 patients with "unstable agina" had an unremarkable clinical course. *Twenty-four patients (12%) had previous myocardial infarcts.* Twenty-five patients (12%) were considered to have symptoms of *stable angina pectoris.* In 73 (36%) the final impression was of *atypical complaints,* most likely of noncardiac origin.

RELATIONSHIP BETWEEN FINAL DIAGNOSIS AND RESULTS
OF THALLIUM-201 SCINTIGRAPHY (Figure 12-2)

All 34 patients determined later to have had acute myocardial infarcts at the time of scintigraphy, had abnormal ^{201}Tl scintiscans: thirty patients showed definite defects and in the remaining four patients the scintiscans were judged as questionable. The two patients with recurrent infarction both had positive scans. Of the seven patients with "unstable angina" who developed acute myocardial infarcts, five had positive scans, and two had questionable scans.

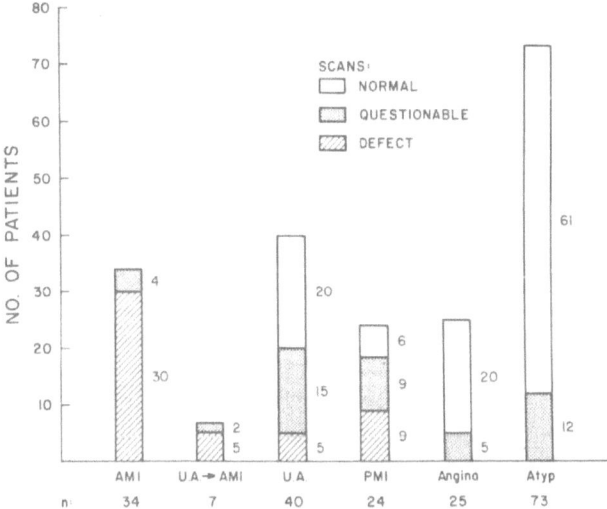

Figure 12-2. Final diagnosis in 203 patients referred to the coronary care unit to rule out acute myocardial infarction and the results of ^{201}Tl scintigraphy on admission. The final diagnosis is based on results of enzyme level determinations, the development of electrocardiographic changes and the reevaluation of the patient's history. Abbreviations: AMI = acute myocardial infarction; PMI = previous myocardial infarction; UA = unstable angina; UA → AMI = unstable angina progressing to acute myocardial infarction; ATYP = atypical complaints. Reproduced with permission from Ref. [3].

Of the remaining 40 patients with uncomplicated "unstable angina", five had positive scans, 15 had questionable scans and 20 had normal scans. Of the patients with previous myocardial infarcts, nine showed ^{201}Tl defects, nine had questionable scans and six had normal scans. None of the patients with stable angina pectoris or atypical complaints had a defect on the ^{201}Tl scintiscans. Five of 25 patients with stable angina had questionable scans; the remaining 20 had normal scans. Of the 73 patients with atypical complaints, 12 had questionable scans and 61 patients had normal scans.

Thus, positive scintiscans were obtained only in patients with acute or previous myocardial infarction or "unstable angina". In this same patient group, questionable scans were obtained in 30 of 105 patients, compared to 17 of 98 patients with stable angina or atypical complaints ($P = $ NS). Normal scintiscans were obtained in 26 or 105 patients who had acute or previous myocardial infarction or "unstable angina", compared with 81 of 98 patients with stable angina or atypical complaints ($P < 0.01$).

The patient group described above represents a common diagnostic dilemma in the coronary care unit or emergency room. Neither the patient's history nor the electrocardiogram permitted a definite diagnosis at the time of admission. Yet, 34 patients evolved acute myocardial infarction and all these patients had abnormal (positive or questionable) ^{201}Tl scintiscans on

228

admission. Diagnostic electrocardiographic changes, if any, occurred in these patients only hours after admission. Figures 12-3 and 12-4 show examples of such patients. These findings are consistent with results reported by Behar et al. [4], who evaluated the electrocardiogram as a decision-making tool in the emergency room. In a consecutive series of patients 35% of those with acute myocardial infarcts showed a normal electrocardiogram initially on arrival in the emergency room.

In addition to the patients with acute myocardial infarcts in our study, there were also 10 patients with "unstable angina" in whom positive ^{201}Tl scintiscans were obtained. Five of these developed acute myocardial infarcts after being admitted to the hospital; a similar progression occurred in two of 22 patients with "unstable agina" who had questionable scintiscans on admission (Figure 12-4). This is consistent with our results in a larger series of patients with "unstable angina", in whom positive studies indicated a

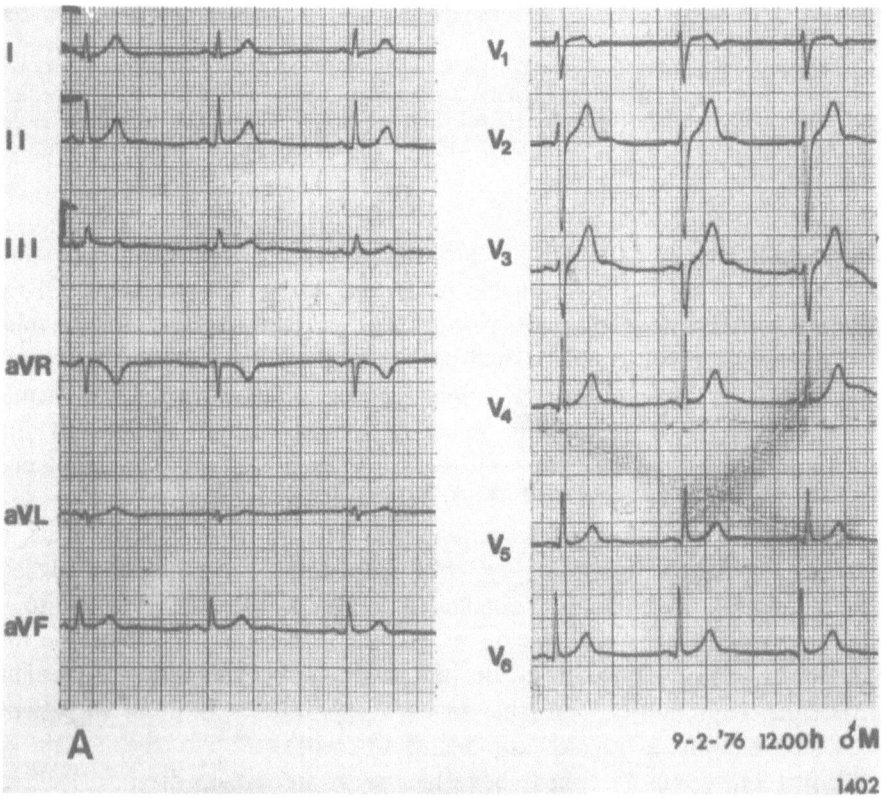

Figure 12-3. (A) Electrocardiogram on admission of a 37-y-old male. The night before admission he experienced recurrent attacks of atypical praecordial pain, which had subsided at admission. Though there is loss of R wave in V_3, this electrocardiogram is not diagnostic for acute myocardial infarction.

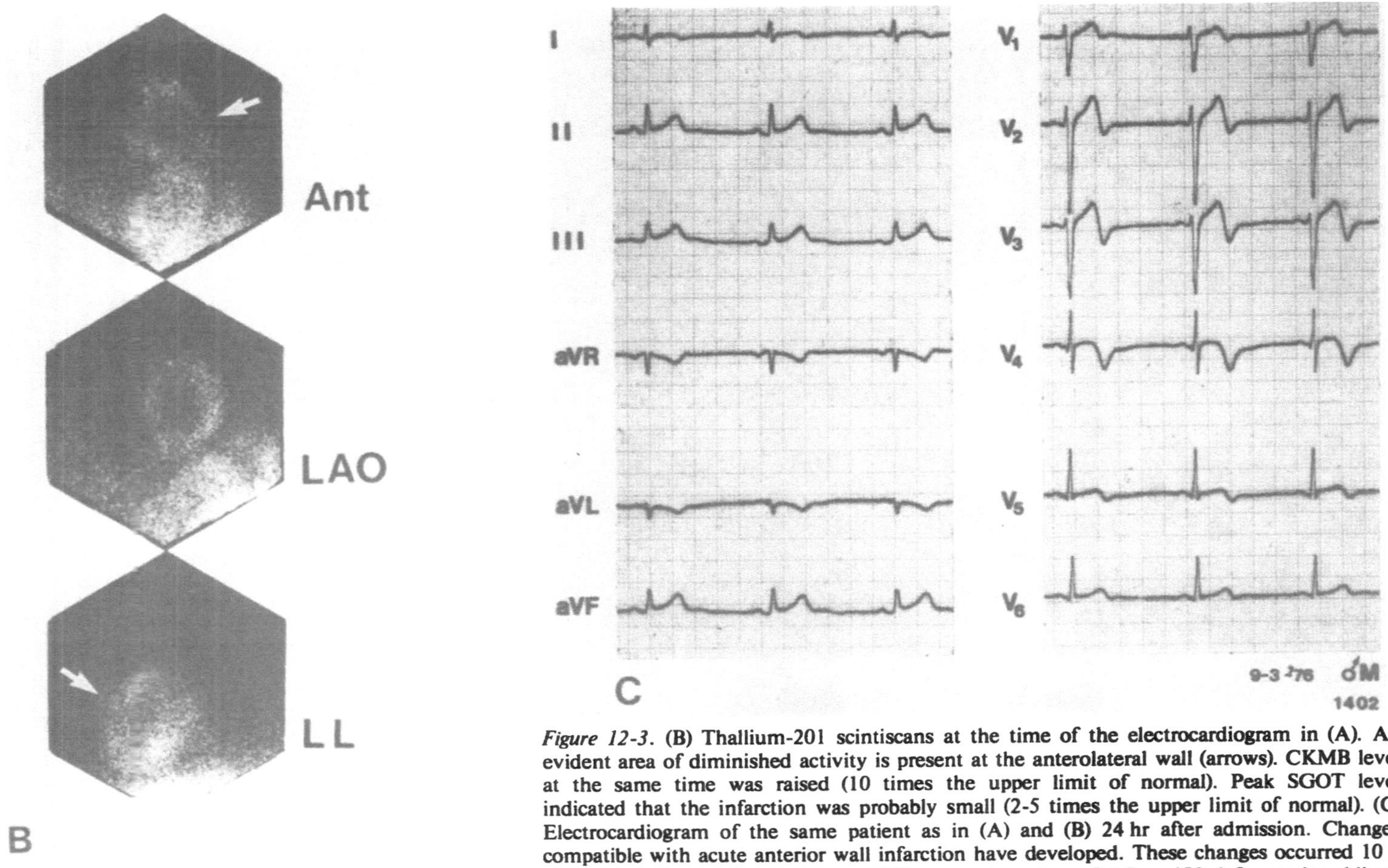

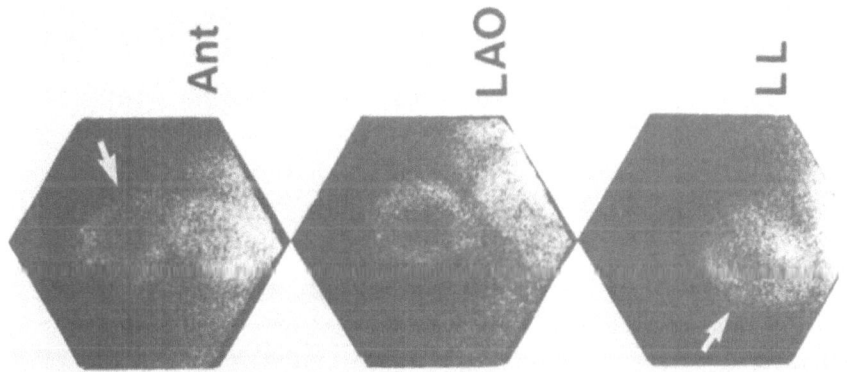

Figure 12-3. (B) Thallium-201 scintiscans at the time of the electrocardiogram in (A). An evident area of diminished activity is present at the anterolateral wall (arrows). CKMB level at the same time was raised (10 times the upper limit of normal). Peak SGOT level indicated that the infarction was probably small (2-5 times the upper limit of normal). (C) Electrocardiogram of the same patient as in (A) and (B) 24 hr after admission. Changes compatible with acute anterior wall infarction have developed. These changes occurred 10 h after admission. Abbreviations: ANT = anterior view; LAO = 45° left-anterior-oblique view; LL = left-lateral view. Reproduced with permission from Ref. [3].

230

poorer prognosis [2]. Thus, the lack of specificity of ^{201}Tl imaging is not necessarily a disadvantage but provides a means to recognize patients at high risk. Moreover, both the presence of an acute myocardial infarction and "unstable angina" are indications for admission to the coronary care unit.

The present series of patients represents a highly selected group of patients in whom neither the electrocardiogram nor the history were diagnostic. Therefore, the value of ^{201}Tl scintigraphy is maximally challenged. It is in this group of patients that a reliable selection method may be of great clinical usefulness. A selection procedure for the coronary care unit or emergency room ideally should be able to detect and differentiate (a) patients with acute myocardial infarcts, (b) patients with previous myocardial infarcts, (c) patients with unstable angina, and (d) patients with noncardiac complaints.

The results of our study indicate that ^{201}Tl scintigraphy might be such a method when positive and questionable scans are considered abnormal.

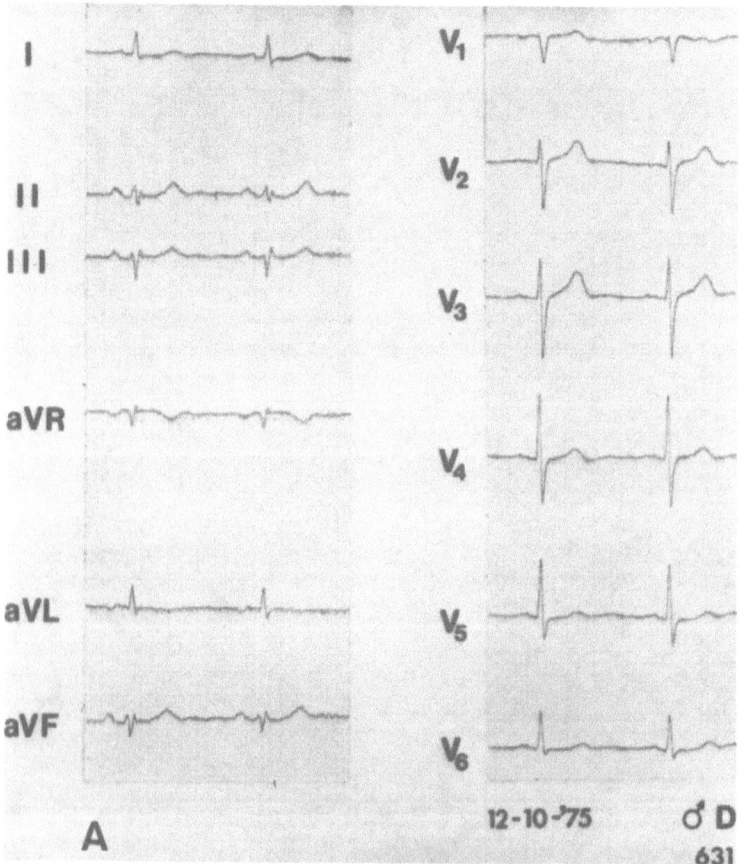

Figure 12-4. (A) Electrocardiogram on admission of a patient with a history of progressive chest discomfort. No diagnostic changes are present.

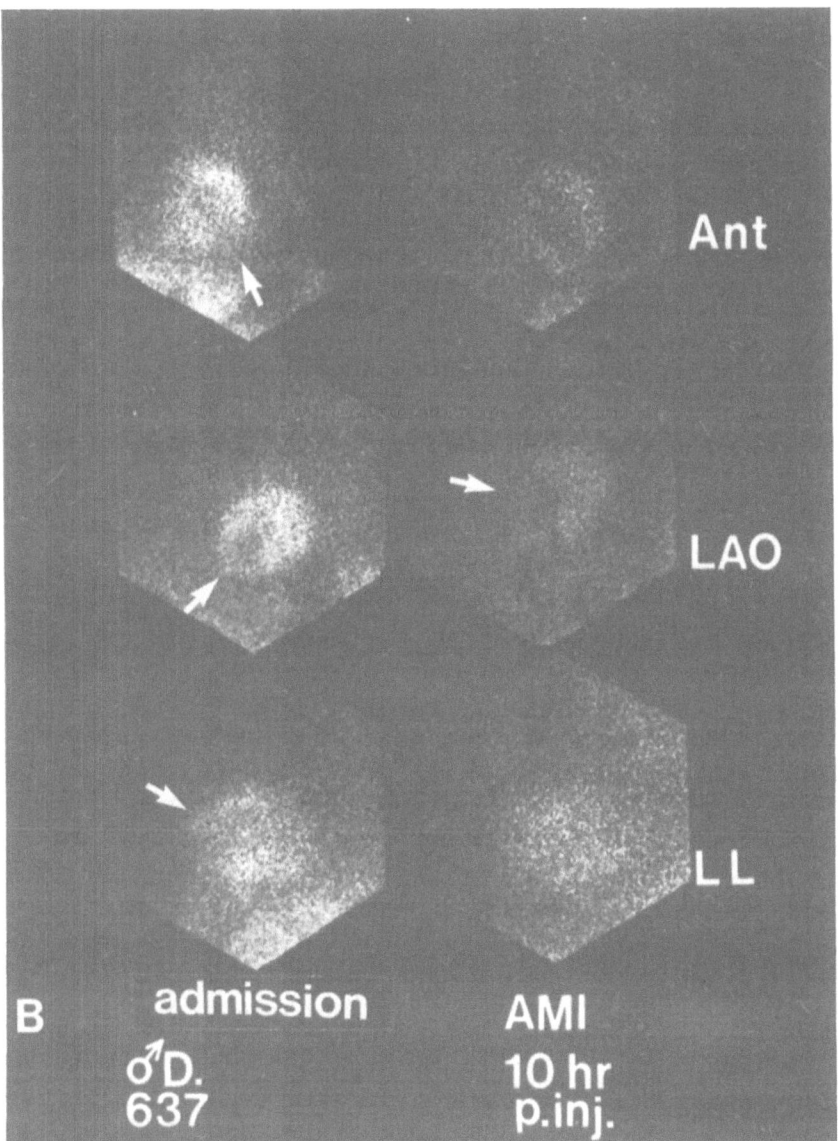

Figure 12-4. (B) Thallium-201 scintiscans on admission (left) and 10 hr later (right), 5 hr after patient developed typical acute chest pain. Admission scintiscans demonstrate a subtle area of diminished activity in the apical-septal region (arrows). The second study is obtained 10 hr after injection of [201]Tl. The left-anterior-oblique view displays a definite septal defect. Thallium-201 apparently has leaked out of the infarcted myocardium.

232

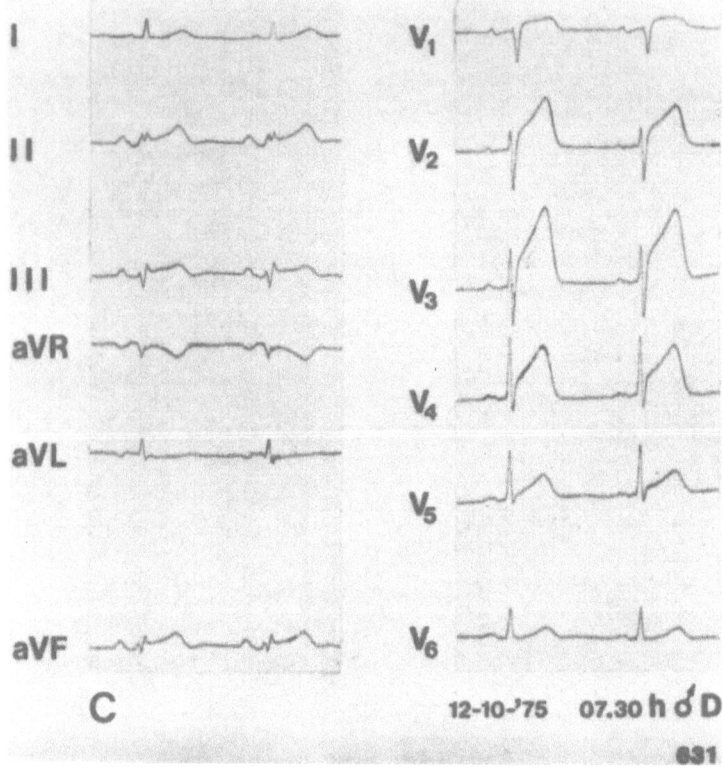

Figure 12-4. (C) Electrocardiogram shorthly after the onset of acute chest pain. ST-segment elevation can be noted in leads II, III, AVF, V_{1-5}.

Potential influence of thallium-201 scintigraphy on CCU admissions

Table 12-2 illustrates the potential influence of ^{201}Tl scintigraphy on the admission policy in the coronary care unit. It seems conceivable that in most

Table 12-2. Evaluation of admission policy in 203 patients: admission based on electrocardiograms and history is compared with that based on ^{201}Tl scintigraphy and related to final follow-up diagnosis (see text)[3]

Admission based on	Destination		Incorrect decision	
	Hospital	Home	Hospital	Home
Electrocardiogram + history	203	—	122 (60%)	—
Thallium-201 scintigraphy	96	107	35 (36%)	20 (18%)
Retrospect diagnosis	81	122		
	(AMI, UA)	(atyp)		

Abbreviations: AMI, acute myocardial infarction; UA, unstable angina; atyp, atypical complaints

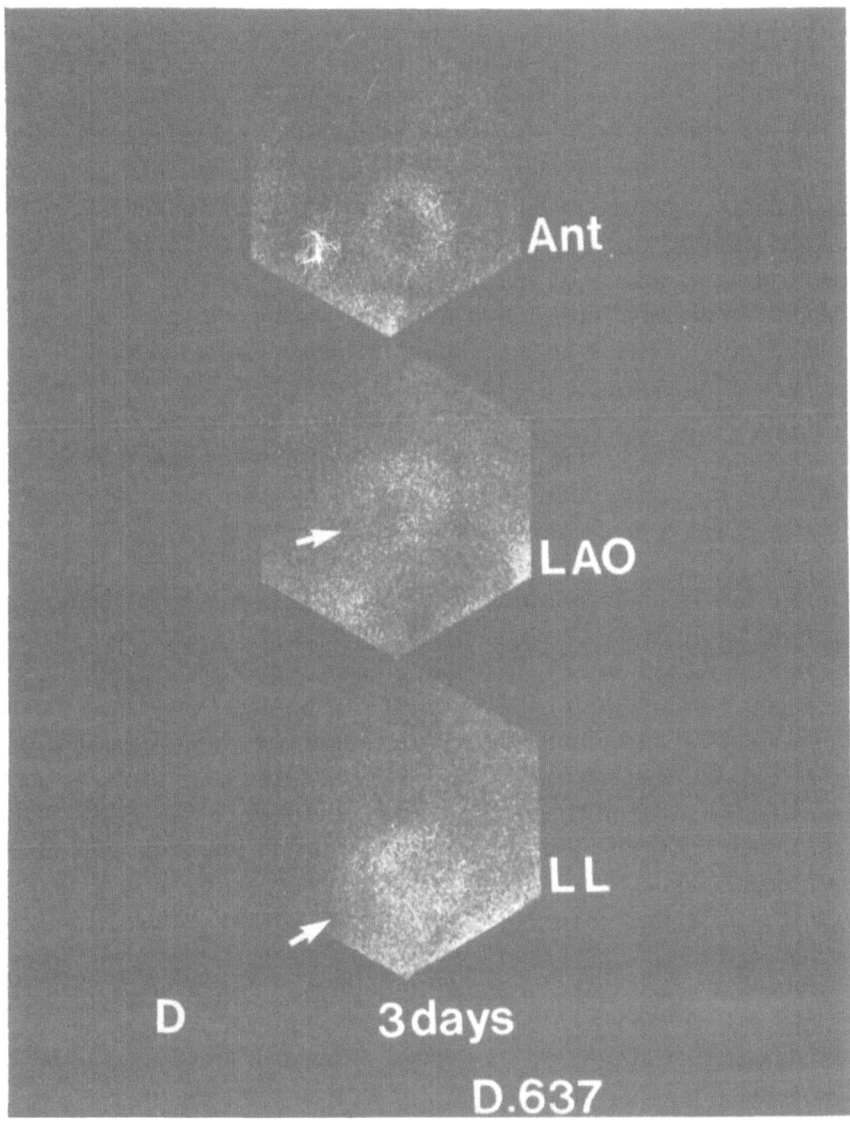

Figure 12-4. (D) Thallium-201 scintiscans (after new injection of ²⁰¹Tl) 3 days after acute infarction. An inferoseptal perfusion defect (arrows) can be noted, similar to the admission study. Abbreviations: ANT = anterior view; LAO = 45° left-anterior-oblique view; LL = left-lateral view.

medical centers the 203 patients included in the study described above would have been admitted to rule out acute myocardial infarcts. Everyone would agree that all patients with acute myocardial infarcts and "unstable angina" should be admitted to a coronary care unit. Consequently in the present study, a total of 81 patients (those who later appeared to have acute myocardial infarcts or unstable angina) had to be admitted to the coronary care unit. Therefore, the remaining 122 patients (60%) were admitted unnecessarily. In contrast, if the results of ^{201}Tl scintigraphy were used as selection criteria, 96 patients with positive and questionable scans would have been admitted and 107 patients with normal scans would be allowed to return home. Therefore, using ^{201}Tl scintigraphy as admission criterion, all patients with acute myocardial infarction, and the majority of patients with "unstable angina" would have been admitted correctly to the coronary care unit, and only 35 patients (18 with previous infarction, five with stable angina, and 12 with atypical complaints) would have been hospitalized unnecessarily. On the other hand, 20 patients with "unstable angina" would have been allowed to return home. However, it should again be emphasized that "unstable agina" in the present context represents a liberal use of the terminology. Moreover all patients with "unstable angina" who had normal scintiscans, had an unremarkable and favorable clinical course. Thus it appears that ^{201}Tl scintigraphy has potential value as a means to help select patients for the coronary care unit.

Since the completion of the above described study, these results have been reproduced in a much larger series of patients in the coronary care unit of the Wilhelmina Gasthuis in Amsterdam, The Netherlands [5]. Moreover, Haft et al. [6] reported recently similar results in 66 consecutive patients admitted to the coronary care unit with chest pain and possible acute myocardial infarction. Thallium-201 imaging in these patients was performed within the first 24 hr after onset of chest pain. Fifteen of 66 patients later proved to have sustained acute myocardial infarction by serial enzymes and electrocardiograms. Eleven (73%) of these had positive scans and four had equivocal or normal images. Thus, these results are comparable to ours and it is conceivable that with earlier myocardial imaging all patients would have been detected.

In view of the high cost of coronary care units, it is mandatory that only those patients with bonafide acute coronary syndromes are admitted. The sensitivity of ^{201}Tl scintigraphy to detect acute myocardial infarcts (88%) indicates that this method might be useful as a selection method for the coronary care unit in the emergency room. The standard electrocardiogram may be nondiagnostic during the early hours of an acute infarction in some patients. In addition, when abnormal initial ventricular activation pattern is present, such as in left bundle branch block, WPW syndrome, or pacemaker rhythm, the electrocardiographic diagnosis of acute infarction is hampered.

On the basis of the present study, the following practical guidelines can be given for the use of ^{201}Tl scintigraphy as a method for triage:

(a) Thallium-201 scintigraphy has to be performed within 6 to 10 hr after the last episode of chest pain.

(b) In the presence of previous myocardial infarction positive ^{201}Tl scintiscans have limited diagnostic value, although the size of scintigraphic abnormality provides clinically useful information.

(c) Negative ^{201}Tl scintiscans obtained within 6–10 hr after acute chest pain, reduce the likelihood of acute myocardial infarction importantly, although acute coronary insufficiency cannot be excluded.

(d) Positive ^{201}Tl scintiscans may represent either acute myocardial infarction, previous myocardial infarction or "unstable angina". Delayed or redistribution imaging 3–4 hr after injection might be helpful in these patients to differentiate between acute ischemia and myocardial infarction [7, 8].

In conclusion, it should be emphasized that the above described study deals with a particular subgroup of patients in whom the history and the electrocardiogram were of little help in clinical decision making. Thallium-201 scintigraphy has to be viewed as an additional but important diagnostic method, along with the history and electrocardiogram, that can improve efficient management of patients with potential coronary artery disease syndrome.

REFERENCES

1. Wackers FJTh, Busemann Sokole E, Samson G, van der Schoot JB, Lie KI, Liem KL, Wellens HJJ: Value and limitations of thallium-201 scintigraphy in the acute phase of myocardial infarction. N Engl J Med 295:1-5, 1976.
2. Wackers FJTh, Lie KI, Liem KL, Busemann Sokole E, Samson G, vander Schoot JB, Durrer D: Thallium-201 scintigraphy in unstable angina pectoris. Circulation 57:738-741, 1978.
3. Wackers FJTh, Lie KI, Liem KL, Busemann Sokole E, Samson G, van der Schoot J, Durrer D: Potential value of thallium-201 scintigraphy as a means of selecting patients for the coronary care unit. Br Heart J 41:111-117, 1979.
4. Behar S, Schor S, Kariv I, Barell V, Modan B: Evaluation of electrocardiogram in emergency room as a decision making tool. Chest 71:486-491, 1977.
5. Lie KI: Personal communication, 1979.
6. Haft JI, Platt RN, Wilson JL, Sturman MF: The value of thallium imaging in early diagnosis of acute myocardial infarction. (abstract) Clin. Res 27:563A, 1979.
7. Pohost GM, Zir LM, Moore RM, McKusick KA, Guiney TE, Beller SA: Differentiation of transiently ischemic from infarcted myocardium by serial imaging after a single dose of thallium-201. Circulation 55:294-302, 1977.
8. Pond M, Rehn T, Burow R, Pitt B: Early detection of myocardial infarction by serial thallium-201 imaging. (abstract) Circulation 56, suppl II, III:230, 1977.

13. TECHNETIUM-99m-PYROPHOSPHATE MYOCARDIAL IMAGING IN PATIENTS WITH ATYPICAL CHEST PAIN

JAMES T. WILLERSON, ROBERT W. PARKEY, FREDERICK J. BONTE, ERNEST STOKELY, SAMUEL E. LEWIS and L. MAXIMILIAN BUJA

Technetium-99m-pyrophosphate myocardial scintigrams may be utilized to help exclude the presence of acute myocardial infarcts in patients with atypical chest pain that are admitted to the coronary care unit. Our previous clinicopathologic correlates have suggested that ^{99m}Tc-pyrophosphate myocardial scintigrams are capable of identifying acute myocardial necrosis with 89% sensitivity and high specificity; this scintigraphic approach has an even higher sensitivity (one approaching 100%) in the identification of acute myocardial necrosis amounting to 3 g or more in weight when serial myocardial imaging is utilized and imaging is performed within the proper time frame (Table 13-1)[1–3]. When two ^{99m}Tc-pyrophosphate myocardial scintigrams are obtained in the first 24 hr to 5 days after acute myocardial infarction, one may be confident that serial negative ^{99m}Tc-pyrophosphate myocardial scintigrams exclude acute myocardial necrosis amounting to 3 g or more tissue with better than 95% sensitivity (Table 13-1)[1, 2]. This, of course, requires optimal imaging technique and imaging within the appropriate time periods after the onset of symptoms (chapters 3 and 7) and some experience so that one may properly interpret the ^{99m}Tc-pyrophosphate myocardial scintigrams.

Thus, patients with other causes for chest pain including mitral valve prolapse, anxiety, pulmonary lesions, gastrointestinal abnormalities with pain referred to the chest, etc. may be excluded from those with acute muocardial necrosis by the proper use and interpretation of this imaging test [1–6].

Table 13-1. Predictive indices for the recognition of myocardial necrosis by ^{99m}Tc-pyrophosphate myocardial scintigraphy for 59 clinical events in 52 patients *

Predictive indices	Microscopic or gross necrosis	Gross myocardial infarct
Prevalence	78%	53%
Sensitivity	89%	94%
Specificity	100%	57%
Predictive value		
Positive scan	100%	71%
Negative scan	72%	98%

* This table is reproduced from the work by Poliner et al. [2]

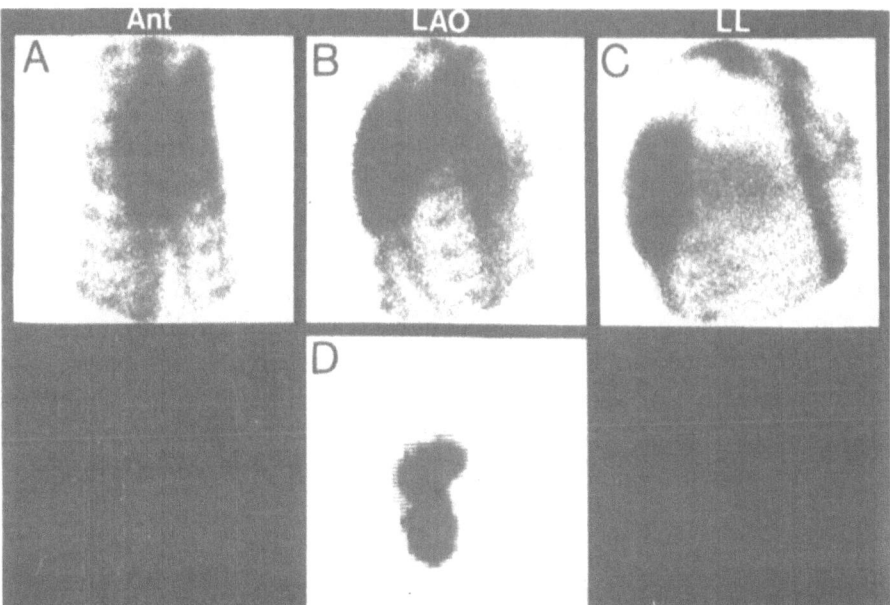

Figure 13-1. The important skeletal muscle damage and myocardial necrosis that occurs in experimental animals receiving multiple episodes of cardioversion across a closed chest wall is demonstrated in this figure. The imaging views are the anterior view (panel A), left anterior oblique (panel B), and left lateral one (panel C). Panel D is an isolated *in-vitro* image of the heart from this experimental animal. Important skeletal muscle necrosis is demonstrated in panels A through C; myocardial necrosis as evidenced by increased ^{99m}Tc-pyrophosphate uptake is shown in panels C and D. Reproduced from Ref. [6] by permission.

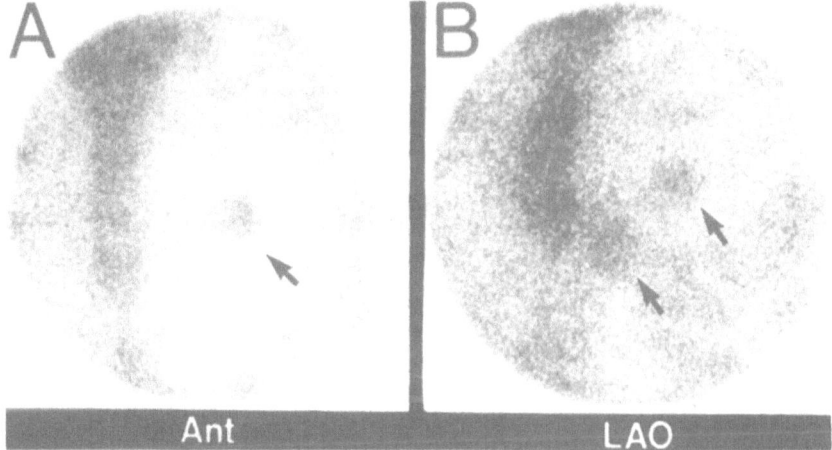

Figure 13-2. The entrance and exit wounds of a bullet passing through the heart of a patient are shown in panel B. This figure demonstrates a ^{99m}Tc-pyrophosphate myocardial scintigram that documents the presence of acute myocardial necrosis as indicated by increased ^{99m}Tc-pyrophosphate uptake both at the entrance and exit sites of this bullet wound. Panel A represents an anterior view and panel B a left anterior oblique view. The entrance and exit wounds for the bullet are best seen in panel B.

It does need to be emphasized, however, that acute myocardial necrosis may occur for reasons other than ischemic heart disease including cardioversion, invasive cardiac tumor, myocarditis, trauma, etc. (Figures 13-1 and 13-2). In these circumstances, ^{99m}Tc-pyrophosphate myocardial scintigrams will be abnormal if more than 3 g of acute myocardial necrosis exist and imaging is performed in the proper time frames [6–8]. In addition, some have suggested that patients with large left ventricular aneurysms commonly have abnormal ^{99m}Tc-pyrophosphate myocardial scintigrams [9]. Our experience has not confirmed this suggestion and in the occasional patient with a left ventricular aneurysm that has an abnormal ^{99m}Tc-pyrophosphate myocardial scintigram, we believe the abnormal scintigram emanates from the margins of the aneurysms where myocardial necrosis and active myocardial ischemia may exist. However, the possibility that calcified, large ventricular aneurysms may also result in an abnormal ^{99m}Tc-pyrophosphate myocardial scintigram needs to be kept in mind.

REFERENCES

1. Buja LM, Poliner L, Parkey RW, et al.: Clinicopathologic findings in patients with persistently positive technetium-99m stannous pyrophosphate myocardial scintigrams and myocytolytic degeneration after acute myocardial infarction. Circulation 56:1016, 1977.
2. Poliner LR, Buja LM, Parkey RW, et al.: Clinicopathologic findings in 52 patients studied by technetium-99m stannous pyrophosphate myocardial scintigrams. Circulation 59:257, 1979.
3. Rude RE, Rubin HS, Stone MJ, et al.: Radioimmunoassay of serum creatine kinase B isoenzyme: correlation with technetium-99m stannous pyrophosphate myocardial scintigraphy in the diagnosis of acute myocardial infarction. Am J Med 68:405, 1980.
4. Buja LM, Parkey RW, Dees JH, et al.: Morphologic correlates of technetium-99m pyrophosphate imaging of acute myocardial infarcts in dogs. Circulation 52:596, 1975.
5. Buja LM, Parkey RW, Stokely EM, et al.: Pathophysiology of technetium-99m stannous pyrophosphate and thallium-201 scintigraphy of acute anterior myocardial infarcts in dogs. J Clin Invest 57:1508, 1976.
6. Pugh BR, Buja LM, Parkey RW et al.: Cardioversion and its potential role in the production of "false positive" technetium-99m stannous pyrophosphate myocardial scintigrams. Circulation 54:399, 1976.
7. Harford W, Weinberg M, Buja LM, et al.: Positive technetium-99m stannous pyrophosphate myocardial scintigram in a patient with carcinoma of the lung. Radiology 122:747, 1977.
8. Willerson JT, Parkey RW, Buja LM, et al.: Technetium-99m stannous pyrophosphate "hot spot" imaging to detect acute myocardial infarcts. In: Nuclear cardiology, p 139, Willerson JT, ed. Philadelphia: F.A. Davis, 1979.
9. Ahmad M, Dubiel JP, Verdon TA Jr, et al.: Technetium-99m stannous pyrophosphate myocardial imaging in patients with and without left ventricular aneurysms. Circulation 53:833, 1976.

CONCLUDING REMARKS

14. MYOCARDIAL IMAGING WITH THALLIUM-201 AND TECHNETIUM-99m-PYROPHOSPHATE IN THE CORONARY CARE UNIT: CONCLUSION

FRANS J. TH. WACKERS and JAMES T. WILLERSON

Since the first reports on successful visualization of acutely infarcted myocardium in patients using ^{99m}Tc-pyrophosphate (1974)[1] and ^{201}Tl (1975)[2], these imaging techniques have been widely employed in patients with acute chest pain syndromes. Not always is the clinical recognition of acute myocardial infarction easily accomplished. The patient's history may be atypical, the electrocardiogram may be nondiagnostic for multiple reasons and the routinely obtained serum enzymes do not always provide absolute certainty for the diagnosis of acute myocardial infarction. Thus, in selected patients there is clearly a place for additional techniques capable of detecting acute myocardial infarction.

Myocardial imaging with ^{201}Tl and ^{99m}Tc-pyrophosphate is a relatively noninvasive technique, requiring only an intravenous injection of the radiopharmaceutical and can be performed at the patient's bedside without major discomfort for the patient.

Each myocardial imaging method has its own attributes and limitations. In the preceding chapters the characteristics of both ^{201}Tl and ^{99m}Tc-pyrophosphate myocardial imaging are outlined. It is critically important to understand the specific temporal sequence and accuracy of each technique so that they can be employed with maximal efficiency.

The two techniques are not just complementary to each other, but they provide different and clinically useful information. Defects on ^{201}Tl scintiscans represent regional disturbances in myocardial blood flow. On one single study, no differentiation can be made between ischemia and necrosis. However, delayed imaging, 2–4 hr after injection[3], may be helpful in assessing the zone of jeopardized ischemic myocardium. On the other hand, cardiac accumulation of ^{99m}Tc-pyrophosphate indicates the presence of myocardial damage and necrosis[4], although this is not specific for loss of myocardium due to coronary artery disease. Since the accumulation of this infarct-avid agent is dependent upon the degree of residual blood flow, the presence and pattern of ^{99m}Tc-pyrophosphate accumulation may provide insight into the pathophysiologic process of development of collateral flow into the ischemic and infarcted area.

The sensitivity of both imaging agents to detect acute myocardial infarction is excellent when scintigraphy is performed within the appropriate time frame after acute myocardial injury. Thallium-201 scintigraphy is extremely sensitive during the acute (6–10 hr) phase after infarction [5], whereas ^{99m}Tc-pyrophosphate scintigraphy yields the highest sensitivity during the subacute phase (24–72 hr) after infarction [6]. False negative results will often be related to the timing of the study after onset of infarction. In addition, false negative results will be predominately obtained in patients with relatively small and nontransmural infarcts.

It is still premature to make definite statements about the validity of estimating the size of scintigraphic abnormalities by either technique, although pathological and clinical data are available suggesting that the relative size of ^{201}Tl defects and the size and pattern of ^{99m}Tc-pyrophosphate accumulation may have prognostic importance. Dual imaging with ^{201}Tl and ^{99m}Tc-pyrophosphate allows definition of old and new myocardial infarction in the same patient. Combined imaging is also extremely helpful during the subacute phase of infarction, especially in patients with small and/or nontransmural infarcts. Particularly in these situations, combination of the two radiopharmaceuticals will result in a more efficient detection of acute myocardial infarction than each imaging agent alone [7].

The detection of right ventricular infarction can also be performed by dual imaging. Using the ^{201}Tl image as an anatomic reference, the eventual extension of myocardial necrosis into the right ventricle can readily be demonstrated on ^{99m}Tc-pyrophosphate study [8]. In patients with the clinical syndrome of unstable angina, ^{201}Tl perfusion defects may be demonstrable in

Table 14-1. Indications for radionuclide imaging in the CCU

Indications for ^{201}Tl

    1. Acute phase (<24 hr) of acute myocardial infarction
    2. Rule out myocardial infarction (<18 hr of chest pain)
    3. Unstable angina
    4. Precise location of acute or old myocardial infarction
    5. Estimation of size of myocardial infarction (acute and old)
    6. Potentially for prognostic reasons (size defect)

Indications for ^{99m}Tc-pyrophosphate

    1. Subacute phase (24-72 hr) of acute myocardial infarction
    2. Differentiation of old versus acute myocardial infarction
    3. Estimation of size of acute infarction
    4. Potentially for prognostic reasons ("persistently abnormal scan" and "doughnut lesions")

Indications for combined imaging

    1. Subacute phase (24-72 hr) of acute myocardial infarction
    2. Right ventricular infarction
    3. Assessment of relative site and size of old and acute myocardial infarction

approximately 50% of the patients, even during the pain free period after an anginal attack [9]. This finding generally indicates severe coronary artery disease and identifies a subgroup of patients at high risk for progression to myocardial infarction and failure to respond to medical treatment. Delayed imaging after 2–4 hr usually will demonstrate filling in of the defects by redistribution of ^{201}Tl, indicating that the initial defect was caused by severe ischemia.

Cardiac accumulation of ^{99m}Tc-pyrophosphate has been reported in one-third of patients with unstable angina pectoris [10]. The pathologic correlate of this scintigraphic finding appears to be progressive myocytolytic degeneration as the result of ongoing myocardial ischemia [11]. In patients with coronary artery spasm, prominent perfusion defects can be demonstrated when ^{201}Tl is injected during chest pain [12], lending support to the hypothesis that these patients sustain important transmural ischemia. The site of perfusion defects on the ^{201}Tl scans provides an indication as to the coronary artery in which spasm has occurred. In contrast to patients with unstable angina, the ^{201}Tl studies immediately after relief of pain may be completely normal or demonstrate reactive hyperemia.

The most important practical application of both ^{201}Tl and ^{99m}Tc-pyrophosphate imaging in the coronary care unit, is in patients in whom acute myocardial infarction has to be ruled out. Usually this involves patients with an atypical history of chest pain and nondiagnostic electrocardiogram, in whom there is a suspicion of acute myocardial infarction. In this patient population both ^{201}Tl and ^{99m}Tc-pyrophosphate scintigraphy are sufficiently sensitive (88% and 89%, respectively) to advocate these techniques as extremely valuable additional diagnostic methods in the coronary care unit or emergency room [13-15]. It should again be emphasized that the timing of scintigraphy after onset of acute chest pain and the appropriate choice of imaging agent, is of crucial importance for optimal results [16]. During the early hours after the acute chest pain ^{201}Tl scintigraphy is the agent of choice, whereas during the subacute phase ^{99m}Tc-pyrophosphate is preferred. Dual imaging may increase sensitivity importantly when small infarction is suspected and/or one needs to distinguish old and new infarcts.

Table 14-1 summarizes the indications for radionuclide imaging with ^{201}Tl and ^{99m}Tc-pyrophosphate in the coronary care unit.

REFERENCES

1. Parkey RW, Bonte FJ, Meyer SL, Atkins JM, Curry GL, Stokely EM, Willerson JT: A new method for radionuclide imaging of acute myocardial Infarction in humans. Circulation 50:540-546, 1974.
2. Wackers FJTh, van der Schoot JB, Busemann Sokole E, Samson G, v Niftrik GJC, Lie KI, Durrer D, Wellens HJJ: Noninvasive visualization of acute myocardial infarction in man with thallium-201. Br Heart J 37:741-744, 1975.

3. Pohost GM, Zir LM, Moore RH, McKusick KA, Guiney TE, Beller GA: Differentiation of transiently ischemic from infarcted myocardium by serial imaging after a single dose of thallium-201. Circulation 55:294-302, 1977.
4. Buja LM, Tofe AJ, Kulkarni PV, Mukherjee A, Parkey RW, Francis MD, Bonte FJ, Willerson JT: Sites and mechanisms of localization of technetium-99m phosphorus radio-pharmaceuticals in acute myocardial infarcts and other tissues. J Clin Invest 60:724-740, 1977.
5. Wackers FJTh, Busemann Sokole E, Samson G, van der Schoot JB, Lie KI, Liem KL, Wellens HJJ: Value and limitations of thallium-201 scintigraphy in the acute phase of myocardial infarction N Engl J Med 295:1-5, 1976.
6. Parkey RW, Bonte FJ, Buja LM, Stokely EM, Willerson JT: Myocardial infarct imaging with technetium-99m phosphates. Semin Nucl Med 7:15-28, 1977.
7. Berger HJ, Gottschalk A, Zaret BL: Dual Radionuclide study of acute myocardial infarction: comparison of thallium-201 and technetium-99m stannous pyrophosphate imaging in man. Ann Intern Med 88:145-154, 1978.
8. Wackers FJTh, Lie KI, Busemann Sokole E, Res J, van der Schoot JB, Durrer D: Prevalence of right ventricular involvement in inferior wall infarction assessed with myocardial imaging with thallium-201 and technetium-99m pyrophosphate. Am J Cardiol 42:358-362, 1978.
9. Wackers FJTh, Lie KI, Liem KL, Busemann Sokole E, Samson G, van der Schoot JB, Durrer D: Thallium-201 scintigraphy in unstable angina pectoris. Circulation 57:738-742, 1978.
10. Donsky MS, Curry GC, Parkey RW, Meyer SL, Bonte FJ, Platt MR, Willerson JT: Unstable angina pectoris: clinical, angiographic, and myocardial scintigraphic observations. Br Heart J 38:257-263, 1976.
11. Buja LM, Poliner LR, Parkey RW, Pulido JI, Hutcheson D, Platt MR, Mills LJ, Bonte FJ, Willerson JT: Clinicopathologic study of persistently positive technetium-99m stannous pyrophosphate myocardial scintigrams and myocytolytic degeneration after myocardial infarction. Circulation 56:1016-1023, 1977.
12. Maseri A, Parodi O, Severi S, Pesola A: Transient transmural reduction of myocardial blood flow, demonstrated by thallium-201 scintigraphy, as a cause of variant angina. Circulation 54:280-288, 1976.
13. Wackers FJTh, Lie KI, Liem KI, Busemann Sokole E, Samson G, van der Schoot J, Durrer D: Potential value of thallium-201 scintigraphy as a means of selecting patients for the coronary care unit. Br Heart J 41:111-117, 1979.
14. Willerson JT, Parkey RW, Bonte FJ, Meyer SL, Atkins JM, Stokely EM: Technetium stannous pyrophosphate myocardial scintigrams in patients with chest pain of varying etiology. Circulation 51:1046-1051, 1975.
15. Poliner LR, Buja LM, Parkey RW, Bonte FJ, Willerson JT: Clinicopathologic findings in 52 patients studied by technetium-99m stannous pyrophosphate myocardial scintigraphy. Circulation 59:257-267, 1979.
16. McKillop JH, Turner JG, Gray HW, Bessent RG, Greig WR: Clinical value of delayed thallium-201 myocardial imaging in suspected acute myocardial infarction. Br Heart J 40:870-873, 1978.

15. SELF-ASSESSMENT QUESTIONS

1. The approximate percentage of injected dose of ^{201}Tl that accumulates in the heart is:
   A) 50%
   B) 10%
   C) 4%
   D) 25%.

2. Which of the following statements describes best the mechanisms involved in myocardial accumulation of ^{201}Tl:
   A) Severely ischemic myocarcial cells possess a high affinity to ^{201}Tl, resulting in a preferential uptake by injured myocardium.
   B) Thallium-201 is predominantly accumulated in the heart by redistribution from the systemic pool. Two hours after injection, the maximal myocardial concentration is reached.
   C) Thallium-201 is accumulated in proportion to regional myocardial blood flow, 88% being extracted by the myocardial cells at each transit.
   D) Thallium-201 is accumulated as a function of regional coronary artery pressure, 40% being extracted only during the first transit.

3. Which of the following statements is true:
   A) Thallium-201 remains fixed to the myocardial cells for 7,5 h after i.v. injection.
   B) Thallium-201 enters and leaves the myocardial cells in a constant dynamic pattern, such that each 70 min half of intracellular ^{201}Tl has been replaced.
   C) Thallium-201 is exchanged with the systemic pool until a static equilibrium is reached. After this ^{201}Tl remains fixed to the cells.
   D) Thallium-201 redistribution depends on serum potassium levels.

4. For ^{201}Tl scintigraphy, multiple views are routinely obtained:
   A) But one single view is usually sufficient since count densities are independent of geometrical considerations.
   B) But the 30° right-anterior-oblique view provides most clinically important information.
   C) These include an anterior view, 45° left-anterior-oblique view and left-lateral view.
   D) These are for each patient individually determined by the anatomy of the heart.

5. Artifactual ^{201}Tl defects make the interpretation of the scintiscans sometimes difficult:

A) To the extent that a new and better radiopharmaceutical is required.

B) However, these artifacts can be suspected since they occur at specific anatomic locations.

C) Computer processing is extremely helpful for correct interpretation.

D) Since they occur mostly in obese females, these patients cannot be studied reliably by ^{201}Tl scintigraphy.

6. Artifactual defects on ^{201}Tl scintiscans are due to:

A) Normal variation in ^{201}Tl accumulation, effect of abnormal size and configuration of the heart, effect of patient positioning.

B) Poor "tagging" of ^{201}Tl to the myocardial cells, indicating abnormal myocardial metabolism.

C) High incidence of false positive ^{201}Tl scintiscans in patients without heart disease.

D) Technically impure ^{201}Tl.

7. A technically correct left-lateral view is important for visualization of the posterior wall. This left-lateral view should be obtained as follows:

A) Patient supine and 10° caudal tilt of detector head.

B) Patient lying on his right side and the detector head above the table parallel to the patient's sagittal plane.

C) Patient lying on his left side and the detector head below the table.

D) Patient supine and the detector head vertical (90°) or across the table.

8. Definitely decreased ^{201}Tl activity in a consistent anatomic area of the left ventricle on three different projections indicates:

A) 95% likelihood of acute transmural myocardial infarction.

B) Probably artifactual defect since no true perfusion defect can be seen in three views.

C) Severe ischemia, acute myocardial infarction or old myocardial infarction, or relative greater myocardial mass in the area with apparently normal ^{201}Tl uptake.

D) High suspicion for cardiomyopathy.

9. During the early phase (<6 hr) of acute myocardial infarction the sensitivity to detect transmural and nontransmural infarction respectively, with ^{201}Tl scintigraphy is close to:

A) 80%, 73%.

B) 100% for both.

C) 75% for both.

D) 53%, 25%.

10. The size of ^{201}Tl perfusion defect in patients with acute transmural infarction:

A) Has no relationship to the actual anatomic size of infarction at postmortem.

B) Is only of significance during the first 6 hr, since the size of defects tends to decrease after this time interval.

C) There is a fair relationship between size of infarction at postmortem and abnormally contracting segment on angiography.

D) Is the most accurate method to determine the size of infarction.

11. Comparing the size of ^{201}Tl myocardial perfusion defects at different time intervals after onset of infarction, it can be noted that:

A) No change occurs and thus there is no reason for early imaging.

B) All patients show dramatic decrease in size of defects.

C) Many patients, especially those with small infarctions, demonstrate a decrease in size of defect. Early imaging in these patients is indicated to avoid false negative results.

D) None of the patients show extension of the perfusion defects.

12. Thallium-201 scintigraphy can be used as a selection method in the emergency room or coronary care unit:

A) Because this method will detect accurately all patients with noncardiac complaints.

B) When performed within 10 hr after chest pain this method will detect approximately 85% of the patients with acute myocardial infarction by definite abnormal ^{201}Tl scans.

C) The method is simple and inexpensive with a high degree of accuracy.

D) Since the method differentiates readily between ischemia and acute or old infarction.

13. Dual myocardial imaging with ^{201}Tl and ^{99m}Tc-pyrophosphate provides clinically important information in selected patients:

A) Technetium-99m-pyrophosphate and ^{201}Tl are injected simultaneously as one bolus. Subsequently the accumulation of each radiopharmaceutical is imaged by changing the energy window from 80 keV to 140 keV.

B) Technetium-99m-pyrophosphate imaging preferably is performed first, followed by ^{201}Tl imaging.

C) Technetium-99m-pyrophosphate imaging is performed on day 1. Only 24 hr later, ^{201}Tl imaging can be performed.

D) Thallium-201 imaging is performed first, immediately thereafter ^{99m}Tc-pyrophosphate is injected. Two hours later imaging can be performed on the 140 keV energy peak of ^{99m}Tc.

14. Dual myocardial imaging with ^{201}Tl and ^{99m}Tc-pyrophosphate during the subacute phase of myocardial infarction:

A) Has no advantage above imaging with one of the imaging agents alone.

B) Exposes the patient to unacceptably high radiation dose.

C) Enhances the sensitivity to detect infarction, especially in patients with small or nontransmural infarctions.

D) May be a cause of infarct extension and/or arrhythmias.

15. The prevalence of right ventricular involvement in acute inferior wall infarction as assessed by myocardial imaging with ^{201}Tl and ^{99m}Tc-pyrophosphate is:

A) 37%

B) 10%

C) 50 – 60%

D) 1 – 2%.

16. Accumulation of ^{99m}Tc-pyrophosphate indicates right ventricular infarction:

A) This occurs almost exclusively in patients with acute inferior wall infarction.

B) Is a typical complication of anteroseptal infarction.

C) Is unrelated to coronary artery disease.

D) All patients are in cardiogenic shock.

17. The presence of previous myocardial infarction limits the clinital usefulness of ^{201}Tl scintigraphy for the detection of acute infarction. What percentage of previous myocardial can be demonstrated on ^{201}Tl scans?
    A) Approximately 66%.
    B) 83%.
    C) 25%.
    D) Depends on size and location of previous infarct: approximately 50%

18. In patients with unstable angina positive ^{201}Tl scans can be obtained:
    A) Only when ^{201}Tl is injected during the anginal episode.
    B) In all patients with significant left main disease.
    C) During the pain free period within 6 hr after an anginal attack in approximately 50% of the patients.
    D) This is an indication that subclinical infarction occurred.

19. Patients with positive ^{201}Tl scintiscans during the pain free period after an anginal attack:
    A) Have increased risk for complications: acute myocardial infarction or failure to respond to medical treatment.
    B) Have no different prognosis compared to patients with negative scans.
    C) Is an indication for intraaortic balloon pumping.
    D) This finding can be discarded as false positive result.

20. In patients with variant angina ^{201}Tl scintigraphy is of clinical value since the perfusion defects:
    A) Provide an indication in which coronary artery vasospasm occurs.
    B) Predicts whether vasospasm occurs in normal coronary arteries or in arteries with significant stenosis.
    C) Is of prognostic value in individual patients.
    D) Can be quantitated more readily than ECG changes.

21. Which radionuclide technique may be useful to identify patients with coronary artery vasospasm:
    A) Technetium-99m-pyrophosphate scintigraphy.
    B) Thallium-201-scintigraphy.
    C) Multiple ECG-gated cardiac blood pool imaging.
    D) Levophase of flow study (first pass).

22. What chamber(s) of the heart are usually visualized on resting ^{201}Tl scintiscans:
    A) Left ventricle.
    B) Left and right ventricle.
    C) Right and left atrium, right and left ventricle.
    D) Left atrium, left ventricle.

23. If no other radionuclide techniques are available, and there is suspicion of predominant right ventricular infarction in a patient in cardiogenic shock, how can ^{201}Tl imaging be helpful? (It is assumed that hypovolumenia has been excluded):
    A) Sometimes the right ventricle is visualized and a perfusion defect in the inferior wall of the right ventricle can be seen.

    B) A normal sized left ventricle with a rather small perfusion defect at the inferior wall provides strong indirect evidence of right ventricular infarction. Sometimes the dilated right ventricle can be seen as a "negative image".

    C) Extensive anteroseptal infarction always involves the right ventricle.

    D) Increased pulmonary uptake of ^{201}Tl.

24. A 53-y-old male experienced prolonged chest pain, with nausea and diaphoresis 3 h before admission. What radionuclide technique would be most useful?
    A) Gated cardial blood pool imaging.
    B) Thallium-201 scintigraphy.
    C) Technetium-99m-pyrophosphate scintigraphy
    D) Myocardial imaging with ^{111}In-labeled leukocytes.

25. A 65-yr-old female was admitted 3 days ago after a prolonged episode of chest pain. The electrocardiogram demonstrated non-specific ST-segment changes with negative T waves in the precordial leads. Cardiac enzymes were only slightly elevated after admission and returned to normal. CKMB fraction was not determined. What radionuclide technique(s) would you request to arrive at a diagnosis?
    A) None, since no technique is sensitive enough at this time.
    B) Dual imaging with ^{201}Tl and ^{99m}Tc-pyrophosphate.
    C) Gated cardiac blood pool imaging.
    D) Technetium-99m-pyrophosphate.

26. A 70-yr-old male, known for years to have hypertension and diabetes, is admitted after a prolonged episode of chest pain. Patient sustained a myocardial infarction 3 yr ago. A radionuclide test is ordered 24 hr after the chest pain, since no diagnostic electrocardiographic changes occurred. Which technique would you recommend?
    A) Thallium-201 myocardial imaging.
    B) Technetium-99m-pyrophosphate imaging followed by ^{201}Tl imaging.
    C) Technetium-99m-pyrophosphate imaging.
    D) Indium-111-labeled white blood cells myocardial imaging.

27. The optimal imaging time for obtaining a ^{99m}Tc-pyrophosphate myocardial scintigram for myocardial infarct detection is:
    A) 3 hr after the onset of symptoms.
    B) 8 hr after the onset of symptoms.
    C) 24-72 hr after the onset of symptoms.
    D) 1 week after the onset of syniptoms.

28. Technetium-99m-myocardial scintigrams identify acute nontransmural (subendocardial)myocardial infarcts as well as they identify acute transmural myocardial infarcts.
    A) True.
    B) False.

29. A limit of resolution of the ^{99m}Tc-pyrophosphate imaging technique for myocardial infarct detection is:
    A) 3 g or more of irreversible myocardial damage.
    B) 10 g or more of myocardial damage.
    C) 1 g or more of myocardial damage.
    D) 30 g or more of myocardial damage.

30. Serial myocardial imaging with ^{99m}Tc-pyrophosphate myocardial imaging technique allows one to determine:
    A) Presence of a new infarct.
    B) To detect the delayed development of an abnormal scintigram in the rare patient in whom this occurs.
    C) Differentiate old from new myocardial infarcts.
    D) Begin to evaluate "persistently abnormal" PYP myocardial scintigrams.

31. Technetium-99m-pyrophosphate concentrates in:
    A) Regions of irreversible myocardial damage.
    B) Regions of reversible myocardial cellular damage.
    C) Areas of no myocardial damage.
    D) Areas of hemorrhage.

32. Persistently abnormal ^{99m}Tc-pyrophosphate myocardial scintigram may indicate:
    A) The presence of ongoing severe ischemic damage.
    B) Abnormalities in function of the sarcoplasmic reticulum.
    C) Increased compliance.
    D) Alterations in coronary perfusion.

33. Abnormal ^{99m}Tc-pyrophosphate myocardial scintigrams may be expected in those circumstances in which:
    A) Irreversible myocardial cellular damage occurs irrespective of the etiology as long as the images are obtained in the proper time frame.
    B) Reversible myocardial damage
    C) With left ventricular hypertrophy.
    D) With right ventricular hypertrophy.

34. The most important determinants of abnormal ^{99m}Tc-pyrophosphate uptake in the heart are:
    A) Presence of myocardial damage.
    B) Some persistent coronary blood flow to the region of damage.
    C) Calcium deposition within the region of irreversible cellular damage.
    D) All of the above.

ANSWERS

1. C	13. D	24. B
2. C	14. C	25. B
3. B	15. A	26. C
4. C	16. A	27. C
5. B	17. D	28. A
6. A	18. C	29. A
7. B	19. A	30. All of the above
8. C	20. A	31. A
9. B	21. B	32. A
10. C	22. A	33. A
11. C	23. B	34. D
12. B		

INDEX